Disease Management

A Systems Approach to Improving Patient Outcomes

WARREN E. TODD
DAVID NASH, MD
EDITORS

FOREWORD BY
SENATOR BILL FRIST, MD

 American Hospital Publishing Inc.
An American Hospital Association Company
Chicago

Library of Congress Cataloging-in-Publication Data

Disease management: a systems approach to improving patient outcomes
/ edited by Warren. E. Todd and David Nash.
    p.   cm.
Includes bibliographical references and index.
ISBN 1-55648-168-3
1. Health planning. 2. Medical protocols. 3. Medical care —
Quality control. 4. Outcome assessment (Medical care) I. Todd,
Warren E. II. Nash, David B.
    [DNLM: 1. Patient Care Planning. 2. Managed Care Programs. W
84.7 D611 1996]
RA394.9.D55   1996
362.1 — DC20
DNLM/DLC
for Library of Congress   96-30138
                                                                            CIP

Catalog no. 067103

©1997 by American Hospital Publishing, Inc.,
an American Hospital Association company

Printed in the USA

𝔸ℍ𝔸 is a service mark of the American Hospital Association used under license by American Hospital Publishing, Inc.

Text set in English Times

4M — 12/96 — 0449

Audrey Kaufman, Senior Editor
Lee Benaka, Nancy Charpentier, and Mark Swartz, Editors
Peggy DuMais, Assistant Manager, Production
Marcia Bottoms, Books Division Director

Contents

List of Figures

List of Tables

About the Editors

Warren E. Todd, MBA, is vice-president of business development of Hastings Healthcare Group in Pennington, NJ, and was formerly vice-president of marketing of the National Jewish Center for Immunology and Respiratory Medicine in Denver. His broad experience in health care has focused on new product and business development, including a business plan for the creation of a national chain of full-service home health care centers. He has also had extensive strategic planning experience involving both inpatient and outpatient services as well as physician recruitment and liaison services for a large regional medical center.

Mr. Todd has been actively involved in disease management for the past 4 years and helped engineer National Jewish's transition from a national center of excellence in severe asthma to a comprehensive asthma disease management program. While at National Jewish, Mr. Todd also developed several major strategic alliances with other national providers of asthma disease management products and services. He has written and lectured extensively on disease management, capitation, and other health care subjects. He is a member of the adjunct faculty of the University of Denver's master's program in public health administration.

Mr. Todd graduated with a bachelor's degree from Northeastern University in Boston and received his MBA from Columbia University. He is also a graduate of the University of Missouri, Kansas City, Henry Bloch School of Business Administration's executive program in managed care.

David B. Nash, MD, MBA, FACP, is the first director of the Office of Health Policy and Clinical Outcomes at Thomas Jefferson University and is associate professor of medicine at Jefferson Medical College. Named by Faulkner and Gray as one of the most influential policy makers in academic medicine, and the 1995 recipient of the distinguished Clifton Latiolais Prize in managed care from the American Managed Care Pharmacy Association, Dr. Nash is nationally recognized for his work in outcomes management, medical staff development, and quality of care improvement. His professional activities include membership on the American Medical Association's Expert Panel on Physician Performance Assessment, membership and post-chairmanship of the Center for Clinical Quality Evaluation (CCQE) (formerly the American Medical Review Research Center), membership on the Joint Commission's Performance Council, and membership and past chairmanship of the Clinical Evaluative Sciences Council of the University Health-System Consortium. Dr. Nash is editor of the *Journal of Outcomes Management* and a member of the *Medical Economics* editorial board. A former Robert Wood Johnson Clinical Scholar, Dr. Nash received his MD from the University of Rochester School of Medicine and his MBA in health administration from the Wharton School at the University of Pennsylvania.

Contributors

Charles E. Barr, MD, MPH, provides medical informatics and clinical expertise to Greenstone Healthcare Solutions, Kalamazoo, MI. Prior to joining Greenstone, Dr. Barr was director of the Center for Applied Medical Informatics at the Michigan State University Kalamazoo Center for Medical Studies. In addition, he was assistant professor, department of internal medicine, at the Michigan State University College of Human Medicine. In addition to his work with Greenstone, he maintains a practice in internal medicine. Dr. Barr also completed a postdoctoral fellowship in medical informatics at Harvard Medical School and Brigham & Women's Hospital.

David B. Bernard, MD, FACP, is senior medical director and director of disease management at the University of Pennsylvania Health System. He is professor of medicine at the University of Pennsylvania School of Medicine. Dr. Bernard was a fellow in quality management, cost-effective practice, and managed care at the University of Pennsylvania. Previously, he was a professor at Boston University School of Medicine, where he held various administrative appointments. Dr. Bernard has written extensively on nephrology.

Stan Bernard, MD, MBA, is associate principal, Health Care and Pharmaceutical Industry at A.T. Kearney. Dr. Bernard previously worked as an executive for six years at Bristol-Myers Squibb Pharmaceutical Company. He served as U.S. director, pharmacoeconomics, responsible for initiating and directing health/disease management initiatives, and as U.S. managed care medical director, the first person to hold such a position in the pharmaceutical industry. Dr. Bernard received his MBA from the Wharton School of Business and his medical degree from Baylor College of Medicine. Dr. Bernard is associate lecturer at the Wharton School of Business where he teaches disease management and pharmaceutical management. Since 1992, Dr. Bernard has served as an expert consultant to the U.S. Agency for Health Care Policy and Research (AHCPR).

Joseph E. Biskupiak, PhD, MBA, is director of technology assessment for Hastings Healthcare Group. In this capacity, he directs research in the areas of clinical outcomes, health service utilization, disease management, and clinical studies. Before joining Hastings, Dr. Biskupiak served as research assistant professor and assistant project director for Jefferson University Hospital in Philadelphia. His responsibilities included assisting new businesses in health care product development and conducting research in the areas of pharmacoeconomics, technology assessment, and health policy. Dr. Biskupiak has authored numerous articles in the scientific field, as well as several textbook chapters on outcomes research and disease management. Dr. Biskupiak holds a BS in chemistry from the University of Connecticut, a PhD in medicinal chemistry from the University of Utah, and an MBA from Seattle University.

Daniel L. Bouwman, MD, MPH, is clinical data manager at Greenstone Healthcare Solutions, Kalamazoo, MI, where he provides extensive expertise in clinical and preventive medicine. Dr. Bouwman came to Greenstone from the Occupational Health & Safety Division of The Upjohn Company, where he practiced occupational medicine and directed or participated in services and projects related to hazardous material, industrial emergency medical services, toxicologic and biological hazards in chemical/pharmaceutical research and production, and occupational epidemiology. In addition, he maintains a practice in occupational medicine and participates in community emergency response programs.

Peter Chodoff, MD, MPH, is professor of anesthesia, Jefferson Medical College; adjunct professor, School of Life Sciences, University of Delaware; and a faculty member of the Medical Scholars Program of the University of Delaware/Jefferson Medical College. He facilitates special projects in the College's Office of Health Policy and Clinical Outcomes, where he also participates in teaching and research. His research interests lie in the relationships among continuous quality improvement, cost-effectiveness, and managed care. Dr. Chodoff's past positions include having served as chief medical officer for the Social Security Administration; medical director of St. Joseph's Hospital, Reading, PA; assistant dean, Jefferson Medical College; and vice-president for academic affairs and for medical education and Research at The Medical Center of Delaware. Dr. Chodoff received his MD from Jefferson Medical College and an MPH from Johns Hopkins University; he completed a fellowship in neuropharmacology at the University of Michigan.

John B. Doyle, PhD, is a principal with Doyle Consulting, Inc., Boulder, CO. Doyle Consulting helps clients maximize health care value by means of care program design, best practices, and outcomes assessment. Dr. Doyle has developed components and evaluated outcomes of several disease management initiatives both in his current capacity and previously with Inter-Study and Park Nicollet Medical Foundation, Minneapolis.

John H. Eichert is president of the Hastings Healthcare Group, Pennington, NJ. Mr. Eichert frequently publishes and speaks on the design, development, and implementation of disease management systems and population-based health care. He codeveloped an innovative patient-directed outcomes management system used for several chronic conditions and is actively engaged in numerous disease management projects.

Dennis P. Kane has over 20 years of experience in health care and has been involved in outcomes research and disease management since 1986. He has lectured internationally on such topics as pharmacoeconomics, drug use evaluations, and research design. Mr. Kane has been involved with Greenstone Healthcare Solutions (GHS), the disease management arm of Pharmacia & Upjohn, Inc., since its inception. He was instrumental in the development of the strategic vision for GHS and the inclusion of prospective health care as a critical component of disease management.

John T. Kelly, MD, PhD, is chief medical officer and senior vice-president of clinical information services at GMIS, a medical information management firm based in Malvern, PA. Previously, he was director of the American Medical Association's (AMA's) Office of Quality and Utilization Management, where he guided the AMA's activities on practice guidelines. Dr. Kelly has written extensively on the development and implementation of practice guidelines. He has served on advisory committees on practice guidelines for the Agency for Health Care Policy and Research and the Institute of Medicine.

Richard A. Kipp, FCA, is a consulting actuary and an associate member with the Philadelphia office of Milliman & Robertson, Inc., where he also serves as research manager. Previously, Mr. Kipp was senior director of actuarial, underwriting, and provider reimbursement at Blue Cross and Blue Shield of New Hampshire–Vermont and manager of actuarial and underwriting at Blue Cross and Blue Shield of Rhode Island. He is a frequent speaker at national meetings on the subject of provider risk taking and disease management.

Sharyn S. Lee, RN, BSN, MS, is the vice-president of sales and development of Interim Healthcare in the Northeast, and regional vice-president of Interim Home Solutions, Danvers, MA. Ms. Lee is responsible for the integration of infusion therapy and high-tech home care and for the development of disease management specialty programs in alternate settings. She also works closely with payers, physicians, managed care executives, and administrators in the development of clinical pathways in alternate care and their integration in home care. Ms. Lee's 20 years of health care experience include joint venture management, faculty positions in colleges in Miami and Boston, and critical care nursing. She has published and lectured extensively on the subjects of alternate care, home care disease specialty programs, and critical pathways.

Howard A. Levin, MD, is a senior health care consultant with the Philadelphia office of Milliman & Robertson, Inc. Prior to that, Dr. Levin was a corporate medical director for U.S. Healthcare, where he served as director of utilization and quality and as vice-president in charge of research and development at USQA, a subsidiary of USHC in Blue Bell, PA. In addition, Dr. Levin was medical director at the San Jose Medical Clinic in San Jose, CA.

Frank Lobeck, PharmD, is responsible for intervention research and design at Greenstone Healthcare Solutions, Kalamazoo, MI. Dr. Lobeck came to Greenstone from The Upjohn Company, where he was a drug information clinical pharmacist. His previous experience includes serving as a mental health clinical pharmacist at the Oklahoma City Veterans Administration Medical Center, where he was responsible for development, implementation, and justification of pharmaceutical care programs. Dr. Lobeck was also clinical assistant professor at the University of Oklahoma College of Pharmacy.

Kent W. Peterson, MD, is an internationally known expert in preventive, occupational, and environmental medicine. In 1984, he founded Occupational Health Strategies, Inc., Charlottesville, VA, which provides management consulting, strategic planning, and health information services to Fortune 500 companies and health care companies. Previously, Dr. Peterson served as manager of preventive and environmental medicine at IBM Worldwide. He has also been corporate medical director at American Standard, and executive vice-president of the American College of Preventive Medicine. He was honored as a Robert Wood Johnson Clinical Scholar at George Washington University, and is board certified in both preventive and occupational medicine. Dr. Peterson is currently president of the American College of Occupational and Environmental Medicine, and a member of the board of directors of the Society of Prospective Medicine. He is a clinical professor of environmental medicine at New York University and holds faculty appointments at Georgetown University and the Federal Executive Institute. He has authored more than 200 books, chapters, articles, and scientific presentations to professional societies.

Julia A. Rieve, RN, BSHCM, CCM, CPHQ, is a specialist in case and disease management systems development, and her services emphasize quality improvement, patient care systems redesign, and cost-effective care management solutions. Ms. Rieve is founder and owner of CQI, a health care management services company. She is a frequent speaker on managed care, case and disease management, quality improvement, and outcomes indicators. In addition, Ms. Rieve recently coauthored a disease management article published in *The Journal of Care Management.*

David R. Smith, MD, is currently commissioner of health for the state of Texas and the state health officer. In that capacity he oversees the operations of the Texas Department of Health (TDH). During his tenure as commissioner, Dr. Smith has prioritized the need for public/private collaboration. The innovative program "Shots across Texas" is but one such model that has been responsible for an almost 100 percent improvement in childhood immunization levels in Texas. Additionally, TDH has initiated a strategy to transition some of the department's medical services to the private/academic sectors. As a former senior vice-president of Parkland Memorial Hospital in Dallas, he oversaw the design and development of a large, integrated, community-based delivery system, The Community Oriented Primary Care Program. Dr. Smith has been asked to serve on many national and international work group commissions and advisory boards, and to provide expert testimony on a variety of health issues before the U.S. Congress.

W. Charles Towner, ASA, is an associate actuary with the Chicago office of Milliman & Robertson, Inc. Previously, Mr. Towner was responsible for health data analysis and development of claims analytical software at the Central States Health and Welfare Fund and at the University of Chicago Physicians' Group.

Marcia Diane Ward, RN, CCM, is market segment manager for IBM Worldwide Healthcare Solutions, Hawthorne, NY. In addition, Ms. Ward serves on the editorial advisory board for the American Health Consultants' publication *Case Management Advisor,* a national newsletter, and the advisory board of the Managed Home Care Congress. She is a member of the American Association of Managed Care Nurses. Ms. Ward is an inactive faculty member of Asher School of Business in Atlanta, where she has taught medical law and ethics, and is a contributing author to case management journals and information technology journals. She codeveloped a disease management track for the Case Management Society of America's annual conference (1996) based on an article she coauthored in the *Journal of Care Management,* October 1995, "Disease Management, Case Management's Return to Patient-Centered Care." Ms. Ward is a strong advocate and educator of the nurse care management process across the entire health care enterprise.

Herbert Wong, PhD, holds the position of senior vice-president of strategic development at Columbia Healthcare Corporation, responsible for strategic planning, training and education, consumer products, and disease management. Dr. Wong received his PhD in sociology with emphasis in multivariate statistics, social psychology, and organizational change from the University of California, Santa Barbara. He did his postdoctoral work at the University of California, Berkeley, in policy analysis. He has published extensively in journals such as *Sociological Inquiry, Quality, Health Care Quality Management, Quality Progress,* and *Training.*

Mark Zitter, MBA, is president of the Zitter Group, a San Francisco–based education and publishing firm focusing on health care outcomes and disease management. The Zitter Group produces the nation's largest outcomes conference as well as several disease management tools. Mr. Zitter has authored four books on health care and has been featured in such publications as *Journal of the American Medical Association, Modern Healthcare, Medical Interface,* and *Newsweek.* A graduate of Stanford and Wesleyan Universities, he has been a guest lecturer at Stanford Business School, Harvard School of Public Health, and Yale Medical School.

Foreword

As we approach the millennium, we find ourselves in the midst of a health care revolution unlike anything we could have imagined. The old systems of medical and health care are eroding, and innovative ones are rapidly emerging. As these systems evolve, new and integrated approaches to care are being developed. Many factors have contributed to these changes, including increasing demands by the stakeholders for both cost containment and proof of quality and value. At the same time, advances in computer technology have provided us with the potential to develop centralized databases which can facilitate better provider and consumer decisions. Because of these changes, we are in reach of significantly advancing the way we approach health promotion, disease prevention, and treatment.

Health care practitioners must reorient themselves if they are to meet the future challenges of our health care system. Specifically, practitioners must learn from one another as population-based data, rather than experiential history, become more widely available and demanded by health care purchasers. Both changes are the results of reorganization of the role of the various stakeholders in the delivery system. The stakeholders have changed: it is no longer just the physician and the patient, but also employers, health plans, and the government who are at the table. The new concept of *disease management* would not have come about without the pressures of cost containment, the integration of health systems, and the need to sustain and improve quality of care. There were good things about the old system, but there were also bad things. Cost was uncontrolled, and quality was measured in only the most primitive of ways.

Disease management, the focus of this monograph, is one of the most promising approaches to health care. It is not a new concept; physicians have always managed disease, but frequently they managed unconnected episodic events without integrating all elements of care that affect the results for the patient. Disease management today is based on outcomes research, a field still in its infancy. It is information driven and continually being improved as more knowledge and health outcomes are analyzed. While disease management might seem to be a simple concept, it is a very sophisticated approach to patient care that requires a knowledge of public health, disease history, health economics, and outcomes research. Integration of the most cost-effective and highest quality care available will provide the best care possible for patients. This is a well-reasoned, timely book which will inform the larger health care discussion as we move into the 21st century.

Bill Frist, MD, U.S. Senator from Tennessee

Preface

It has been 5 years since the Boston Consulting Group first popularized the term *disease management,* thereby helping to launch a potentially powerful new concept in health care delivery. Today, we are in a position to assess the preliminary results of a plethora of first-generation disease management programs created during what might best be viewed as the discovery phase of the disease management era. As with anything new, it is always helpful to revisit the initial efforts of those organizations that had the courage to explore new means of delivering health care and to enhance future programs with lessons learned from these early explorers.

The Systems Approach

Disease Management: A Systems Approach to Improving Patient Outcomes was conceived as a vehicle to help bring systems thinking and organizational structure to what appeared to be a frenzy of well-intentioned efforts to more effectively coordinate the delivery of health care to patients. The book will serve as a guide for the design, development, and implementation of new disease management and total health management systems. While this intention of providing a systematic approach to the development of disease management initiatives is still valid for those organizations just beginning to examine the potential of disease management, you may also use the contents to revisit existing disease management initiatives that have not fully measured up to their original expectations. One of the basic messages of this book is that the development of true disease management *systems* is a process that is much more complex than "programs" that consist of loosely integrated interventions. It appears that many have discovered just how complex this process can be, given the cross-functional and cross-organizational teamwork needed to literally reengineer how health care is delivered.

Disease Management consists informally of four different sections. The first, comprising chapters 1-6, deals in some detail with the process of developing disease management programs. After chapter 1 addresses the forces driving disease management, chapter 2 outlines a systems approach to the design, development, and implementation of disease management initiatives. This important chapter provides the infrastructure for much of what follows in the rest of the book. The remainder of the first section focuses on four critical components of disease management systems — outcomes analysis and measurement, actuarial considerations, disease considerations, and the importance of clinical practice guidelines.

The second section, chapters 7-10, addresses how disease management will impact several important sectors and stakeholders — the pharmaceutical industry, managed care organizations, case management, and home care. The third section consists of a single chapter, chapter 11, which addresses the critical need for development of strategic alliances to help insure the success of disease management systems. Finally, the last "section," chapter 12, explores the evolution of disease management into total, population-based health management.

How to Use This Book

The ultimate challenge of this book is to help you devise and implement a disease management system or systems that will both improve health care delivery and reduce costs. The system you develop will provide a sense of stability for patients as well as the members of your organization, and at the same time will make it natural and easy to continue evolving toward the goal beyond disease management — total health management systems. For disease management should be regarded as an evolutionary step, a way for organizations to learn to walk before they run.

Managers and practitioners at different stages of implementing a disease management system will use *Disease Management* in different ways. If you now operate within a traditional case management system, whether one that seems to function efficiently or one that has been buffeted by the same market and industry forces that have pushed other organizations toward disease management, the book provides a general introduction to the concept and a recipe for preparing a disease management system from the ingredients available within your organization. Reading the accounts of experienced and expert commentators, you may find that you are already moving in the direction of disease management, or, you may be surprised by the extent to which the systems approach redefines the roles and relationships in the health care field. As John H. Eichert, Herbert Wong, and David R. Smith promise in the second chapter, such a change requires a myriad of skill sets: "The systems approach at the heart of disease management involves not only the practicalities of cost analysis, outcomes measurement, and so forth, but also the intuitive human relations side of gaining buy-in among stakeholders and helping adjust the attitudes of everyone from patients to providers to payers to managed care organizations."

If you and your organization have already taken some steps in the direction of disease management—or, perhaps, in the direction of what you thought was disease management—you would not be alone if you had found the challenge of rebuilding the health care delivery system to be steeper than you anticipated. After those few tentative steps toward change, the organization may have slid back into its old ways or into a disorganized limbo. Comprehension of the logic behind the disease management concept may have been at fault; previous to this book, the literature on the subject was confusing and definitions were left vague. A breakdown in finances, alliances, staff morale, patient satisfaction, or, most troubling, actual quality of care might have suggested to you that you are not ready for disease management. You can view the contributors to this book as trusted and experienced colleagues who can restart your motivation, pinpoint the trouble spots, and equip you for a more organized and systematic foray into the unfamiliar territory. If you and your associates read *Disease Management* and internalize its objectives, then at least you will be operating under the same assumptions about what you want to accomplish.

If your organization has already implemented a full-scale disease management program, then *Disease Management* will be of use as a maintenance toolbox. You have already come to realize that these systems, once in place, do not automatically run themselves. Disease management is an inherently dynamic concept; the cost of the freedoms it brings is eternal vigilance. By comparing your successes and failures to those of other organizations, you may hit upon ways to fine-tune your program or to prepare it for approaching the next hurdle, the transition from disease management to health management.

Health management has to wait until disease management is in place. For health management to be not just an abstract notion but a realistic destination, not just the same old thing with a new name but, in the words of Kent Peterson and Dennis P. Kane, "the optimization of clinical, financial, and quality-of-life outcomes accomplished by management of the entire range of health risk for a population," the structures supporting disease management must first withstand a series of external and internal disruptions. With *Disease Management: A Systems Approach to Improving Patient Outcomes,* the authors extend to you a manual for coping with these disruptions and leading your health care organization on the complex and challenging path ahead.

Chapter 1

A New Paradigm in Health Care Delivery: Disease Management

Mark Zitter, MBA

For most of the 20th century, health care has emphasized acute medical treatment. Reimbursement has favored hospitalization and physician visits and has been less generous to most long-term care, home health, and preventive services. Further, each service typically has been delivered, billed, and reimbursed separately. This functional and financial separation of treatment components has inhibited optimal care by encouraging each provider segment to focus on the patient only within the context of that component. This, in turn, has led to higher systemwide costs, even though—and perhaps *because*—various individual components may be comparatively efficient.

This book addresses a relatively new concept in health care delivery called *disease management.* Over the past several years, disease management has grown to become almost a household word in the health care industry as payers, providers, pharmaceutical companies, consultants, and almost every segment of the industry have begun to explore the potential for this phenomenon. This chapter focuses on defining disease management and discusses whether it can fulfill its promise of a new generation of value and accountability for the industry. The evolution of disease management also is explored with emphasis on what forces have driven the amazingly widespread acceptance of this approach to health care delivery.

Before explaining what disease management is and how it can benefit health care organizations, it is necessary to understand how care has been delivered historically and why change is needed.

• The Traditional Component Management Model

Health care in the United States has historically been delivered via a "component-style" system of individual providers and payers that has been characterized by a high degree of fragmentation and consistently misaligned reimbursement priorities. The traditional components of this type of delivery

1

system have included physician office visits, outpatient treatment, inpatient hospitalization, home care, long-term care, and so forth. Although each component of this system might strive to deliver cost-effective care, providers did not address the long-term cost of care across settings, and, more importantly, the patient's quality of life was not necessarily maximized. In fact, as the following example demonstrates, the system components were frequently at odds.

Assume that a moderately asthmatic patient is admitted to a hospital emergency room and is treated effectively, efficiently, and pleasantly. Many would say that this patient has received good-quality health care. However, this may not be true at all. There is an excellent chance that the patient in question may have "lost control" of his or her disease due to (1) a failure to monitor lung capacity, (2) underuse of inhaled steroids, (3) a poor understanding of what to do when the disease flared up, or (4) some combination of these issues. It is likely that, prior to this incident, the patient's physician did not follow the most widely accepted asthma management guidelines, that the pharmacist did not fully explain the proper times for and doses of medication, and that the patient was unaware of what he or she could do to minimize the likelihood of hospitalization. The *hospital staff* may have done a great job, but the *health care system* probably failed the patient.

In short, it is likely that the patient in this hypothetical example was a victim of the traditional *component management system*. Component management derives from both providers and payers viewing health problems through the specific window of care for which they are responsible. Hospital-based providers focus on what occurs within the inpatient setting, not before or afterward. Pharmacy directors attempt to minimize the pharmacy budget regardless of the impact on total system costs. Insurers reimburse for a drug used in the hospital but do not cover the same medication for the same illness once the patient walks out the door. Even more crucial to the overall effectiveness of care, the reimbursement mechanisms of this system do not reimburse providers for patient education. Who is responsible for patient education in a component-style system of health care delivery? No one — because no one is reimbursed for providing it!

From a quality standpoint, the component management approach is inferior. Rather than specifically designing treatment plans to prevent or minimize the impact of a disease, providers tend to organize their activities into reimbursable packages. Ironically, research also now shows the limits of component management as a cost-containment strategy. *Optimizing any component of care separately from other components often generates higher systemwide costs.*

Some of component management's most dramatic failures to limit total costs involve pharmaceutical therapy. An early observational study by Stephen Soumerai and his colleagues at the Harvard School of Public Health analyzed the effect of a payment cap on Medicaid drugs — a classic component management tactic — instituted by the state of New Hampshire during the 1980s. The program cost more in outpatient services than it saved in drug use. Prescription costs for mental disorders dropped an average of $5.14 ± 0.67 per patient per month during the payment cap, but outpatient mental health service expenses rose $139 per month, or $1,530 during the 11-month cap period.[1] Similarly, when Louisiana's Medicaid program omitted certain powerful drugs from its formulary, medication costs dropped by 13 percent, but physician services rose 29 percent and inpatient mental health services increased 39 percent.[2] These are only two examples of how the historical component style of health care delivery, while attempting to be more cost-effective in one area of patient care, significantly increased both costs for another area and total costs.

Component management frequently is compared to squeezing a balloon at one end: The air just pops up somewhere else. However, a more apt analogy would be squeezing a balloon in one place and seeing the balloon expand at another point by *twice the size of the air originally displaced*. If the objective is to minimize total health care costs, the squeezing of one component at a time may be counterproductive.

Increasingly, health care professionals and policy makers are realizing that the component management approach to patient care serves the industry poorly for several reasons:

- It emphasizes medical treatment over prevention, thus skewing priorities for both how health care is delivered and how much is paid to whom, leading to a system that is more "sickness care" than "health care."
- It reimburses disproportionately for the most expensive services in the most expensive settings (that is, acute inpatient care), thus encouraging overtreatment in costly settings and undertreatment elsewhere.
- It lacks incentives for providers to understand and treat the entire disease process, because each provider can only affect — and be reimbursed for — events within a given setting or budget category.
- It leads to an uncoordinated delivery system that lacks care continuity for patients. It fails to recognize the interrelation of health services and total health costs — for example, how mental health care or pharmaceutical resources may improve overall health and thus reduce other expenses.
- It frequently pits patient-focused providers (who may want to provide or prescribe treatment beyond their component) against budget-oriented managers (who are reluctant to provide services for which they will not be reimbursed).

Ironically, because component management does not focus on system-wide results, it often increases total treatment cost with no corresponding health benefit. It is a system well designed to create cost without necessarily improving patient outcomes.

• The Disease Management Approach

Fortunately, another concept of health care delivery is emerging in this country. It has been referred to collectively as *disease management* and is generally defined as a comprehensive, integrated approach to care and reimbursement based on a disease's natural course. The goal of disease management is to address the illness or condition with maximum effectiveness and efficiency regardless of treatment setting(s) or typical reimbursement patterns. This approach emphasizes management of a disease in a manner that focuses both clinical and nonclinical interventions when and where they are most likely to have the greatest positive impact. Ideally, disease management prevents exacerbation of a disease and the use of expensive resources, making prevention and proactive case management two important areas of emphasis in most disease management programs.

Disease management is similar enough to several related approaches that an argument can be made for shared nomenclature. *Population-based care,* as practiced by Group Health Cooperative of Puget Sound and other organizations, is based squarely on disease management principles. The Lovelace Clinic's *episodes of care* project clearly is also a disease management program, as is the *systems management approach* promulgated by the National Pharmaceutical Council and others.

The Evolution of Disease Management

Elements of disease management have been practiced by individual providers for years. However, comprehensive, concerted disease management programs have been untenable due to the following:

- The fragmented health care delivery system
- Reimbursement policies that reinforce and reward component management
- Insufficient data collection
- Information management systems that frequently are incompatible with each other
- Administrative and financial separation of provider budget elements
- Lack of disease maps and economic models for many conditions
- Lack of outcomes and health economic research on which to base treatment strategies
- Lack of guidelines and treatment algorithms, and inexperience in implementing those that exist
- Medical training that emphasizes component management

The development of managed care and integrated delivery systems, combined with burgeoning health care costs, has made the disease management approach more practical and appealing. Perhaps the earliest example of disease-focused work, as well as use of the disease management nomenclature, started in the late 1980s at the Mayo Clinic. Work accelerated in 1990 when Mayo and John Deere's Heritage Health Plan formed a partnership in which Mayo agreed to help build a clinic and implement its disease management concept on a broader scale for Deere employees.

Today, a number of forces are acting to accelerate the growth of disease management programs. These forces include:

- Rapid health system integration, which facilitates care across treatment settings
- Improvement in health care information systems, which allows better patient identification and targeting, decision support, and computerized prescribing
- Growth in capitation as a reimbursement mechanism, which provides incentive to find the most cost-effective treatment regardless of setting
- Proliferation of outcomes studies that assist with cost identification and guide therapeutic choices
- Development of more and better practice guidelines, which suggests improved therapeutic strategies
- Growing sophistication in utilization review and formulary enforcement tactics, both of which enhance compliance with treatment algorithms
- Providers' increasing experience with quality improvement techniques, which facilitate analysis and implementation of disease management strategies
- Substantial investment of resources by large health care organizations, which increases the amount and quality of approaches being devised and tested

• Key Success Factors for Disease Management

Although chapter 2 addresses the process of developing and implementing disease management programs in considerable detail, a number of important basic "ingredients" to all programs are worth introducing here.

Understanding the Course of the Disease

The key to managing a disease condition is understanding its causes and patterns of manifestation. For example, some chronic diseases, such as asthma, are marked by acute episodes, frequently referred to as "cost drivers," which cause the greatest health risks and cost spikes. In the case of asthma, misdiagnosis can also be an important cost driver in that misdiagnosis of the disease can result in significant and unnecessary long-term costs. At the National Jewish Center for Immunology and Respiratory Medicine, up to

20 percent of chronically ill asthmatics referred to the facility for treatment do not suffer from asthma but from another illness called vocal cord dysfunction, which mimics asthma but requires a very different treatment regimen. For diabetes, the short-term costs of intensive management may be more than offset by long-term cost savings. A well-constructed model of the disease is essential to provide the best and most efficient care (see figure 1-1).

Targeting Patients Likely to Benefit from Intervention

Most disease management initiatives are drawn up in the hope of improving care and reducing long-term costs. Realistically, this means that successful programs must identify those patients who are most likely to generate expenses for the system and target them for intervention. Analyses of populations of asthmatic and diabetic patients typically find that a small proportion of severely ill patients account for most systemwide costs in each population. For example, the 22 percent of asthmatics classified by one insurer as severely ill accounted for nearly 85 percent of costs, which averaged $4,347 per patient annually. Mild asthmatics, who accounted for approximately 60 percent of the insured population, represented less than 10 percent of expenditures, or $115 per patient per year (figure 1-2). Similarly, one large health maintenance organization (HMO) found that 4.9 percent of its diabetic members accounted for approximately 91.9 percent of its costs for treating that disease.[3]

The good news is that the relatively small number of sickest patients in most populations can often be identified and targeted for interventions that will have the greatest chance of affecting health and cost, and thus the highest likelihood of being cost-effective. A wide variety of criteria, such as the following, may be used to target patients for disease management programs:

- Demographics: age, sex, race
- Severity of illness/disease subcategories
- Compliance behavior
- Historical cost profile
- Frequency of recurrence
- Seasonality
- Other epidemiological markers

Targeting can be tricky, but the field is evolving: U.S. Healthcare, a large managed care organization (MCO), found that it could identify more than two-thirds of its diabetic members via visit encounters and almost half via either pharmacy data or claims data.[4]

Figure 1-1. A Disease Cost Model for Depression

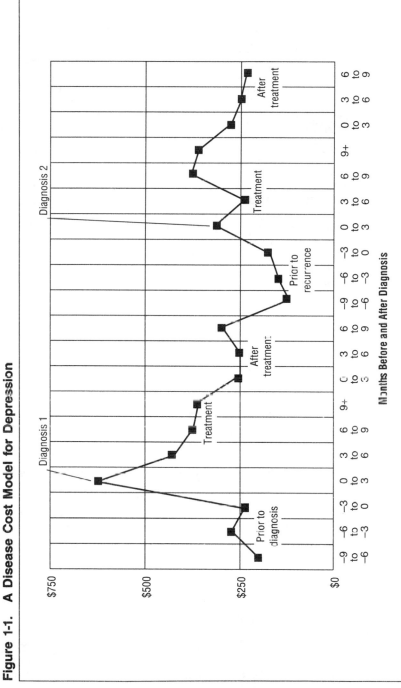

Source: Adapted from BCG.

Figure 1-2.   Cost Profiles of Asthmatic Patients, by Disease Severity

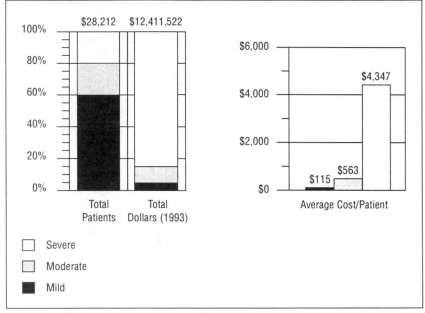

Source: Blue Cross of Western Pennsylvania.

Focusing on Prevention and Resolution

A true disease management program for many chronic diseases must focus
first on prevention and then on swift and effective resolution of acute episodes. A disease management program for asthma might involve lifestyle
and medication education for patients and families to minimize acute episodes, such as the highly successful program at National Jewish Center for
Immunology and Respiratory Medicine in Denver. In another instance,
prevention-oriented education and peer counseling might be central to an
AIDS program, whereas prevention of nosocomial pneumonia might include
elements as mundane as encouragement for both patients and providers to
wash their hands frequently. Many interventions essential to prevention or
swift resolution are not currently reimbursed under traditional health insurance plans.

Increasing Patient Compliance through Education

For chronic diseases — the central focus of many disease management activities — patient behavior often is the key determinant of illness manifestation.
This is particularly true for such asymptomatic conditions as hypertension

and hyperlipidemia. When noncompliance with therapy is a major risk factor, a disease management program will provide education to that effect and incentives to comply. These might include mailings, videos, telephone prescription-refill reminders, transportation to provider sites, electronic pillboxes, and print materials explaining the rationale for compliance even when no symptoms are apparent. The targets for such programs include not only patients, but families, providers, and lay caregivers. As suggested in the following section, disease management typically includes a heavy dose of education, prevention, and wellness activities.

Providing Full Care Continuity

A stroke victim may be cared for at home or in a hospital, nursing home, or rehabilitation facility during the course of a few months. This provides frequent opportunities for drug interactions, falls, and other misadventures. A disease management program might employ aggressive case management — a frequently used disease management tool — to plan and monitor treatment across all of these settings. The goal would be to avoid problems and to determine how to keep the patient out of the expensive (and typically less desirable) settings. This might involve anything from home nursing visits to assistance with grocery shopping, as well as helping the family support the patient's daily activities. Many organizations have found this emphasis on care continuity beneficial. Kaiser Permanente found that case management improved functional status and reduced risk factors in patients following heart attacks.[5] The Pennsylvania-based Guthrie Clinic has found that it can release patients who have undergone hip replacement surgery directly to their homes 90 percent of the time — double the national average — by using a care map and aggressive follow-up services.[6]

Establishing Integrated Data Management Systems

The importance of sophisticated delivery capabilities and data systems to the successful implementation of disease management programs cannot be overstated. Such technological advances as computerized patient records and automated surveys will be necessary to make access to and analysis of data possible. Perhaps the single greatest obstacle to the success of the disease management movement is the current lack of integrated data management systems. Such systems allow providers to track progress of patients across care settings, allow continuous and ongoing improvement of treatment algorithms, and assist greatly with diagnosis and care approaches through application of expert system techniques. The consolidation of many sectors of the health care industry, especially integrated delivery systems, offers hope that these systems will become available, as organizations design and implement new information systems that can be accessed and used by all members (such as acute care hospitals, home care agencies, and ambulatory centers that belong to the same network).

• The Impetus behind Disease Management

It would be heartening to know that the force behind disease management came from concerned clinicians seeking better patient outcomes — heartening, but untrue. In fact, this relatively new approach was born of business pressures, market consolidation, and questions about quality of care that were too great to ignore.

Cost-Containment Pressures

As with most major changes in health care over the past few decades, a primary motivator in the evolution toward disease management has been cost. That is because health expenditures have risen far faster than general inflation. Between 1965 and 1993, U.S. health care costs rose from $41.6 billion to $884.2 billion — a 2,206 percent increase — whereas the consumer price index increased only 358 percent.[7] This caused health care's share of the gross domestic product to rise from 5.9 percent to 13.9 percent.[8]

But the aggregate figures do not tell the whole story. Among those feeling the pinch most acutely were employers, who in 1993 paid 31.2 percent of the nation's health care bill.[9] Between 1970 and 1990, although wages grew just 1 percent ($116 in 1989 dollars), health benefits per employee grew an astonishing 163 percent ($1,066 in 1989 dollars).[10] In 1995 General Motors incurred an expense of $5.4 billion, or an average of about $1,200 per vehicle assembled in the United States, that could be attributed to the cost of health benefits.[11]

As government and private purchasers faced burgeoning medical costs, pressures for cost containment and health system reform intensified. Over the past two decades, the Health Care Financing Administration (HCFA) has introduced such measures as a prospective payment system (PPS), a resource-based relative value scale (RBRVS), and peer review organizations (PROs) to contain costs and reduce inappropriate care. Employers have formed scores of business health coalitions, many of which negotiate with health plans and other providers for rate discounts. A wide variety of plans to change health care delivery and financing are currently being debated in federal, state, and regional forums — all with the need to rein in soaring health costs as their premise.

These cost pressures have caused providers and purchasers alike to examine how health care is organized and delivered, thus paving the way for disease management. In the past two years, MCOs have reduced premium increases to single-digit levels; unless new ways are found to further reduce costs, these organizations will either experience sharply reduced profit margins or be forced to resort to significant price increases (see chapter 8). Price pressures have also had considerable influence on the revolutionary shift of pharmaceutical and pharmacy benefit management companies into disease management (see chapter 7). In short, many organizations envision disease management as a major opportunity to help keep health care cost increases in the single digits.

Questions about Quality

Rising cost and reduced profit margins are not the only factors encouraging adoption of a disease management approach to health care delivery. Higher costs have caused purchasers to ask increasingly tougher questions regarding the value they get for their dollar. The results have been disturbing.

Inappropriate Care

High-quality treatment must not only be done well, it must be necessary. When researchers at the RAND Corporation in Santa Monica, CA, evaluated several common medical procedures for appropriateness, they were surprised to find substantial rates of inappropriate care. Scientists judged 23 percent of tympanostomy tube insertions for children younger than 16 years to be inappropriate and another 35 percent to be equivocal.[12] Additionally, 16 percent of women underwent hysterectomies for reasons judged to be clinically inappropriate — 25 percent for uncertain reasons.[13] Rates of inappropriate care for coronary angiography, carotid endarterectomy, and upper gastrointestinal tract endoscopy varied from 15 percent to 40 percent.[14] Purchasers concluded from this research that elimination of such wasteful treatment could save significant money without harming quality.

A Dearth of Medical Evidence

Although most Americans believe that medical practice is firmly grounded in scientific research, this generally is not the case. According to the Office of Technology Assessment, only about 10 percent to 20 percent of all medical tests and procedures have been proven effective in clinical trials. This leaves a great number of current medical practices that are of uncertain benefit — at substantial cost.

Variations in Treatment Patterns

Concerns about the necessity and effectiveness of care are augmented by the obvious disagreement among practitioners and providers. Pioneering research conducted by John Wennberg and his colleagues at Dartmouth consistently found wide regional variations in treatment rates for numerous medical procedures:

- In Iowa, more than 60 percent of men in one area received a prostatectomy by the age of 85, compared to less than 15 percent of men in another area.
- In Maine, 70 percent of women over age 70 in one hospital area underwent hysterectomies, compared to only 20 percent in a nearby region.
- In Vermont, the chances that a child's tonsils would be removed varied from 70 percent in one town to just 8 percent in another.

Other researchers have found the same diversity in costs. For example, 1989 per capita Medicare expenditures in Miami ($1,874) were more than double those in San Francisco ($872) for the same year, although there is no evidence that older Miamians differ in health status from older San Franciscans.[15]

Managed Care Growth and Consolidation

Another factor driving the rapid acceptance of disease management is the continued growth and consolidation of the managed care industry. In 1976, only 6 million people, or 2.8 percent of the U.S. population, were enrolled in HMOs.[16] By 1993, that figure had risen to 45.2 million covered lives, or 17.5 percent of the population.[17] Tens of millions more lives were covered by preferred provider organizations (PPOs) and point-of-service (POS) plans.[18] This trend is accelerating, fueled in part by the movement of Medicare and Medicaid enrollees into managed care (figure 1-3).

The growth of managed care and its increasingly pervasive impact on how health care is delivered has facilitated disease management in at least two ways. First, prepayment, which is essential to most managed care arrangements, provides strong incentives for a disease management approach. Providers who assume the risk inherent in prepaid contracts have reason to deliver efficient and effective care. Inefficient care directly reduces provider profits, and ineffective care often will lead to follow-up corrective care, which also reduces the bottom line. Further, prepayment eliminates the incentives found in traditional fee-for-service (FFS) reimbursement to perform more tests and procedures. Thus, a prepaid health plan has solid financial reasons to provide the most effective care at the lowest possible cost—a characteristic of good disease management.

Second, MCOs typically cover both inpatient and outpatient care and may pay for home care, rehabilitative services, wellness care, and even long-term care. Disease management usually involves chronic care that may require a variety of services delivered in multiple settings. An MCO's involvement

Figure 1-3. Managed Care Growth

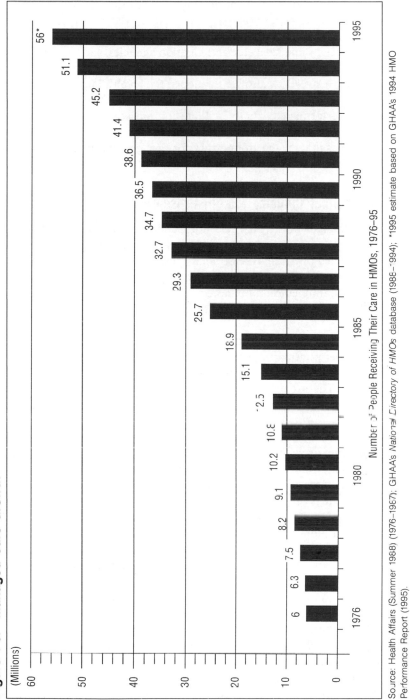

Number of People Receiving Their Care in HMOs, 1976–95

(Millions)

1976: 6
6.3
7.5
8.2
9.1
1980: 10.2
10.8
12.5
15.1
18.9
1985: 25.7
29.3
32.7
34.7
36.5
1990: 38.6
41.4
45.2
51.1
1995: 56*

Source: Health Affairs (Summer 1968) (1976–1987); GHAA's *National Directory of HMOs* database (1988–1994); *1995 estimate based on GHAA's 1994 HMO Performance Report (1995).

with or ownership of significant portions of the continuum of care is far more conducive to disease management than to the FFS system.

With the growth of managed care has come a corresponding growth and acceptance of managed care accreditation agencies, such as the National Committee for Quality Assurance (NCQA), which inspects and certifies the quality of HMOs. NCQA also has developed the Health Plan Employer Data and Information Set (HEDIS), a standardized method for HMOs to collect and report performance data to facilitate comparisons between plans. This and other new "report card" initiatives have forced many MCOs to quickly begin activities that lay the groundwork for first-generation disease management programs.

Pharmaceutical Industry Margin Pressures and Integration

Profound changes in the pharmaceutical industry also have advanced the field of disease management. Until the last several years, pharmaceutical firms considered physicians their primary customers. Doctors wrote prescriptions for which patients either paid out of pocket or charged to an insurance plan. Manufacturers attempted to persuade physicians to prescribe certain medications through well-funded promotional and advertising campaigns.

The rise of managed care, including pharmacy benefit managers (PBMs) and mail-order pharmacies, dramatically altered this situation. MCOs have the size and purchasing clout to negotiate aggressive bulk discounts on pharmaceuticals. The use of formularies by HMOs is on the rise, from 66 percent in 1990 to 89 percent in 1993; three-fourths of these formularies are closed (that is, restrictive).[19] Along with telephone reminders and other techniques, this has allowed MCOs to shift pharmaceutical market share. Suddenly manufacturers find that their seller's market has changed to a buyer's market. The proportion of prescriptions filled through managed care arrangements rose from 25.4 percent in 1990 to 48.6 percent in 1995. By 2000, the figure is projected to rise to 77.3 percent.[20] In addition, the accelerated shift to generic pharmaceutical products has eroded margins in the industry even more. It is expected that by the year 2000 as many as 200+ patented prescription drugs with sales of over $22 million will go "off patent." As discounts have increased and prices have leveled off, many pharmaceutical executives expect margins on their traditional business to decline.[21]

The industry has responded with stunning moves toward integration and consolidation. Several companies have merged (including Hoechst Roussel with Marion Merrell Dow, Glaxo with Burroughs Wellcome, Syntex with Hoffman La Roche) or formed strategic alliances to gain the research and marketing clout that comes with size. Vertical integration — characterized by both the acquisition of prescription benefit management companies and the development of freestanding disease management divisions as subsidiaries of the industry leaders—has also been widespread. Chapter 7 details the impact of these changes in the pharmaceutical industry.

Both the declining attractiveness of traditional drug development and the restructuring and vertical integration/horizontal expansion of the industry have plunged manufacturers into the field of disease management. Organizations no longer want to be considered drug manufacturers but prefer to be thought of as health care companies. Strategies to effect this image change range from value-added disease management programs wrapped around pharmaceutical products and acquisition of niche players to stand-alone offerings sold outright to MCOs and employers—in effect, entirely new, profit-seeking business lines. Whatever the form, the pharmaceutical industry is investing hundreds of millions of dollars annually in an effort to develop and implement disease management programs.

The Growing Use of Practice Guidelines

At the heart of the disease management approach is a systematic way of treating patients with similar characteristics. This may take the form of practice guidelines, treatment algorithms, clinical pathways, or some combination. Although the use of a guideline is not in and of itself a disease management program, it typically is an essential element of such an approach.

The health care system is growing increasingly familiar with such techniques. According to the American Medical Association (AMA), approximately 2,000 guidelines (which they call *practice parameters* or *clinical practice guides*) have been developed by national medical specialty societies and government agencies. Thousands more have been created by state medical groups, private companies, utilization review firms, and individual providers of all kinds. Enlightened purchasers have begun to insist on guideline use: In Minnesota, a group of large employers awarded a large, multi-year contract partly on the basis of the winning provider group's commitment to create and implement 16 practice guidelines during the program's first year.[22]

MCOs are using practice guidelines increasingly to enhance care quality, reduce treatment variation, and cut costs. Eighty-two percent of HMOs surveyed by the Group Health Association of America encourage providers to follow specific clinical practice guidelines to increase the likelihood that members will receive top-quality care. Of these HMOs, 85 percent have staff who are formally assigned to the development and implementation of guidelines. Fifty-six percent of respondents reported that they used guidelines developed internally. More than 40 percent of the HMOs promoting guidelines adapted them from those published by the federal Agency of Health Care Policy and Research, and 81.6 percent modified versions of other guidelines developed externally, such as those created by professional societies and medical specialty associations.[23]

Preliminary research has demonstrated the effectiveness and cost-saving potential of adherence to practice guidelines.[24] Clearly, providers' and purchasers' growing experience with practice guidelines is yet another factor facilitating the move toward disease management (see chapter 6).

Increasing Availability of Outcomes Research

Fueling the development of condition-specific disease management strategies is the burgeoning published literature on patient outcomes and cost-effectiveness. The 21 pharmaceutical manufacturers responding to the *1995 Pharmaceutical Outcomes Activities Study* by The Zitter Group and Technology Assessment Group expected to conduct approximately 280 pharmacoeconomic studies that year, the majority of which presumably could be used in the development of disease management programs. This growing body of research, which covers nearly all medical conditions and a wide range of therapies, expands the knowledge base essential for the creation of sound disease management strategies (see chapter 3). Without meaningful outcomes-measurement systems, disease management programs will likely be very short-lived.

• Health Care Industry Acceptance of Disease Management

Various segments of the health care industry have begun to adopt disease management, and the number of disease management programs continues to expand at an increasing rate. A recent industry report identified more than 130 disease management programs in more than eight major therapeutic categories.[25] Table 1-1 lists seven areas in which companies have invested substantial resources. As noted in the last section, the growth of disease management has been especially rapid in the pharmaceutical industry.

Table 1-1. Proliferation of Disease Management Programs

Type of Program	Number of Programs
Metabolic disease	21
Asthma/respiratory	25
Cardiovascular disease	26
Cancer	9
Infectious disease	10
Gastrointestinal disorders	4
Neurological disorders	21

Source: POV Inc., July 1995.

Pharmaceutical Manufacturers

As suggested above, pharmaceutical manufacturers have aggressively entered the disease management fray. As larger PBMs and managed care customers have exacted increasingly steep discounts, pharmaceutical manufacturers have sought new ways to differentiate their product offerings and new vehicles to earn profits.

Although the evolution of pharmaceutical industry strategy may have taken years, a study conducted in 1991 for Pfizer, Inc., by the Boston Consulting Group (BCG) is largely recognized for the "birth of disease management." This study recommended that the pharmaceutical industry take a hard look at the 93 percent of health care costs for which they were not traditionally responsible, because the prognosis for pharmaceuticals, which account for 7 percent of health care costs, was poor and getting worse. Essentially, this study recommended that pharmaceutical manufacturers redirect their expertise/resources into the "management of diseases." Originally, this recommendation was implemented via a very narrow use of more aggressive and proactive patient prescription utilization programs that many viewed as new marketing initiatives. In recent years, these first-generation disease management programs have broadened and become far more comprehensive. The early programs emphasized chronic conditions that rely heavily on pharmaceutical therapy, such as asthma, diabetes, hypertension, ulcers, and migraine.

Today, pharmaceutical executives speak of turning their organizations from drug companies into health care companies. The 1995 survey by The Zitter Group and Technology Assessment Group found that most pharmaceutical firms surveyed had staff formally assigned to disease management activities, with an average of 11 full-time equivalents per firm.[26] Because several of the firms with the largest disease management programs declined to respond for proprietary reasons, these figures probably significantly understate actual industry activities.

Major companies tend to pursue one of two distinct approaches to disease management, although some follow both simultaneously. First, some offer disease management services as an adjunct to a medication in an effort to enhance sales and/or profits for that product. In this situation, pharmaceutical manufacturers will offer a package that will help customers better manage patients suffering from a particular illness, in the hope that the client will use more of its product. The package usually involves a medication distributed by the manufacturer as well as a variety of other value-added services designed to improve outcomes and reduce costs for that disease state.[27] The second common approach used by pharmaceutical manufacturers involves getting into health and disease management as a separate business. Several companies have created separate divisions intended to offer disease management services on a full-fee basis. Services might include outcomes measurement, data collection and analysis, formulary design, physician education, patient information, or other elements. Chapter 7 details the role that pharmaceutical manufacturers and prescription benefit management companies have played in the rise of disease management.

Pharmacy Benefit Management Companies

Pharmacy benefit management companies have experienced tremendous growth over the past five years. They have been highly successful in helping large employers achieve significant reductions in payments for prescription drugs. Unfortunately, as with pharmaceutical manufacturers, increased competition and reduced profit margins have forced PBMs to identify new sources for cost reduction and differentiation. Disease management has represented one of their major strategies. This strategy hinges on the assumption that their past investment in sophisticated computer systems will provide the infrastructure needed to further reduce costs for either medications (which PBMs manage) or more expensive health care services (which other entities manage). Interestingly, the latter often involves an *increase* in the drug budget that is more than offset by a decrease in other costs. Usually the assumption is made that health outcomes are improved or (at least) remain constant while overall costs drop.

Given the early stage of disease management implementation by PBMs, the jury is still out regarding the long-term success of the strategy. There is evidence, however, that at least one large PBM has been able to move market share toward its owner (a pharmaceutical manufacturer), although it is not clear that this shift resulted directly from activities.[28]

Managed Care Organizations

The involvement of MCOs in disease management is the result of a very natural evolution of the industry. The original concept of an HMO was to focus on the *maintenance* of a member's health, on the core principle that healthier members would be less expensive. Unfortunately, over the past decade, most HMOs (now more broadly referred to as MCOs) failed to focus sufficient resources on health maintenance. Chapter 8 discusses MCOs' evolution toward disease management. As both providers and payers, MCOs have great incentive to improve outcomes and reduce costs. A 1994 study of MCOs found that more than half of the responding 62 major MCOs were either implementing, developing, or seriously considering disease management programs.[29]

For example, the Mayo Clinic has developed disease management strategies — listed in figure 1-4 — for more than a dozen disease conditions, including uncomplicated cystitis, hypertension, breast cancer, low back pain,

Figure 1-4. Elements of Disease Management at the Mayo Clinic

- Primary care practice guidelines
- Information systems
- Continuous quality improvement
- Resource management techniques
- Information management
- Specialty care management
- Hospital management
- Emergency room management

- Pharmacy management
- Diagnostic utilization management
- Case management
- Patient education
- Primary care teams
- Triage system/telephone system
- Benefit design

Source: Nesse, R. E., and Angstman, G. L. *Disease Management Strategies: A Foundation for Health Systems Integration,* unpublished paper.

diabetes, and asthma. Group Health Cooperative of Puget Sound has also implemented disease management for diabetes through its population-based care approach. An expert team developed evidence-based guidelines that focused on planned patient assessments, improved clinical care, and systematic patient education, and included elimination of such previously routine measures as hospitalization of newly diagnosed diabetics. Other managed care disease management leaders include the Lovelace Clinic and its "Episodes of Care" program, Harvard Community Health Plan, Kaiser Permanente, and U.S. Healthcare.

Other Health Care Organizations

Several other industry segments are also getting heavily involved in disease management. Home infusion providers, traditional national nursing agencies, and newly formed disease management companies are all investing in the people and systems necessary to pursue disease management on a national scale. The breadth and scope of disease management is reflected in Value Health's annual report, which devoted its entire essay section to the topic, referring to it as "the holy grail of health care" as it relates to both cost and quality, and proclaiming it an important part of the company's future strategy.

A fast-growing pool of niche players is also emerging in the disease management game. Some of these are focusing on the management of such rare chronic diseases as hemophilia and cystic fibrosis. Caremark, prior to the sale of its infusion business to Coram Healthcare, had established care networks that provide comprehensive services to patients suffering from hemophilia, HIV/AIDS, and kidney failure, and had pursued disease management through its PBM.[30] Quantum Health Resources and Accordant Health Services, Inc., have also established disease management initiatives focused on rare chronic diseases such as hemophilia and cystic fibrosis. Others have developed specialized physician networks and disease management systems for more broad-based diseases such as asthma and diabetes. For example, Diabetes Treatment Centers of America has established direct relationships with endocrinologists and diabetologists to provide diabetes disease management care.[31] Numerous small companies, many focusing on providing treatment algorithms and services for just one disease, are proliferating. Although it is too early to gauge the success of any of these specific efforts, collectively they attest to the growing belief in the disease management approach.

• Potential Benefits of Disease Management

Proponents of the disease management approach believe that it holds substantial promise to improve health outcomes while reducing costs. A variety of experience, research, and analysis supports this belief.

The National Asthma Education Program (NAEP), a branch of the National Heart, Lung, and Blood Institute, issued guidelines for the treatment of asthma in 1993. The guidelines recommend an integrated "bundle" of interventions that go well beyond traditional acute care, such as creating a written treatment plan for each patient and training asthmatics in the use of a peak flow meter. Because research has demonstrated the effectiveness and cost-saving potential of this approach, virtually all asthma disease management programs developed to date are based at least in part on these widely accepted guidelines.

Based on an extensive study of current health care practices, BCG has estimated the possible savings of using disease management for asthma and depression. By educating patients in the proper use of steroids and educating physicians in early identification of asthmatics and appropriate specialist referral, BCG estimates that a systemwide approach to managing asthma could save approximately 25 percent of costs. Similarly, a depression disease management program could focus on early diagnosis and treatment, compliance enhancement, minimization of recurrence, and other activities. The company's analysis suggests that such an approach might reduce net system costs by 10 percent to 20 percent.[32]

Trigon Blue Cross and Blue Shield of Richmond, VA, developed an asthma disease management program centered on a one-page summary of NAEP's treatment guidelines. The summary was distributed to all plan physicians. The preliminary results are promising: After the first year, functional status scores for severe asthmatics rose from 41 percent to 46 percent on the Health Status Questionnaire. Also, average annual office visits dropped from 3.4 to 2.6 per asthmatic, and emergency room visits sank from 1.0 to 0.6.[33]

Value Health, a large MCO, has also made a significant investment in disease management. Based on experience and a review of existing research, the company believes that its diabetes disease management program can achieve the following improvements:

- A 50 percent reduction in lower-extremity amputations
- A 70 percent reduction in episodes of ketoacidosis
- A 50 percent reduction in end-stage renal disease
- A 60 percent reduction in diabetes-related blindness
- A 40 percent reduction in days lost from work[34]

Each of these examples illustrates the promise of disease management to improve health outcomes and save total costs.

• Generations of Disease Management Programs

Disease management continues to evolve. The rapid growth of the field has contributed to the confusion about what disease management really is (and is not). In the rush to embrace this new framework, the label has been applied to a variety of activities that clearly differ from traditional medical care but do not necessarily reflect new principles. As the field has developed, programs have become better defined and more comprehensive.

The First Generation: Picking Off Care Elements

Early disease management programs simply offered one or more services that were outside typical medical care and could be useful in addressing an illness. As mentioned above, many of these first-generation programs were motivated by the need to meet HEDIS–like quality report card requirements developed by national accreditation agencies and employers. However, there was no comprehensive approach to combating the entire spectrum of a disease or even attacking the primary cost drivers. For example, one program sponsored by a pharmaceutical manufacturer used telephone reminders to encourage all hypertensive patients to refill their prescriptions. By zeroing in on medication compliance, a major issue in controlling blood pressure, the program demonstrated savings in physician and hospital visits and overall treatment costs.[35] However, only hypertensive patients receiving medication were contacted, patients were not targeted by severity of illness, treatment appropriateness was not considered, and no health outcomes were measured (only resource consumption). In short, only the medication compliance element was addressed.

The Second Generation: Targeting Patients for High-Impact Interventions

Before long it became clear that more severely ill patients not only need more care, but that their high costs mean greater opportunity to save dollars.

The next generation of disease management programs targeted the sickest patients and/or those at greatest risk of generating high costs and intervened where impact would be greatest. For example, a prototype second-generation program for depression would educate primary care physicians about detecting depression, educate depressed patients regarding the importance of medication compliance, and follow up proactively with patients after their first episode to address recurrences before they became catastrophic. Most current disease management programs are at this stage.

The Third Generation: Truly Integrated Care

The next generation of disease management will fully integrate care and reimbursement and will resemble some of the disease management programs described in this book. Programs will be population based and will identify all patients suffering from or at risk for a given disease; they then will be stratified according to the severity of their illness or health risk. Different strategies will be employed according to the risk and cost profile of each patient. All significant elements of care will be addressed, with treatment centrally coordinated across care components. An example might be an asthma program that would categorize all asthmatic patients into mild, moderate, and severe groups. All patients would receive education, a written care plan, and basic treatment, but the severely ill would spend one-on-one time with a health educator, keep an electronic journal of peak flow readings that is tied into a provider office, and receive home visits from a care manager on a regular basis. These visits might include an environmental analysis of the home environment to detect factors that might exacerbate the illness. Such a program would use health and cost metrics to track results and calculate cost–benefit on an ongoing basis. A few of the leading disease management programs are approaching this third stage.

The Fourth Generation: Health Management

Perhaps someday we will reach a true health management model. As addressed in chapter 12, the ultimate extension of disease management, health management, will focus more on optimizing health than on treating existing disease. This will involve a serious commitment to lifelong health education aimed at prevention, as well as strong incentives for maintaining a safe and healthy lifestyle. Genetic markers and periodic health assessments will help providers target individuals most in need of personalized health education and behavior modification programs. Providers will consider an individual's total health picture rather than focusing on each disease separately. Preventive health resources will be allocated based on who is most likely to respond and benefit. The foundation for health management will be the prevention of disease and accidents; this will involve a less medically oriented approach to health than our current system employs. Chapter 12 details the current status of prevention initiatives in this country and discusses the issues/obstacles that will influence the evolution of our health care system into true health management.

If the United States does make this transition, health plans will eventually compete based on their success in maintaining health given the risk inherent in their member population. Illness that occurs will be treated via a third-generation disease management model, modified to better reflect comorbidity issues. The degree to which this health management paradigm will be adopted depends on America's ability to make substantial changes in reimbursement, medical training, information system capabilities, and — perhaps most important — public attitudes towards health, medical providers, and personal responsibility.

• Disease Management: The Opportunity

Disease management is not a panacea for America's health care woes, and its potential currently far exceeds its demonstrated effectiveness. However, there are at least three reasons to believe that the disease management approach will spread in prevalence and impact:

1. It has a theoretical model that fits the evolving health care system better than the component management approach does.
2. There is preliminary evidence in a variety of disease states that the model has great potential for both improved health outcomes and reduced costs.
3. Scores of major health care organizations from various industry segments have invested substantial resources in disease management.

America's health care leaders are positioning themselves to operate and succeed in a health care system increasingly focused on preventing and addressing specific diseases regardless of care setting or budget component. They are analyzing their entire member populations, targeting high-risk patients for the most aggressive intervention, and developing information systems and measurement techniques to assess the impact of their efforts. The future belongs to these progressive organizations, who will be best prepared to efficiently maximize the health of all Americans in the next millennium.

References

1. Soumerai, S., McLaughlin, T. J., Ross-Degnan, D., Casteris, C. S., and Bollini, P. Effect of limiting Medicaid drug-reimbursement benefits on the use of psycho-

tropic agents and acute mental service by patients with schizophrenia. *The New England Journal of Medicine* 331(10):650–55, 1994.

2. Moore, W. J., and Newman, R. J. U.S. Medicaid drug formularies: do they work? *Pharmacoeconomics* 1992 (suppl. 1):31.

3. Hanchak, N. A. The epidemiology of costs of diabetes mellitus, US Quality Algorithms. *Quality Monitor* 2(1):5, Winter 1995.

4. Hanchak, p. 4.

5. DeBusk, R. F., Miller, N. H., Superko, H. R., Dennis, C. A., Thomas, R. J., Lew, H. T., Berger, W. E. III, and others. A case-management system for coronary risk factor modification after acute myocardial infarction. *Annals of Internal Medicine* 120(9):721–29, May 1, 1994.

6. Robert Michaels, MD, telephone conversation with author, Apr. 20, 1995.

7. Consumer Price Index Detailed Report. US Department of Labor, Bureau of Labor Statistics, May 1996, table 24, pp. 64–65.

8. McDonnell, K. Employee Benefit Research Institute, Washington, DC. *Issue Brief No. 164,* Aug. 1995.

9. McDonnell.

10. Presentation by Ian Morrison, National Managed Health Care Congress, Washington, DC, Apr. 1994.

11. Duane Poole, General Motors, letter to author, Oct. 6, 1995.

12. Kleinman, L. C., Kosecoff, J., Dubois, R. W., and Brook, R. H. The medical appropriateness of tympanostomy tubes proposed for children younger than 16 years in the United States. *JAMA* 271(16):1250–55, Apr. 27, 1994.

13. Bernstein, S. J., McGlynn, E. A., Siu, A. L., Roth, C. P., Sherwood, J. W., Keesey, J. W., Kosecoff, J., and others. The appropriateness of hysterectomy. *JAMA* 269(18):2398–402, May 12, 1993.

14. Leape, L. L., Park, R. E., Solomon, D. H., Chassin, M. R., Kosecoff, J., and Brook, R. H. Does inappropriate use explain small-area variations in the use of health care services? *JAMA* 263(5):669–72, Feb. 2, 1990.

15. Welch, W. P., Miller, M. E., Welch, G., Fisher, E. S., and Wennberg, J. E. Geographic variation in expenditures for physicians' services in the United States. *The New England Journal of Medicine* 328(9):621–27, 1993.

16. *Health Affairs,* Summer 1988.

17. Group Health Association of America. National Directory of HMOs database. Washington, DC: Group Health Association of America, 1995.

18. Jon Gabel, GHAA, telephone conversation with author, Oct. 2, 1995.

19. Marion Merrell Dow. *Managed Care Digest, HMO Edition.* Kansas City, MO: Marion Merrell Dow, 1994.

20. IMS America. *The Retail Method of Payment Report.* Plymouth Meeting, PA: IMS America, 1995.

21. *Statistical Abstract of the United States,* p. 490.

22. Tom Pavey, Minneapolis/St. Paul Business Health Care Action Group, telephone conversation with author, Sept. 20, 1995.

23. Group Health Association of America. *1994 HMO Performance Report.* Washington, DC: GHAA, 1994.

24. Trigon blues see swift results with one-page version of national asthma guideline. *Report on Medical Guidelines & Outcomes Research* 6(17):9, Aug. 24, 1995.

25. Point of View, Inc. *Disease Management . . . and Its Impact on Business Strategy for the Health Care Industry,* Woburn, MA: POV, July 1995.

26. The Zitter Group and Technology Assessment Group. *1995 Pharmaceutical Outcomes Activities Survey.* San Francisco: The Zitter Group, 1995.

27. *F-D-C Report* 56(28), July 11, 1994.

28. Browning, E. S., and Burton, T. M. Lilly's PCS receives Rx: a write-down. *Wall Street Journal,* July 30, 1996, p. C-1.

29. The Zitter Group. *Disease Management Study.* San Francisco: The Zitter Group, 1994.

30. Caremark. *Annual Report.* Lincolnshire, IL: Caremark, 1994.

31. Bob Stone, Diabetes Treatment Centers of America, telephone conversation with author, Oct. 6, 1995.

32. Boston Consulting Group. *The Changing Environment for U.S. Pharmaceuticals.* Report prepared for Pfizer Pharmaceuticals, Apr. 1993.

33. *Report on Medical Guidelines & Outcomes Research.*

34. Value Health. *Annual Report.* Avon, CT: Value Health, 1994.

35. Sclar, D. A., and others. Effect of health education on the utilization of HMO services: a prospective trail among patients with hypertension. *Primary Cardiology* 18(S1): 30–35, 1992.

Chapter 2

The Disease Management Development Process

John H. Eichert, Herbert Wong, PhD, and David R. Smith, MD

The new paradigm of disease management, outlined in chapter 1, has been so well received by various segments of the health care industry that implementation has frequently run well ahead of thoughtful design and planning of the systems and infrastructure needed to ensure successful implementation. Fueled by the pressure of powerful forces within the industry, the evolution of the health care system as a whole, and a high level of interest, disease management has taken on almost revolutionary proportions. Unfortunately, this rush to explore the potential of disease management has resulted in the development of many *programs* rather than *systems*.

The design, development, implementation, and ongoing improvement of disease management systems are complex and time-consuming undertakings requiring substantial resources and commitment from organization leaders. This chapter outlines a comprehensive process for creating a disease management system. The processes described address the organizational/structural elements needed for successful implementation, as well as the clinical, medical, and financial approaches to develop systems designed to lower total treatment costs and improve overall quality of care. The processes are broad guidelines meant to be flexible and adaptable to the individual organizations attempting to implement a systems approach to disease management.

• A Health Care System in Transition

As discussed in chapter 1, health care experts and progressive health care management organizations are recognizing the need for systems-based disease management designed to reduce preventable morbidity and mortality from specific diseases and to improve the health status of populations. They recognize that each disease has its own characteristic pattern of cost elements (that is, specific components of cost), a different and varying set of cost occurrences (that is, the components that exist within a given episode of illness), and a complex range of available therapies and interventions.

To make rational choices among therapeutic options, these organizations understand they must focus on the interactions of cost and clinical quality drivers over the entire course of the disease and throughout all elements of the system. They recognize that a spectrum of health risks for each population influences how resources are consumed. They also understand that, as a greater percentage of plan members are capitated globally, they must begin to focus on disease management and, eventually, health management strategies that reduce long-term demand on the system.

As the market shifts from the old, fragmented, fee-for-service (FFS) "sick care" system to the new, integrated, cost-based "health care" system, all components of the system must also reinvent themselves to remain competitive. This transition will be forced to accelerate over the next few years, because the FFS base of most health care delivery systems will be substantially eroded by Medicaid and Medicare reform. Plans funded almost entirely by Medicaid and Medicare will realize that the reduction in FFS revenues will have a domino effect, significantly impacting all other provider networks. Therefore, reinventing business and marketing strategies becomes necessary for survival and increases the need to balance the old and the new while remaining flexible enough to evolve as the market changes.

This transitional period, or bifurcation, is characterized by individual, organizational, and system confusion, chaos, fear, and anxiety.[1] The numerous conflicting events occurring simultaneously are at the root of these transitional emotions. Many individuals and organizations are paralyzed as they wait for the market to stabilize. Meanwhile, their market share declines and profits erode.

Market transition is being driven by a number of factors that must be considered when designing a disease management system:[2]

- The shift from revenue- to cost-based reimbursement
- Advances in information systems and technology
- The need to control total health care system costs, not individual component costs
- The increasing number of capitated lives that enable plans/systems to employ population-based strategies that can reduce risks and short- and long-term costs
- The growing influence of payers and demands for increased savings in both the short and long term
- The need for accountability

A disease management strategy will begin to surface when a systems-thinking mentality takes hold, disease management principles are agreed on and adopted, and key elements have begun to be created. But strategy must match the structure, skills, and culture of each organization in the health

Figure 2-1.   The Evolution of Managed Care and Disease Management

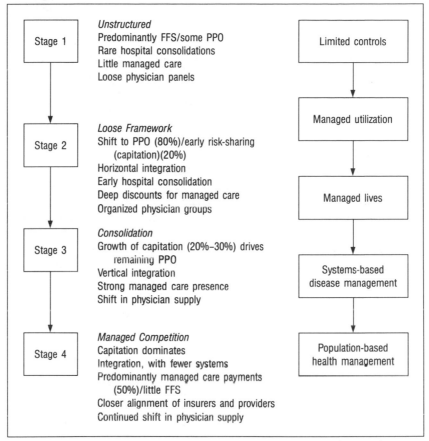

Source: Wong, H. *Welcome to Systems Thinking*. Austin: Quantum Solutions, Inc., Sept. 1993.

care system. Success will never be achieved without this alignment. *Structure* should support the strategy; *skills* will enable successful implementation of the strategy; and a receptive *culture* will encourage the systems approach disease management needs to emerge and thrive as a practical reality.

Disease management strategy must be matched with the stage of managed care evolution within each metropolitan or regional market. Mistiming the strategy can mean partial or complete failure because the infrastructure of the marketplace and the reimbursement incentives are not yet placed properly to support the effort.

The evolving managed care marketplace currently includes the four stages shown in figure 2-1.[3] A systems approach to disease management needs to be designed, developed, and implemented at critical junctures during this evolution.

The complete shift from component management to disease management will not happen overnight. Health services are undergoing a major evolution as they gradually move from managing the individual episode of illness to managing the course of the disease (diagnosis to outcome, whether cure, resolution, or death) and to regulating the overall health of a member population. The key to success with population-based disease management is the systematic oversight of total members/covered lives, from birth to death.

Getting started on the path toward an integrated system of health management is often a difficult task. Success depends on identifying key leverages in the health system and on focusing resources early. These actions will yield timely results. The difficulty in identifying the leverage action is compounded by the lack of an integrated communications data system, the inability to enlist the collective support of the provider network, and a rapidly changing market.

Over the next three years, physician integration will be the most difficult and important task for health care systems throughout the United States. Although individual practice associations (IPAs) for capitated contracting are common in some areas on the West Coast, they are still forming in the rest of the country and are struggling to learn the process. In stages 2 and 3 of the evolutionary model (see figure 2-1), the task of aligning physician incentives becomes very important. The questions are:

- How do we bring certain physicians into the IPA while excluding others?
- What are the criteria for inclusion/exclusion?
- What are legal implications of that process?
- How do we communicate critical outcomes information and educate physicians about appropriate interventions?
- How are the revenues divided between primary care and specialists?

In order for systems-based disease management to work, these issues must be resolved.

In addition, given the lack of data, an organization will not be able to jump from discounted FFS (stage 2) to global capitation (stage 4). The presence or lack of an integrated information systems infrastructure will dictate the ability, speed, and effectiveness at which health plans and systems make the transition.

Experimentation and the ability to learn quickly from success and failure will characterize the successful integrated health system. Health plans will need to experiment with "bundling" services around diseases and procedures. The first step, of course, is actually developing and implementing a disease management system — which is the focus of the rest of this chapter.

• Developing a Disease Management System: Process Overview

Developing a systems strategy for disease management in an increasingly complex, transforming environment means more than continually assessing where you are, where you want to be, and how you plan to get there. Any strategic approach must also consider the implications of creating and packaging a broad range of new products and services in an environment that is intensely competitive with rapidly maturing product life cycles.

To design, develop, and implement a disease management system, it is helpful to use a systems-thinking model developed by Quantum Solutions Inc. and illustrated in figure 2-2 that is based on the organizational principles of Peter M. Senge and the continuous quality improvement (CQI) concepts of W. Edwards Deming, Philip Crosby, and Dr. Joseph Duran.[4] To adapt the general systems model to disease management in particular, each

Figure 2-2. Systems-Thinking Model: The Disease Management Process

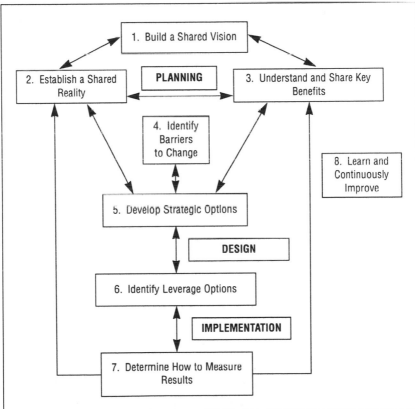

step in the process of system development incorporates four key elements: (1) disease management strategy, (2) organizational culture, (3) structure, and (4) skills, as illustrated in the "organizational tetrahedron" in figure 2-3.

The Steps in the Process

The following steps are covered in detail later in the chapter, but brief descriptions are given here to illustrate the systems model:

1. *Build a shared vision.* Create a common vision about the mission or purpose of the disease management system. Note the word *shared* in this step. It is critical to consolidate all stakeholders' points of view about their vision of disease management in an effort to reach a vision of the system that everyone believes in and is willing to work toward achieving.
2. *Establish a shared reality.* Reach a common understanding of where your organization is today in managing a particular disease or population of people. For example, you need to determine how health care is delivered, how much it costs for a given disease or population, and where opportunities for change will result in measurable improvements in clinical outcomes or lower total system costs.
3. *Understand and share key beliefs.* Establish a shared understanding and acceptance of key beliefs, or assumptions, within your organization about how and how much disease management can improve your quality of care and reduce costs. Shared assumptions are the key goal of this step.

Figure 2-3. Organizational Tetrahedron

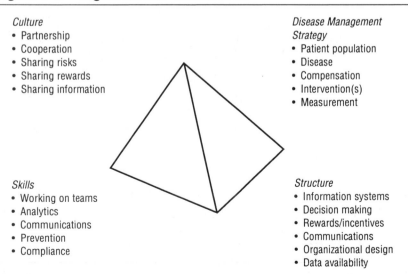

Culture
- Partnership
- Cooperation
- Sharing risks
- Sharing rewards
- Sharing information

Disease Management Strategy
- Patient population
- Disease
- Compensation
- Intervention(s)
- Measurement

Skills
- Working on teams
- Analytics
- Communications
- Prevention
- Compliance

Structure
- Information systems
- Decision making
- Rewards/incentives
- Communications
- Organizational design
- Data availability

4. *Identify barriers to change.* Pinpoint barriers to change, such as lack of knowledge, insufficient information, inadequate information systems, poor-quality or insufficient data, lack of provider cooperation, misaligned incentives and rewards, inadequate reimbursement, and poor communications systems. These problems frequently hinder successful implementation of disease management systems.

5. *Develop strategic options.* Define what options exist for making improvements in the management of a population or disease, either in reducing total cost or in improving quality or increasing patient and provider satisfaction.

6. *Identify leverage options.* Pinpoint critical junctures in disease treatment, that is, points where the greatest change can be achieved with the least expenditure of resources. Many organizations elect to start their disease management efforts with a pilot program, or beta site, to determine whether they have selected the best option and to gain insight into the effect of their plan.

7. *Determine how to measure results.* Determine critical outcomes to measure the impact of your actions and to challenge your reality, vision, and key beliefs. Measurement is the key to success in disease management. If you do not make a commitment to incorporate measurement systems into your plan, you cannot expect to change the system in any meaningful way. Furthermore, if you do not communicate the results in a timely fashion to those involved in the delivery of health care, you will not effect change.

8. *Learn and continuously improve.* Incorporate data collection and data analysis to evaluate the impact of your intervention(s), to capture and communicate key learning, and to apply CQI principles to your disease management plan. Initial success may consist of process improvements, with real clinical or economic outcome changes occurring later. Therefore, it is important to incorporate both process and outcomes measures in your plan. Continuous improvement is another hallmark of disease management and must be incorporated into your plan to be successful.

• Key Points for Organizational Change to Disease Management

A disease management strategy necessitates a redesign of the organizational system, creating a transformational bridge from the old to the new. It must be a flexible, dynamic, and comprehensive organizational system that is able to continuously gather information from its environment, process the information, quickly begin appropriate action, and monitor input on costs and quality.

There are three key focal points to consider when creating and implementing innovative disease management strategies for a rapidly changing market: the culture, structure, and skills resident in the organization.

Creation of a Responsive Culture

Culture is an organization's vision, values, and norms. To be successful in today's market, organizations need flexibility in their thinking and in the infrastructure that supports disease management products and services. One of the key necessities of culture is the ability to manage change. Change management is enabled by speed, the ability from the top to make quick decisions; and the simultaneous ability to receive input and evaluate it. The flip side of speed is being able to tolerate mistakes and to learn from them.[5] (Recall that culture is one of the four elements on the organizational tetrahedron in figure 2-3.)

An example of the cultural shift necessary to successfully transform from a component management organization to a systems management organization is how your organization views suppliers. In the old component culture, the focus was on minimizing the individual expense of a particular item used in managing a disease (for example, drugs). In the new systems culture, the supplier may be viewed more as a partner and the particular item it supplies is viewed within the context of its value in the overall treatment of disease. The relationship with the supplier is therefore less adversarial and more collaborative.

A similar situation is the relationship between the managed care organization and the provider. In the old component culture, the provider was viewed as an adversary rather than a partner. In the new culture, the provider is part of the health care team and an integral part of the solution, rather than the problem. This new partnership can be structured within existing contract language, as can performance measures.

Key cultural norms for successful disease management are:

- Cooperation and collaboration
- Teamwork
- Communication and information sharing
- Decision making driven by data rather than opinion[6]
- Delivery of high-quality, cost-effective health care
- The sharing of a common language (definitions and principles of disease management)
- Commitment to pinpointing mistakes

Most of these norms are already familiar to those who have been involved in continuous improvement.

Creation of a Viable Structure

Closely related to culture, *structure* drives and reinforces the organization's behavior. Cooperative networks, "virtual departments" (groups that form around a new product and disappear as the product matures), free-flowing information, and team-centered reward systems characterize the new model required for health care today. Information enables sound decision making and gives the ability to decide what should be centralized and decentralized. Some of the key structural requirements for successful disease management initiatives are:

- Consistently strong support from top-level management
- Information systems linking all elements of the health care system, providing data collection, data management, data analysis, and data communications throughout the continuum of care
- The ability to share cost information across all components of the health care system (cost transparency) complete with standards providing for the format, content, and structure of disease-associated cost information[7]
- The ability to measure outcomes at the point of care, that is, clinical, quality, and patient and provider satisfaction
- Aligned rewards and incentives for patients, providers, and plans
- Communications systems enabling dialogue among patients, providers, and plans
- Quality data and information about the disease, for example, medical/ clinical, costs, utilization, pharmaceutical, and laboratory
- Organizational structure that incorporates all the key elements for total patient care across the continuum of care for the targeted disease with protocols for referring patients from one setting to the other; for example, inpatient, home care, long-term care, ambulatory care, primary care, and specialist care
- Decision-making processes for disease management, for example, evidence-based clinical practice guidelines and protocols
- Cost-control tools for the disease, for example, formularies, utilization review, report cards, and performance reviews

As evidenced by this list, the structural elements of a disease management system are more cost conscious than are the cultural elements.

Development of Requisite Skills

Skills fuel an organization's strategy, culture, and structure. In a world of product fragmentation and short product life cycles, skills at individual, team, and organizational levels must focus on knowing how to manage a business in the midst of constant change and uncertainty. Some of the crucial skills for disease management include working on multidisciplinary, cross-functional teams; data analytics; patient communication; prevention; wellness; and compliance enhancement.

As new strategies are forged, it is critical to consider both clinical and organizational issues. Building new clinical management strategies or implementing component programs without focusing on the organization's supporting culture, skills, and structure would significantly diminish the chances for successful transformation to a disease management systems approach. Additionally, the transformation can be slowed by the evolving complexities of cross-functional teams and of an expanding system. The inherent struggle is that the more complex a system becomes, the longer it takes to make decisions.

A systems approach to the management of disease is at the heart of the emerging health care system. The strategy required to achieve this vision will need to provide effective processes to successfully transition today's fragmented, revenue-based health care delivery model to an integrated system that provides full continuity of care. This strategy will be wedded to an information infrastructure that will be needed for decision support, outcomes measurement, and quality improvement.

To help explain how to move an organization toward these changes, the following sections take a more comprehensive look at each of the eight steps in the process of developing a disease management system.

• Step 1: Build a Shared Vision

The vision of a disease management system incorporates several key components that will be refined and completed as all players in the industry work to develop a total systems approach to managing disease and eventually optimizing health. The vision must be shared by all stakeholders in the disease management process. Therefore, it may take some time to gain agreement. It is very important to have a shared vision, because it is the blueprint that provides your organization with a sense of purpose and direction. The vision statement should range in length from a few sentences to a page and describe what your disease management system will look like. You should look forward anywhere from 3 to 10 years and envision what the disease management system will look like in the future. It is important to recognize that it takes time to build a disease management system that evolves from a component orientation to an integrated system of health care. Your disease management vision may also evolve over time as you learn from experience or as your organization changes in response to the competitive environment.

You have an option to create your vision either before or after the assessment of where you are today (completed during step 2). It really does not matter when you create your vision, as long as you do so before developing strategic options. Many organizations leap from an assessment of their current disease management system directly to implementation of programs. This is unwise, because disease management is not a program or isolated set of interventions, but an integrated system of interventions, measures, and continuous improvement processes to facilitate learning and evolution.

Continuity of care is the cornerstone of this type of system—through it all components are linked into an integrated whole, eliminating duplication of care and unnecessary practices and procedures. For any single disease, continuity of care includes interventions at every stage in the health care continuum—prevention and wellness programs, primary care and diagnosis, acute care and chronic care, rehabilitative care and supportive care. Figure 2-4 illustrates the steps in the continuum and how they coincide in an ongoing cycle.

Continuity of care will marry information tools to all players involved with the patient. Building continuity can take years and is often the last limiting step in the development of comprehensive disease management systems. This approach encourages conservation and more efficient use of resources by ensuring that everyone who treats the patient will observe a coherent, unified treatment plan. The result will be lower overall use of services, more efficiently managed resources, reduced duplication of efforts, better disease prevention and improved health promotion, and a focus on "health care" versus "sick care." Ultimately (perhaps over several years) this will provide greater marketability to payers due to lower long-term costs and increased patient satisfaction. Savings may also be seen on the job in better attendance, improved functionality, and reduced workers' compensation.

Figure 2-4. Continuum of Care

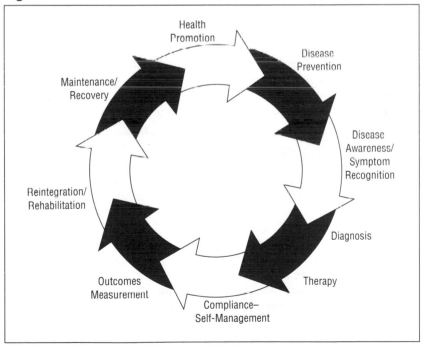

Other important elements of a disease management vision are:

- *Identifying at-risk populations prospectively* to focus resources on primary prevention of disease and on secondary prevention of disease complications to avoid unnecessary resource consumption
- *Tracking the natural history of the disease* over time to help identify, quantify, and track typical cost and quality drivers and how they change over time as you implement your disease management system
- *Implementing disease and health processes* that drive diagnosis and treatment based on the natural course of the disease rather than on reimbursement
- *Implementing patient-centered versus product-centered information systems* to track patient usage of health care resources at the point of care and throughout the continuum of care (These systems will aggregate individual patient data and allow populationwide analysis.)
- *Instituting evidenced-based guidelines* to help focus limited resources to fund the most powerful and cost-effective interventions regardless of treatment method, setting, or reimbursement
- *Realizing that disease management interventions will cut across care settings*
- *Instituting ongoing measurement and feedback* of clinical, economic, organizational, and behavioral outcomes to nourish CQI processes and foster a learning organization
- *Aligning reward incentive systems* for patients, providers, and plans

Another important element of your vision is the characteristics you will use to guide the developmental efforts. Considering that disease management uses an integrated system of interventions to optimize clinical, economic, and quality outcomes for a specific disease, you can group the characteristics of your system into these three core categories.

Clinical Considerations

From a clinical standpoint, important characteristics of disease management are that it does the following:

- Addresses total patient care outcomes
- Provides proactive care management
- Minimizes preventable disease
- Minimizes disease-related complications
- Provides performance measures for evaluating clinical effectiveness
- Uses direct measurements of current care patterns
- Facilitates early recognition and proper diagnosis of disease
- Maximizes clinical effectiveness

- Maximizes the efficiency of care
- Eliminates ineffective or unnecessary care
- Streamlines the care process and reduces variation in practice patterns
- Optimizes the use of cost-effective diagnostics and therapeutics
- Provides customized interventions targeted to specific problems
- Provides incentives for performance

Economic Considerations

The important economic characteristics of disease management are that it achieves the following:

- Provides performance measures of economic outcomes
- May provide risk assessment at both the population and disease level to prospectively identify high-risk individuals
- Focuses on total treatment cost, instead of one component
- Optimizes the balance between cost and quality
- Is accountable through the measurement of effectiveness and outcomes

Quality Considerations

In terms of quality, the important characteristics of disease management are:

- It may afford an opportunity to reward patients and health professionals for better compliance or improved outcomes.
- It provides performance measures of satisfaction and quality.
- It includes a CQI process.

As you construct your vision statement, make sure that you note those particular aspects that need to be critical elements of your disease management strategy in steps 5 and 6. Your vision sets the target and, based on where your organization is currently, your strategies will address gaps and deficiencies that need to be assessed to effect improvement.

An important note of caution is in order: There will be a great deal of tension created between vision and reality if there is too much distance between the two.[8] The temptation will be to contract your vision to relieve this tension rather than stretching the organization. No doubt you will need to compromise along the way, but the purpose of the vision statement is to generate creative tension by providing a compelling goal for the organization.

• Step 2: Establish a Shared Reality

Understanding the clinical, economic, organizational, and behavioral aspects of disease management is the most time-consuming and revealing exercise in the process of developing a systems approach. Gaining a shared reality, or a common understanding, about the current health care approach for a given disease or population is a critical success factor for effective implementation. All stakeholders (primary care physicians, specialists, hospitals, home care, long-term care, purchasers, health plans, patients) must be involved in establishing the baseline against which all future efforts will be measured. This shared reality provides information in a number of important areas:

- Understanding how care is currently delivered, illustrating care processes with care maps and disease treatment models
- Assessing the present state of clinical knowledge about the disease or condition
- Identifying where resources are currently consumed (for example, outpatient, inpatient, drugs)
- Assessing institutional resources and structures currently available for the disease or condition
- Determining total treatment costs
- Determining ease and accuracy of diagnosis
- Analyzing the complexity of pathology
- Assessing chronic, or lifelong, disease management issues
- Considering Agency for Health Care Policy and Research (AHCPR), National Institutes of Health (NIH), *Guide of Clinical Prevention Services,* or other guidelines
- Assessing the severity and impact of disease, or condition, on the patients affected
- Identifying common cost elements (for example, drugs, physician office visits, diagnostic tests, hospitalization)
- Defining and describing "best practices"
- Creating a descriptive overview of the disease, or condition, with data regarding prevalence and cost, including age, gender, comorbidity, predisposing factors (genetics, lifestyle)
- Summarizing key leverage points, or opportunities for improvement in managing the disease (for example, compliance, prevention, acute flareups, rapid resolution, and high-risk patients)[9]
- Assessing availability of effective treatments and therapies
- Including the disease, or disease processes, in Health Plan Employer Data and Information Set (HEDIS) 2.0/2.5 performance measures
- Assessing current knowledge, attitudes, and practices of providers and patients across the continuum of care

    As you gain a greater understanding of the current system of care for the targeted disease, it is important to identify key leverages for improvement (see step 6). In addition, your goal is to identify a target population of individuals with the disease that are driving costs. For many diseases, a small proportion of patients (about 20 percent) accounts for a large proportion of the total health care costs (about 80 percent).[10]

Figure 2-5 provides a more detailed breakdown of costs. In a typical population, 5 percent of the members (most of whom are severely, chronically ill) consume 60 percent of the health care costs, 45 percent of the members consume 37 percent of the costs, and the remaining 50 percent of the population accounts for only 3 percent of the costs. To achieve the greatest impact on costs in the most efficient manner, it is critical to target the high-utilization/high-expenditure group for early prevention and treatment interventions.[11]

To get the required information, several methods — such as the ones shown in figure 2-6 — will need to be employed. These include primary market research with patients and providers (focus groups, telephone interviews, one-on-one interviews, surveys); analysis of claims data for both inpatients and outpatients; private and public databases; literature review (clinical, economic, satisfaction); and expert panels or advisory boards. Other important information that needs to be included in this analysis is medical condition information (diagnoses data using ICD-9-CM; procedure data using ICD-9, CPT-4, HCPCS; drug identification with NDC number; and severity indicators); cost data, such as billed charges, allowed amounts, reimbursed

Figure 2-5. Use of Health Care Services by Percentage of Population

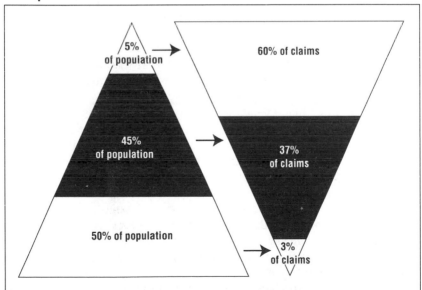

Source: Unpublished data from Value Health Sciences, Inc., Santa Monica, CA, June 1995.

Figure 2-6. Data Sources for Developing Disease Models

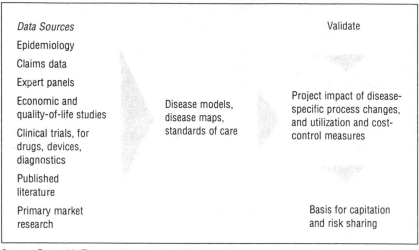

Data Sources		Validate
Epidemiology		
Claims data		
Expert panels		
Economic and quality-of-life studies	Disease models, disease maps, standards of care	Project impact of disease-specific process changes, and utilization and cost-control measures
Clinical trials, for drugs, devices, diagnostics		
Published literature		
Primary market research		Basis for capitation and risk sharing

Source: Costa, M. The use of actuarial modeling in disease management. Paper presented
Oct. 1994.

amounts, and patient cost sharing; provider information; and payer information, such as type of plan, type of coverage, and secondary coverage.

Human Resource Needs

The reality step in the process requires a number of disciplines in order to
be successfully completed. The talents and resources required include:

- A project leader who is responsible for project completion and outcomes
- A project team facilitator to assist the team with issue resolution, deci-
  sion making, project follow-up, and project management
- Clinicians/providers involved in patient care
- Actuarials, or evaluation and quantification of risk-taking issues and dis-
  ease cost structure
- Information systems, including database development, data collection,
  data integration, and data management
- Market research, including primary and secondary research such as on-
  line search capability
- Data analysis, mathematical modeling, and statistics
- Care process mapping, disease modeling
- Guideline development, assessment, and measurement
- Understanding, interpretation, and measurement of outcomes (clinical,
  economic, quality)
- A reimbursement specialist who understands payment mechanisms, pay-
  ment options, and plan types

These disciplines may come from both within and outside the organization. Disease management is a team effort and cannot be achieved without the cooperation and collaboration of stakeholders throughout the continuum of care, as well as the assistance of many outside experts with resources and expertise in areas important to successful development and implementation.

Research and analysis need to focus on several different levels of the disease management process. Figure 2-7 shows that the highest level of assessment is at the national level, where you establish baseline clinical practice standards, disease economics, and epidemiology for the country at large. With the national picture as your baseline, the next level of assessment is at the organizational or system levels, where you compare the national baseline against your organization. Levels three and four, respectively, are the provider and patient practice and behavior patterns within your organization. It is important to note that comparison with the national baseline may not be valid if there are specific regional variations in disease prevalence or treatment approach. For competitive reasons, you may want to compare your organization to the national, regional, and local baseline practices and costs. If another organization in your city has lower costs and better documented outcomes, it is important for you to focus on that versus the impersonal, abstract national baseline.

From these analytical steps, you should be able to accomplish the following:[12]

- Identify the appropriate disease areas for improvement and determine whether the management of the disease represents a significant problem.
  - Determine whether you can identify a reasonable patient study group.
  - Identify disease areas representing high costs.
  - Determine whether educational and clinical programs exist with proven effectiveness in improving outcome.
- Determine baseline clinical practice patterns.
  - Gain consensus from patient care team on the definition and description of how care is currently delivered.
  - Develop clinical criteria for optimal diagnosis and treatment throughout the continuum of care.
  - Identify current published guidelines as starting point for collecting best practices.
  - Measure current practice norms and care processes.
  - Establish national practice norms.
  - Establish a system to track how well each phase of the process is carried out.
- Complete an overall economic analysis of the disease(s).
  - Identify all areas of resource consumption.
  - Estimate cost of each component.
  - Track cost in conjunction with baseline.

Figure 2-7. Developmental Research Guidelines

1. Establish Baseline: National/Regional
   - Clinical modeling
   - Economic modeling
   - Quantify current costs
   - Project future costs
   - Best practices
   - Practice variability
   - Interventional assessment
   - Cost/quality drivers
   - Opportunities/leverages
   - Risk factors
   - Prevalence/incidence
   - Provider/patient behaviors
   - Database development
   - Structural support
   - Skill asessment

Compare

2. MCO/IDS Assessment
   - Marketplace dynamics
   - Marketing strategy
   - Organizational design
     - Provider networks
     - Provider incentives
   - Performance report card requirements
   - Information systems
   - Cost controls
   - Plan sponsors
   - Benefit plans
   - Member demographics
   - Resources/capabilities
   - Costs vs. national average
   - Current DSM efforts
   - Business potential
   - Contract status

Compare

3. Provider Assessment
   - Current practice
   - Patient selection
   - Patient follow-up
   - Communications
   - Multidisciplinary teams
   - Incentives
   - Care processes
   - Skill assessment
   - Continuity of care
   - Compliance with established standards, guidelines, and so on
   - Patient management tools
   - Practice variation

Compare

4. Patient Assessment
   - Compliance
   - Lifestyle behaviors
   - Health beliefs
   - Access to heath care
   - Insurance coverage
   - Risk assessment
   - Risk stratification
   - Behavior modification
   - Incentives

—Identify all related costs.
—Focus on total costs, not component costs.
- Identify key patient segments and critical leverages that have a signifi-
cant impact on clinical quality and total costs.
    —Direct resources to high-cost, high-incidence diseases or patient popu-
    lations at high risk.
    —Identify and track key patient groups, their resource consumption, and
    utilization patterns.
    —Identify all critical junctures (leverages) that result in poor quality of
    care, high costs, and/or lack of patient satisfaction.
    —Evaluate interventional strategies to reduce or eliminate failure points.
    —Develop measurement tools to assess the impact of each improvement.
- Create platforms for disease management programs, or interventions, that
have the potential to make a significant impact, that is, development of
processes and operational mechanisms to more efficiently and effectively
manage the disease (care guidelines, reminder tools, flowcharts, educational programs, decision-support tools).
- Identify performance measures (cost, utilization, patient and provider satisfaction, quality, functional status, morbidity, mortality) for ongoing evaluation of the effectiveness of the disease management effort. You will need
to select explicit, objective, and measurable outcomes.

The reality step in the process is the most time-consuming and requires
a significant resource commitment by top-level management. In addition,
defining how your organization currently delivers health care for a defined
population, disease, or condition must be accomplished with the cooperation and collaboration of everyone involved with the delivery and reimbursement of health services. Other resources, such as information systems, data,
and analytic models, must be located within the organization, developed
from scratch, or outsourced. No doubt, you will run into many barriers,
beliefs, and assumptions about disease management and systems development that will inhibit the achievement of "shared reality." These beliefs and
barriers are discussed in the next two steps in the process.

• Step 3: Understand and Share Key Beliefs

At this point in the process, you have established a common understanding
of your current practices, costs, and organizational dynamics that contribute to both clinical quality and total disease management costs. In the process
you probably uncovered some key assumptions, or beliefs, that stakeholders
have about disease management. These assumptions limit or expand what
is possible to achieve with a systems approach to disease management and
are critical to expose and to challenge. If these beliefs limit the effort due

to skepticism, confusion, and apprehension, then the disease management effort will stumble in the implementation phase. If you choose to avoid beliefs now, you will run into them again later and have to backtrack your efforts in order to be successful.

Another important aspect about this step is that almost everyone involved in the process of delivering health care will not explicitly tell you what their assumptions and beliefs are about disease management and managed care. As you embark on establishing a picture of the current situation and ask questions about how care is currently delivered and what can be improved, your audience will present both spoken and unspoken beliefs about what is possible and impossible to change. You will have to listen carefully to the information being provided and in many cases interpret a belief that underlies a statement or position.

Collect key beliefs about disease management strategy, organizational structure, skills, and culture. You may want to keep the following in mind as you explore beliefs:

Disease Management Strategy

- What disease management strategies physicians believe to be effective (or ineffective) and why
- Physician beliefs about the effectiveness of guidelines
- Providers' belief (or lack thereof) in patients' ability to effectively self-manage the targeted disease
- The level of provider acceptance of a systems approach to disease management as more effective than the traditional component approach
- The extent to which physicians and planning teams believe that each is interested in achieving better quality in addition to lowering costs
- Providers' feelings about sharing risk and whether it is an effective compensation system to help motivate them to lower risk and improve quality
- The perception and acceptance of decision-support tools provided to help standardize care
- Provider attitudes toward the effectiveness of prevention efforts and the role they will have to play in prevention and wellness
- The information currently available to determine cost and quality, and whether it is accurate, relevant, and meaningful

Organizational Structure

- Assumptions about the fairness or effectiveness of the incentive and reward system for a given disease
- Provider beliefs about the patient population that may affect their acceptance of risk sharing or capitation (severity of illness, patient mix, and so forth)

- Key stakeholders' view of what it is possible to achieve given the current structure and how they think the system should be structured
- The relative role of the specialist versus the primary care physician
- The effectiveness of the current care paths and the possible need for process changes

Skills

- Patients' self-knowledge regarding their need for education
- Patients' level of satisfaction with the information they receive from their physicians
- Providers' attitudes toward improving their communication skills
- Stakeholders' buy-in to the belief that a multidisciplinary, cross-functional team will yield better results and a lower cost, as well as improve team skills that will yield a benefit to their patients
- Providers' understanding of the role they have to play in improving patient compliance

Culture

- What the stakeholders in the health care process believe is the norm in your organization, and what they believe is rewarded
- Stakeholders' ability to work together as a team
- Specialists' level of acceptance of primary care physicians' increased role
- How guidelines have worked in the past, and whether providers believe that the organization will reinforce their use

In considering all of these points and exploring everyone's beliefs, you may run across some common ones about disease management, including:

- "Disease management is not new; we have been practicing it for years as physicians."
- "Data are not available to complete a meaningful economic analysis."
- "I don't believe the data are accurate."
- "My patient population is unique and cannot be compared to national 'norms.'"
- "Information systems in this organization are inadequate, and until they are improved, disease management will go nowhere."
- "Guidelines are like 'cookbook medicine' and are not meaningful to my practice."
- "Managed care is not interested in improving quality. They are a bunch of accountants who do not know anything about medicine and are just trying to reduce costs."

- "My patients are already compliant. Even if they weren't, it isn't my responsibility to help them improve."
- "If patients want to change, they will."
- "I can reduce total system costs by lowering the individual cost of each component."
- "My job is to manage the pharmacy. I can't worry about whether a drug increases or decreases costs somewhere else in the system."

As you hear these beliefs, record and consolidate them to determine overall theme(s). It will be important to address each belief both collectively and individually with key stakeholders in order to have a successful disease management system. In many cases, these beliefs are a result of organizational design or incentive systems and can be overcome by reconfiguring these structural elements. In other cases, education may need to be implemented to change assumptions.

Regardless of their origin, it is very important to identify beliefs about disease management, managed care, and the perceived effectiveness of interventional approaches prior to implementing your plan, so that those that are barriers to success can be addressed and those that are keystones for strategic design can be tested, challenged, refined, or reinforced through experience. Testing your key assumptions and beliefs about what drives cost, quality, or satisfaction is one of the important outcomes measurement tasks in this process.

• Step 4: Identify Barriers to Change

The gap analysis is also a very important step, because it quantifies and clarifies organizational and individual deficiencies that must be addressed in order to effectively and efficiently change the way care is delivered. Typical information or knowledge gaps include the following:

- Insufficient data
- Lack of data collection and data reporting standards across the organization; for example, there is no standard for the format, content, or structure of disease-associated cost information[13]
- Incompatible data sets
- Inadequate communication networks for data sharing, information dissemination
- Inadequate information systems for data collection, data analysis, data management[14]
- Poor-quality data; for example, claims data are often inaccurate or do not provide a complete picture[15]
- Inadequate skills for data analytics, disease modeling

- Lack of outcomes information and/or the ability to interpret outcomes data
- Insufficient skills in structuring clinical and economic outcomes trials
- Inability to measure change at the point of care
- Lack of knowledge about the natural course of a disease
- Inadequate information about optimal clinical practice, or insufficient evidence to support optimal care guidelines (health plans and providers do not always know what works)
- Diagnosis and treatment decisions driven by reimbursement schedules rather than by the disease process[16]
- Misalignment of incentives and rewards among plan, provider, and patient[17]
- Conflicting goals among payers, providers, and suppliers[18]
- Incomplete continuity of care systems; for example, lack of home care, sufficient specialty networks, and so forth
- Determining which enrollees in a plan are affected, or at risk, for the targeted disease[19]

Some gaps, or issues, must be addressed prior to implementing a disease management system. For example, if your organization cannot provide continuity of care throughout the natural evolution of the disease process, you will need to enhance your capabilities. If information systems are inadequate for data collection, data management, and data reporting, you will need to upgrade, improve, or install sufficient health information systems. If rewards and incentives continue to reward utilization (FFS or discounted FFS), it will be necessary to change the incentive system so that all stakeholders are rewarded for lowering total system costs and improving total quality through cooperation and collaboration. In other cases, changes in the organization will be an integral part of your disease management plan with organizational programs rolling out in advance of clinical programs.

Disease management is not viewed equally by all players in a health care system. Many problems exist that have yet to be solved; for example, point-of-care patient treatment data to support disease management interventions, the distribution of risk among the various stakeholders involved in care, and ownership of the patient information involved.[20] Other issues you will face include the following:

- Academic medical centers within the plan may be resistant, and often unable, to comply with managed care cost-control measures, standards of care, or outcomes measurement.
- Individual providers within the system (for example, specialists, hospitals) may cause significant resistance as streamlining operations and redesigning care processes threatens their patient volume.
- Regulatory issues remain unresolved for suppliers of health care products, who may need to establish a direct line of communication with patients

using their products, and patient confidentiality often conflicts with efforts to share information.

There will be no shortage of barriers, issues, and excuses—some real, some perceived—waiting to derail the disease management process. The efforts to build a comprehensive, integrated system of care take time and must incorporate strategies to overcome these obstacles.

• Step 5: Develop Strategic Options

It is important to understand the difference between *programs* and *systems*. Whereas individual programs include discrete components of disease management, systems have been created to link all of these components into a continuum of care. In a component-based program, the reward is defined as a change within that specific component (for example, rebates, compliance programs, formularies). In a fully linked interventional system, the reward is defined by the results (for example, improved patient, provider, health, or system outcomes). The graph in figure 2-8 illustrates the evolution from individual disease management programs to fully integrated systems and how rewards must evolve in parallel.

As you consider the strategic options available for developing a disease management system, it will be important for you to understand the potential

Figure 2-8. Evolution of Disease Management

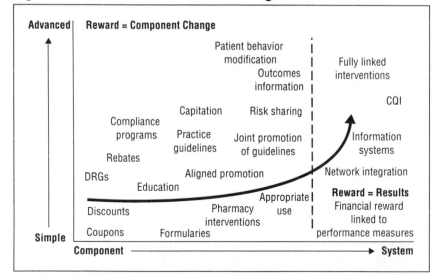

Source: Luginbill, R. Strategy and marketing in the era of integration and consolidation. Conference paper presented in Philadelphia, Oct. 1994.

elements, or components, of a system and what elements must be included in order to build a system rather than simply a program. In order to help increase the level of understanding about the range of possible interventions in disease management, this section provides descriptions of some programs that could be incorporated into a system and how the pieces can fit together.

Strategic options target three core stakeholders in the disease management process—the patient, the provider, and the system (plan or payer). The disease management system brings together this diverse set of constituents and links them into a system. There are five core segments within the system targeting these three constituents, all of which must be linked and include a CQI process:

Patient and Provider

- Outcomes-based behavior modification and education for both patients and providers (for example, continuing medical education [CME], continuing education [CE] programs for providers; and patient education, patient lifestyle and behavior modification programs, and patient self-care tools for the patient)
- Provider-focused clinical interventions and decision-support tools (for example, best practice guidelines, drug formularies, care process maps, referral guidelines, patient communication aids, and so forth)

System

- Information systems for ongoing monitoring, measurement, and communication (for example, point-of-care decision-support tools, performance reporting, outcomes data collection, analysis, and reporting)
- Financial and clinical outcomes research (for example, retrospective, current, and prospectively defined outcomes research focused on costs, utilization, quality, and satisfaction)
- Organizational structure, skills, and culture that support and facilitate systems management of disease (for example, continuity of care, provider networks, financing mechanisms, information systems, communication systems)

Tied into all segments of disease management is CQI. Without ongoing improvement and feedback, we would not have a system, but a static, turnkey program of discrete, finite components. CQI measurement and management elements can include:

- Information systems for data collection and analysis
- Communication systems for ongoing feedback
- Outcomes research and measurement systems

All of these elements appear in figure 2-9, which shows the necessary components for disease management systems.

Clinical/Medical Elements of Disease Management

Clinical/medical elements that can be considered part of the disease management system include various tools that enhance clinical decision making, facilitate communication with patients, and focus resources on specific cost and quality drivers for any given disease. The following elements encourage continuity of care and provide the "tool set" to effectively manage patients within a system:

- *Best practice clinical guidelines* link specific decisions across the spectrum of health care settings — outpatient, inpatient, home care, alternative-site care, nursing home, and so forth. Guidelines should be based on research or evidence and be supported by consensus among all health care providers who interact with the patient.
- *Risk-assessment tools* help prospectively identify individuals at risk for specific diseases or complications. These tools may also target lifestyle and health behaviors that adversely affect clinical outcomes and quality of life.
- *Point-of-service clinical-support tools* lead providers through guidelines, protocols, formularies, drug information, and prescriptions. Education and diagnostic support reduces practice variabilities and enhances compliance with standards.
- *Disease process maps* illustrate the path patients take through the health care system. These maps form the basis for process redesign efforts that increase collaboration, enhance communication, and reduce waste by showing where duplication or unnecessary or inappropriate health care processes occur.
- *Disease models* illustrate the alternatives available for the management of patients with a specific disease/condition. These aid in decision making by providing outcomes probabilities and economic consequences for each decision.
- *Epidemiologic profiles* provide an overview of the logical, natural progression and history of the disease from prevention, diagnosis, treatment, maintenance, and recovery.
- *Patient communication tools* enhance providers' ability to create and sustain meaningful dialogues with patients afflicted with specific diseases/conditions.
- *Diagnostic aids* improve early detection and recognition of disease and monitoring for compliance.

Figure 2-9.   Key Elements of a Disease Management System

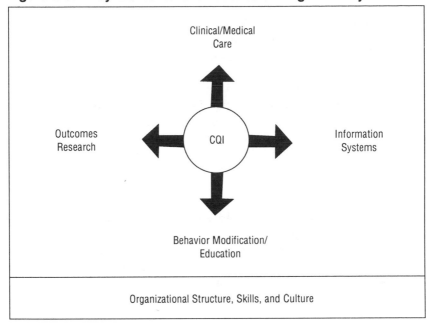

Data, Information Systems, and Technology Elements of Disease Management

Functional disease management will require the ability to quantify, track, and control cost and quality drivers in both the inpatient and outpatient setting. Therefore, a key element of a system must be the ability to make data available to benchmark baseline economic costs. Information systems that track a patient across all segments of the health care continuum need to be developed and instituted. Linkages must be created to track data from physicians' offices to inpatient and outpatient services.

It is important to realize that some cost savings for good disease management may be realized outside of the system through better job attendance and improved work performance. Data repositories will form the foundation for ongoing management of clinical practice and costs.

Data will need to be collected, integrated, analyzed, managed, and communicated:

- *Data collection:* This captures a variety of information across all segments of the health care system for ongoing measurement, analysis, and reporting. This aspect of a disease management system will enable the ongoing monitoring of clinical, economic, and quality outcomes measures. Also available will be point-of-service medical encounter data, electronic data interchange, and linked systems centered on the patient, not the transaction.

- *Data integration:* The ability to consolidate information from several different sources into one database. Data to be integrated may include clinical information, medical encounter/claims, patient outcomes, patient demographics, Medicare cost reports, MEDPAR and Medicare billing information, ICD-9 discharge information, CPT information, Uniform Billing information, diagnosis-related group (DRG) information, financial information, pharmaceutical prescribing information, HEDIS Behavioral Risk Factor Survey, and clinical laboratory findings.
- *Data analysis:* Data will help determine the economic impact of physician practice patterns, patient behaviors, and organizational design. Analytical information can:
  - Recognize over- and underutilization at disease-specific levels
  - Provide a global view of disease-specific practice patterns, linking all services to the patient
  - Disclose variable costs of delivering care to a patient
  - Examine prescription drugs used to treat patients with a specific disease
  - Measure differences in prescription drug impact on global treatment costs
  - Detect off-label drug use
  - Help ensure patient compliance with medication
  - Share data with patients to help modify their behavior
  - Reveal readmission rates for given procedures within a disease
  - Help forecast costs
  - Identify prospective high-risk patients, high-risk behaviors
  - Point out prevalence rates and case-mix complexities
- *Data management:* Effective management means coordination and proper use of large databases. It will aid in generating management reports, inputting raw data, and protecting confidentiality. It will also yield information about: physicians' individual practice patterns versus best practice, medical capitation performance, physician group composition, best practice evidence, prescription drug performance, high-cost patient identification, clinical data (patient registry), electronic data interchange, inpatient/outpatient distribution, geographically distributed utilization rates, and payer distribution.

Education and Behavior Modification Disease Management Elements

Most diseases can be more effectively managed if providers and patients are equipped with relevant information to guide their decisions. This will necessitate training to acquire and apply new knowledge and skills for health improvement. Education will be linked to clinical decision-support tools to deliver tailored instruction based on the provider's specific needs. The time lag between action, feedback, education, and learning will be decreased as the information and technology systems detailed above become more widely used.

Didactic, unilateral education must give way to interactive, problem-based education using adult learning principles. Education and training as part of disease management is characterized by its focus on specific costs or quality drivers and the commitment to measure the impact of these efforts on outcomes. Educational and skill-enhancement elements must be made available to providers as well as patients and their families or caretakers. Educational elements for providers, administrators, and health managers include:

- *CE/CME programs* that provide specific instruction targeted to cost and quality drivers within a given disease/condition. Results could be measured as part of outcomes studies. Health promotion and disease prevention become more important in disease management within a capitated health care system.
- *Administrative training* to give nonclinicians the background they need before taking their first job.
- *Risk management skills* to enhance the provider's ability to manage outcomes based on health status, health risk assessment, and population-based patient management principles. As credentialing of providers becomes more prevalent, decision-making and decision-support skills become increasingly important.
- *Multidisciplinary, cross-functional team experience:* As the health care system consolidates and integrated systems of health care are created around diseases, conditions, and populations, providers will need to work effectively as team members rather than as independent practitioners.
- *Systems-thinking skills* to increase understanding of the interrelationships of the entire health care system and to learn how to work as part of the system.
- *Population-based skills* and health strategies to prevent epidemics.

Educational needs for patients, families, and caretakers include:

- *Compliance training* to help patients understand why it is critical to follow provider directions for prescriptions and therapies. This should provide patients with incentives to comply with instructions, improving prevention, diagnosis, treatment, and maintenance behaviors.
- *Self-management skills* to help reduce demand and increase self-efficacy. These programs offer training and skill development targeted to specific patient behaviors that drive increased cost or poor clinical outcomes. Self-management skills also target psychosocial, behavioral, and lifestyle factors that affect disease progression, treatment outcomes, cost of care, and quality.

- *Medication information* about both prescription and over-the-counter medicines to help patients manage their medication more effectively, thereby minimizing side effects, improving compliance, reducing complications, and avoiding drug-to-drug interactions.
- *Disease- or condition-specific information* to increase knowledge and understanding. Information services should be provided directly to patients to facilitate informed choice, reduce demand on providers, and enhance diagnosis and treatment.

Evaluating Strategic Options

The options for the interventional design of your system and the focus of the disease management effort will be based on your assessment of "reality" (step 2); the key beliefs, or assumptions, within the organization (step 3); the gap analysis (step 4); and the vision (step 1). The primary objective of step 5 is to profile *all* your options for changing the current system and *not* to choose a specific strategy. This comes in the next step, "Identify Leverage Options." In most organizations, the pressure to do something outweighs the necessity to evaluate all options before implementation. From a systems-thinking point of view, this tendency to move quickly without first considering the implications over time leads to "fits-and-starts," confusion, inconsistency, and ultimate failure of the system to perform up to expectations.

With each strategic option comes potential risk and reward throughout the organization. Change is not always good, and change for the sake of change is counterproductive. Each strategic option must have measurable endpoints to help judge the effectiveness of the effort, and systems in place to enable ongoing measurement and feedback to all stakeholders in the process. How you sequence your effort is very important because many changes need to be carried out in a linear fashion, while others can be rolled out in parallel. Interventions targeted to one audience may be ineffective unless a simultaneous initiative is focused on other key constituents in the health care process targeted for change.

• Step 6: Identify Leverage Options

The concept of leverage may be new to most organizations; however, when faced with making fundamental changes in the system of health care with limited resources, leverage becomes a key for success. The *American Heritage Dictionary* defines *leverage* as "the power to produce an effect by indirect means." In the context of disease management, leverage involves the selection of strategies that produce significant change with limited resources, or, what changes you can make in one component of the system that will create change in another component as a matter of course. Wherever you choose to focus your strategy, try to target the root cause of system failure rather than the ancillary problems. Treat the cause—not the symptoms.

Leverage strategies most frequently targeted to critical junctures in disease management have a significant impact on quality and/or costs. These include high-cost, high-prevalence diseases; high-risk patient groups; and decision points in clinical management that are subject to variability in practice and result in poor outcomes. Zitter talks about compliance, acute flare-ups, prevention, high-risk patients, and rapid resolution as cost drivers in disease management.[21] These may be the leverage points in the disease management effort depending on the disease selected. Other leverages may include:[22]

- Coordination of care
- Increasing accountability
- Aligning incentives
- Knowledge or information about optimal care
- Ability to measure quality
- Performance reports
- Transparency of cost information
- Preventable hospital treatment
- Availability and quality of data
- Large number of people affected
- Highly visible costs per patient
- Availability of proven treatment guidelines
- Availability of analytical models to identify treatment patterns
- Large fixed-treatment costs (for example, drugs)
- Impact of teaching patients self-care skills

Identifying where you can direct a system of interventions that results in significant and measurable change will help you choose leverage strategies for disease management. Performance models that can help you select strategic options can be developed using existing data and experimental decision models to predict the outcome of a change prior to implementation. You may elect to use an actuary to help you develop these predictive models prior to making a decision about where to start your disease management efforts.

Leverage actions may also occur in sequence, like cascading dominoes. Prior to implementing an interventional program, it may be important to increase the educational level of the target audience so it can realize the full benefit of the intervention. In this case, education is considered a lever for change because without prior knowledge the target audience is not prepared to utilize the interventional program provided. For some organizations, changes in structure are the leverage action—new reporting structures, revised compensation systems, updated or new information systems, and/or new decision-making processes.

• Step 7: Determine How to Measure Results

Defining key indicators for measurement in baseline data analysis and for ongoing documentation of care improvement is critical to any disease management system. Indicators that are important to measure include functional health status, disease severity, clinical outcomes, clinical processes, quality of life, patient satisfaction, utilization, and costs/economics.

Outcomes measurement and management is crucial to the success of any disease management system. For example, assessment of compliance, clinical and/or economic success, and complications can provide valuable feedback information and can help develop pathways to handle noncompliance and treatment failure. Specific outcomes measures can include:

- *Clinical outcomes:* Patients, providers
- *Economic outcomes:* Events (hospitalizations, office visits, ALOS); productivity (lost workdays); health-related quality of life
- *Organizational outcomes:* Care processes; collaboration, communication; marketing/profitability; member attraction, member retention
- *Behavioral outcomes:* Patient and/or provider compliance, patient self-management, health-seeking behavior
- *Quality outcomes:* Patient satisfaction, prevention

• Step 8: Learn and Continuously Improve

At this point in the process you have achieved the following: gained consensus in the organization around your vision for the disease management effort; established and gained agreement on how health care is currently delivered and on the specific clinical, economic, behavioral, and organizational needs for improvement; gained agreement about the key beliefs and assumptions about what can be achieved with a systems approach to disease management; identified gaps and issues critical to the success of the system; evaluated the range of strategic options available for implementation; and selected a course of action that will achieve the desired results in the requisite period of time.

Now is the time to evaluate the impact and implications of your course of action and measure the results. This is a step in the process that is often overlooked because it means going back to challenge the vision, reality, and beliefs that form the foundation for your disease management plan. This is where learning takes place and you have the opportunity to make improvements in the system, eliminate components that are not working, add elements missed the first time around, and communicate the results to all stakeholders in the system. Step 8 is really the beginning of the process — not the end. The point was made earlier that disease management is not a program, but a process, a continually improving process that absolutely requires feedback, information, and communication.

The quicker your organization cycles through these eight steps, the more effective you will be in coping with rapidly changing markets and increasingly competitive environments. The faster the information is available to the organization (the closer to real time), the more relevant and meaningful the experience will be. Speed, flexibility, and the willingness to act, measure, learn, and improve are keystone characteristics of an effective disease management system.

• Summary

As with any new movement, disease management has its adherents and detractors. And, like any enthusiastic adherents, those who wish to quickly implement disease management and place themselves one step closer to total health management may leap too far before they look.

Although there are only eight basic steps to designing and implementing a disease management system, after reading this chapter, you should recognize that each of these steps involves a great deal of work. Nothing happens overnight, and a shift in care delivery as dramatic as disease management will illustrate this rule to many providers.

The systems approach at the heart of disease management involves not only the practicalities of cost analysis, outcomes measurement, and so forth, but also the intuitive human relations side of gaining buy-in among stakeholders and helping adjust the attitudes of everyone from patients to providers to payers to managed care organizations.

Acceptance and implementation of disease management will grow as health delivery integration accelerates; information systems and databases evolve; capitation becomes more prevalent; outcomes measurement proliferates; practice guidelines prove valuable; utilization reviews and formularies grow more sophisticated; providers gain expertise in outcomes measurement and quality improvement; manufacturers and managed care organizations learn to share risk; and employers demand greater quality and lower costs.

These changes are already occurring — some are even well developed and noted by the media, government, and the population as a whole. A true, functional, working disease management system cannot be far behind.

References

1. Eichert, J. Why wait for health care reform? *Pharmaceutical Executive* 13(10): 96–102.
2. Eichert.

3. How markets evolve. *Hospitals & Health Networks* 69(5):48, Mar. 5, 1995.

4. Senge, P. M. *The Fifth Discipline: The Art and Practice of the Learning Organization.* New York City: Doubleday/Currency, 1990.

5. Wong, H. *Keys to Thriving in Health Care Reform.* Austin: Quantum Solutions, Inc., 1993.

6. Brown, R. A. Implementation issues in disease management programs: a pharmaceutical company perspective. *Medical Interface* 8(5):60–69, Apr. 1995.

7. Datamonitor Pharmaceutical Reports. *Disease Management, The Way Forward?* London: Datamonitor, 1995, p. 42.

8. Koestenbaum, P. *Leadership: The Inner Side of Greatness.* San Francisco: Jossey-Bass, 1991, pp. 219–45.

9. Zitter, M. Disease management: a new approach to health care. *Medical Interface* 7(8):70–76, Aug. 1994.

10. Zitter.

11. Unpublished data from Value Health Sciences, Inc., Santa Monica, CA, June 1995.

12. Gonzalez, E. R., and Crane, V. S. Designing a disease management program: how to get started. *Formulary* 30:326–40, June 1995.

13. Datamonitor Pharmaceutical Reports.

14. Brown.

15. Scott, L. Disease management faces obstacles. *Modern Healthcare* 25(24):30–33, June 12, 1995.

16. Zitter.

17. Brown.

18. Scott.

19. Scott.

20. Datamonitor Pharmaceutical Reports.

21. Zitter.

22. Datamonitor Pharmaceutical Reports, p. 69.

Chapter 3

Health Outcomes: Measuring and Maximizing Value in Disease Management

John B. Doyle, PhD

One of the steps outlined in chapter 2's description of a development process for disease management systems is ensuring that organizations have a very clear definition of what the outcomes of the disease management initiative(s) should be. In the case of one large managed care organization, the decision was made to build its own disease management capabilities rather than carve out services to a pharmaceutical company. In explaining this decision, a medical director from the managed care firm is quoted as saying: "They're going to push their drug, no matter what they say about wanting to lower overall costs."[1]

There is no denying that *financial* outcomes — increased revenues for the provider, reduced costs for the payer — are and should be key drivers for disease management. However, as with all health care services, disease management must also justify its existence in terms of *health* outcomes. Does the investment in time and money pay off in terms of better patient/member health?

The *value* of health care can be thought of as the amount of health achieved per dollar spent. The purpose of this chapter is to help providers of health care *maximize the value* of a disease management through the strategic application of outcomes assessment. The key premise underlying the chapter is that an explicit specification of desired and actual outcomes should provide the basis for designing and implementing disease management initiatives.

This chapter focuses specifically on the role of *health* outcomes in disease management. Like all business, health care has long been successful in *measuring* financial outcomes: sales, costs, profits. More recently, health care has become more proficient at *managing* financial outcomes through such means as capitation, aligned incentives, and demand management. Too often disease management is bought and sold as strictly a financial risk management tool. Here, the measurement and management of health outcomes is presented as a balancing force in establishing the value of disease management.

The chapter is organized into three main sections. First, an overview of health outcomes offers some working definitions of key concepts and how they relate to disease management. Second, the text explores how a thorough orientation to outcomes can be used to design value-maximizing disease management programs. Third, a section on impact assessment describes the core components of outcomes measurement systems and the primary uses of health outcomes data. A composite case example is used to demonstrate a number of the process steps discussed throughout the chapter.

• Health Outcomes: Core Concepts

To frame the discussion of health outcomes in disease management, this section offers some definitions and ways of categorizing outcomes. Three "gray areas" — satisfaction, utilization, and compliance — are discussed in terms of their relationships to health outcomes. The section concludes with some common aspects of disease management that call into question some of the traditional thinking in the health outcomes measurement field.

Definition of Outcome

The meaning of the term *outcome* depends largely on perspective. In health care, everyone is either a provider — someone who delivers care or arranges to have it delivered — or a consumer — someone who uses or purchases care. From the provider's point of view, an outcome is the result of a process; for example, the process of performing hip replacement surgery should result in reduced pain and improved mobility for the patient. A provider may regard a disease management program as "well managed" if its processes consistently generate the expected results. In contrast, a consumer may view outcomes as the capabilities of goods and services available in the marketplace; for example, someone with a bad hip may "buy" a provider's service based on the promise of diminished pain and improved function without necessarily knowing how the provider intends to achieve those outcomes. A disease management program may be regarded as a "good buy" if its package of services provides sufficient value for a price that is acceptable.

As suggested in chapter 2, the successful design and implementation of disease management initiatives has a great deal to do with the degree to which the programs *truly* recognize and deal with the different "viewpoints" of *all* the stakeholders. In the historically disjointed style of health care delivery, little if any consideration has been given to integrating divergent stakeholder viewpoints. In the final analysis, *a successful disease management program is one whose component services maximize the outcomes that are valued by a significant number of potential customers, or stakeholders, at a price they are willing to pay.* This outcomes-based definition should drive the design, operation, and measurement of any disease management initiative.

Types of Health Outcomes

Many different types of health outcomes can be enhanced by a disease management program. Several useful taxonomies have been put forward for categorizing types of outcomes — figure 3-1 summarizes some of the classic lists in an overview by Brook and colleagues.[2] Lohr has noted that most health outcome classifications derive from a sickness model rather than the more currently accepted wellness model.[3] However, in the context of *disease* management, the sickness model is not inappropriate: A "good" disease management program alleviates or eliminates the adverse health consequences of the disease.

Outcomes and the Disease Sequence

In deciding which outcomes to maximize in a disease management program, it is helpful to consider the sequence of events by which a disease affects

Figure 3-1. Outcomes Taxonomies

Donabedian:	*White:*
Recovery	Death
Restoration of function	Disease
Survival	Dissatisfaction
	Disability
Sanazaro and Williamson:	Discomfort
Patient end results:	
Longevity	*Starfield:*
Physical abnormalities	Resilience
Psychological abnormalities	Achievement
Physical symptoms	Disease
Psychological symptoms	Satisfaction
Individual function	Comfort
Process outcomes:	Activity
Attitudes toward physician care	Longevity
Attitudes toward condition	
Compliance	
Risks	
Hospitalization	
Costs	
General improvement	
General deterioration	
General condition unchanged	

Source: Adapted from Brook, R. H., Davies-Avery, A., Greenfield, S., Harris, L. J., Lelah, T., Solomon, N. E., and Ware, J. E. Assessing the quality of medical care using outcome measures: an overview of the method. *Medical Care* 15(Suppl.): Sept. 1977.

health (table 3-1). The sequence begins predisease with *health risk*. Chapter 12 addresses the importance of "health management" and the potential evolution of disease management systems into health management systems. Once the disease occurs, its *physiologic manifestation* becomes subjectively evident to the individual in the form of *symptoms,* and to outside observers as *signs.* Symptoms and signs in turn may have an adverse effect on the patient's *functional status* and consequently on overall *quality of life.* Examples of outcome measures associated with each step in the disease sequence for coronary artery disease are shown in the third column of table 3-1.

A disease management program can be created to halt or reverse disease or its impact at any stage in the disease sequence. For example, a program for managing coronary artery disease could encourage aerobic exercise as a preventive measure, strive for more cost-effective uses of invasive cardiovascular surgery, or help get heart attack patients back to work more quickly. The approach chosen should measure outcomes that are directly related to the focus of the interventions. The case example introduced later in the chapter illustrates how a hypothetical disease management development team decided which outcomes to measure.

Gray Area Measures

Most of the outcome categories presented in figure 3-1 can be readily classified as health outcomes, measuring the impact of health care on patients'

Table 3-1. Causes and Consequences of Disease States

Disease Sequence	Definition	Illustrative Outcome Measure (Coronary Artery Disease)
Health risk	Factors that increase the likelihood that a person will experience the onset or exacerbation of a health condition	Cigarette Smoking
Physiologic status	Description of the person's physical and chemical functioning	Degree of arterial blockage, as measured by angiogram
Symptoms	Subjective indications of disease as perceived by the patient	Chest pain
Signs	Objective indications of disease as perceived by an examiner	Sweating
Functional status	A person's ability to perform normal activities and roles	Ability to climb a flight of stairs
Quality of life	A person's overall sense of well-being	Self-reported satisfaction with physical, social, and financial aspects of life

health status. However, some of the listed measures are not true health outcomes. These "gray area" measures are process based and fall into three main areas: satisfaction, utilization, and compliance.

Satisfaction

Patient satisfaction is often regarded as a health outcome. However, many satisfaction measures focus largely on service quality: waiting time, practitioner's bedside manner, and so on. This is satisfaction with the *process* of care. Patients' satisfaction with their health *outcomes,* or how much they feel they have been helped by the care they have received, is measured in some satisfaction surveys.[4]

Utilization

Sanazaro and Williamson's outcomes taxonomy (see figure 3-1) includes a category called "process outcomes." Two subcategories merit further attention as gray area measures: hospitalization and costs. These two measures — and other related measures of utilization — are often treated as proxies for health outcomes. However, they are at best rough approximations of true health outcomes. For example, a reduced frequency of asthma emergency room visits may indicate that fewer persons are reaching dangerous levels of severity.[5] However, factors other than better health can reduce emergency room utilization rates: Patients with asthma may be inaccurately coded as having "recurrent obstructive airway disease"; or patients may be triaged to urgent care, where the intensity and cost of care may equal that of the emergency room. Either of these tactics can artificially improve a so-called outcome measure without having any appreciable positive impact on either patient health or the cost of care. Therefore, providers and consumers of disease management should exercise caution in equating reduced utilization with better health outcomes. It is usually necessary to measure both utilization and health outcomes in order to determine whether a disease management program is truly cost-effective.

Compliance

Sanazaro and Williamson's taxonomy also lists compliance as a process outcome. Certainly compliance with care is not a true health outcome, in that compliance is not a direct measure of health or its consequences. However, compliance is the result of a health care intervention and can lead to better health outcomes. Later in this chapter, compliance is classified as an important "intermediate outcome," useful in evaluating the means by which a disease management program can improve health outcomes.

Health Outcomes in Disease Management

Measuring health outcomes in disease management poses some unique challenges, especially for the significant proportion of disease management initiatives that deal with chronic illnesses across the continuum of care.

Episode versus Disease Management

Most people with chronic diseases experience periodic flare-ups of their condition. It is important to distinguish the outcomes of treating acute episodes from the outcome of treating the condition itself. Acute outcomes are easier to understand: The patient is sick, gets treated, and feels better. However, the success of disease management cannot be judged solely by its success in helping patients recover from acute flare-ups. Disease management makes patients "better" in a subtler way: Patients may have better health between episodes; they may experience fewer, less severe acute episodes; or their health may deteriorate less rapidly over time.

Encounter-Centered versus Patient-Centered Measurement

Most outcomes data are captured during an encounter. For example, a hospital discharge abstract indicates whether the patient left the hospital alive or dead, or a medical record may record a patient's lab values at the time of an office visit. For most patients suffering from a chronic disease, formal encounters with the health care delivery system are relatively rare occurrences. To construct a more complete picture of the impact of a disease state — and of disease management — on people's lives, health outcome measures should be patient centered rather than encounter centered. That is, the effort should be made to evaluate patients' normal health status and the extent to which their condition affects their lives. Toward that end, it is appropriate to measure outcomes that reflect an extended time period, for example, mortality rate three years following diagnosis, or the extent to which a patient's work productivity has been limited over the past six months.

Individual versus Population Health

The acute health outcomes model discussed previously also looks for improvement in individuals' health attributable to an intervention. However, from a population perspective it may not be clear that each of these interventions is appropriate. Thus, it may be better to evaluate outcomes for chronic conditions from a population health perspective, for example, by assessing the average health status of persons with the disease or the percentage of patients who are able to perform their jobs with high productivity. A population health perspective is also more appropriate when disease management functions in a capitated environment. In a capitated managed care world, the overall goal is frequently that of achieving "good" health outcomes for a clinical subpopulation, regardless of whether everyone within that subpopulation has become a "patient" by accessing the traditional clinical care delivery system.

• Outcomes-Based Program Design and Development

For a disease management program to succeed, those responsible for designing and developing it need to know what the program is expected to achieve and how to achieve it. A thorough orientation to and understanding of health outcomes should enhance success by helping the program designers specify goals and objectives, create the overall program design, and optimize program components. This section addresses a number of the key concepts that should be considered in the *design* of an outcomes-based disease management program, as well as specific steps that should be followed in the *development* of the program. A *hypothetical osteoarthritis management program* illustrates a number of the core health outcomes concepts developed throughout the rest of the chapter. Although the case example is a fabrication, it represents a composite of the author's experiences with various organizations that have developed disease management initiatives.

Establishing Outcomes-Based Goals, Priorities, and Objectives

A successful disease management program is one that achieves desired outcomes. To maximize success, the program's top management should define goals and values, set priorities, and establish objectives based on an explicit consideration of what health outcomes they hope to achieve. Only then should management proceed with actually building and implementing the program.

Defining Goals and Values

What does a disease management program hope to accomplish? Frequently, programs are launched without top management ever answering this question. High-level discussion of value should seek consensus on the relative importance of financial goals versus health-related goals for the disease management program. The balance point between these two types of goals can be set in a variety of ways. For example, any of the following value statements could form the basis for a disease management initiative:

- Reduce the overall cost of health care.
- Reduce the overall cost of the disease, including financial impact on the employer, the family, and society.
- Reduce the overall cost of care without adversely affecting patient health.
- Improve patient health.
- Improve patient health without increasing costs.
- Simultaneously reduce cost and improve health.
- Maximize population health within a fixed medical loss ratio.

Defining the value of the disease management program is not simply a marketing ploy; it is the first and most important step in establishing health outcomes objectives and accountability criteria for the program. As illustrated by the range of options listed, the process of defining the specific goals and values of the program touches on many basic, even ethical, issues. Chapter 2 suggests that the value definition stage of program development demands a true organizational "reality check." The program cannot fully succeed unless everyone agrees on what constitutes success.

Specifying Health Outcome Priorities

Once the organization's senior management establishes the balance between health-related goals and financial goals, the disease management program designers need to identify which specific health outcomes they most want to affect. The purpose of outcomes discussion at this stage in development is to prioritize the health-related goals of the program, for example, by deciding the relative importance of alleviating symptoms, versus improving lab values, versus reducing mortality rates. This list of priorities should result from a thorough consideration of all major health outcomes that could conceivably become the focus for a disease management initiative. Chapter 5 addresses some of the disease state considerations that can influence the selection of outcomes targets.

Setting Outcomes-Based Objectives

An accountable disease management program should measure its success against reasonable but rigorous health outcomes performance criteria. Once management has set the *general* health outcomes priorities, the next step is to set specific outcomes-based objectives based on a variety of criteria. The selection of these criteria will depend on the individual goals of the organization, for example:

- *Competitive positioning:* Outcomes will surpass those of any other program.
- *External standards:* Outcomes will meet or exceed the target specified by national expert panels, accrediting bodies, or other recognized authorities.

- *Customer expectations:* Outcomes will meet or exceed targets specified by key employers in the marketplace.
- *Continual improvement:* The present year's outcomes will exceed those of the prior year by at least 5 percent.

Case Illustration

The following case example provides a theoretical illustration of the steps involved in developing and establishing a disease management program, with an emphasis on outcomes measurement. It appears throughout the chapter to give readers an idea of the steps as a continuous process.

BigHealth is a large integrated delivery system located in a medium-sized metropolitan area. It was experiencing a rapid shift in payer demand, from discounted fee-for-service to capitated contracts. In order to manage the financial risk, BigHealth's executive leadership council asked its financial and clinical managers to identify those disease states that presented the greatest opportunities for cost containment. A cross-functional planning team came up with key criteria for identifying an opportunity, including total cost of care, average cost per patient, variation in cost per patient, and perceived variation in clinicians' practice patterns. Osteoarthritis, the most prevalent form of arthritis, emerged as one of the 20 highest-rated opportunities.

An osteoarthritis management team was assembled, with representatives from rheumatology, orthopedics, primary care, rehabilitation, pharmacy, operations, and BigHealth's largest managed care payer. Top management charged the team with proposing a disease management program that would reduce the average cost of patient care.

The clinicians on the osteoarthritis team expressed mixed feelings about the mission: While appreciating that their incentives were now aligned with cost containment, they felt compelled to do everything in their power to make each patient as healthy as possible. The payer representative asked, "Does that mean you want to perform joint replacements on every arthritis patient?" The rheumatologist and orthopedist acknowledged that, even without capitated contracts, there is an implicit rationing of effective but high-cost procedures. After some heated debate, the team defined a core *goal/value statement:*

> To create a health management program that reduces the average cost of care while increasing the average health of our population of osteoarthritis patients.

In presenting its revised goal/value statement to top management, the team noted that the term "population of patients" trod a middle ground between an individual patient perspective and a covered lives orientation, which might require proactively seeking out persons with arthritis who had *not* sought care from BigHealth. Top management agreed and gave its go-ahead for further development.

The osteoarthritis team then sought agreement regarding which health outcomes were the most important in contributing to the "average health" (from the goal/value statement) of the osteoarthritis population. After conducting discussions with the relevant clinical subspecialties, the team decided to focus its work on two health outcomes *objectives* for BigHealth's population of osteoarthritis patients:

- Reduce the average frequency and severity of joint pain by 5 percent over the next year.
- No one will be unemployable due to osteoarthritis.

The team agreed that, although patient satisfaction and radiological joint evaluations were very important, they were not as critical to patient well-being as pain management and productivity.

Outcomes-Driven Program Design

There is a considerable difference between setting outcomes objectives and achieving them. Disease management programs should be designed to achieve objectives. More specifically, they should be designed to maximize *health return on investment* (ROI), that is, to maximize achievement of the program's defined health objectives given the amount of money to be invested in the program. Successful programs focus on specific opportunities to enhance health ROI.

Once overall program objectives have been set, the program design can be guided by an explicit attempt to maximize health ROI. The following five steps are suggested as a guide to the development of an outcomes-driven disease management program. Although a number of these steps have either been discussed or implied in chapter 2, they are presented here in a more outcomes-oriented context.

Step 1

Define a targeted financial investment, or *budget,* for the program. In disease management, as in any other endeavor, a multitude of factors can influence the budgeting process, including discretionary dollars available, expected return on investment, and politics. A budget sets limits; it is the responsibility of the program designers and managers to maximize outcomes within those limits.

Step 2

Identify *high-leverage opportunities* for achieving program objectives. As identified in chapter 2, every disease has specific cost drivers, or high-leverage areas of intervention in the disease process that will generate the greatest cost savings. There are also health drivers, which can produce the greatest impact on health outcomes. Designers of disease management programs should focus on those stages in the disease sequence and in the continuum of care that afford the greatest opportunities for improving high-priority health outcomes.

Step 3

Identify candidate *best practices* to use as interventions at leverage points. Disease management programs consist of components; components are made up of specific care practices, or *interventions*. An outcomes-driven approach to program design ideally relies heavily on evidence-based best practices.[6] Effective programs are built on practices and/or interventions that have been shown, by means of outcomes research, to achieve the program's high-priority objectives. For example, clinical research indicates that, of the products currently on the market, inhaled corticosteroids or cromolyn sodium are the pharmaceuticals of choice for patients with moderate to severe asthma.[7] An asthma management program should encourage appropriate prescribing and patient compliance consistent with this evidence-based best practice.

Step 4

Define effective *tactics* for implementing the selected best practices. An outcomes-driven tactical framework is presented later in this chapter.

Step 5

Evaluate pro forma health ROI, or the likely impact versus cost of implementing selected best practices. From a design perspective, not every best practice/intervention is "best" in terms of maximizing management's health ROI. Program designers must establish a *pro forma impact assessment* for each best practice considered for incorporation in the disease management program. The pro forma should include:

- An estimate of the expected health outcomes of each practice/intervention
- The strength of the evidence supporting the outcomes estimate
- The expected cost of implementing the practice/intervention

The evidence-based approach to best practices sets the upper limit on what can reasonably be expected in terms of health ROI from the disease management program.

New programs should be designed from the ground up using an explicit orientation to health return on investment. Where design options exist, components with a known higher health ROI should be chosen. In many cases subjective data may need to be used in making these decisions in first-generation disease management programs. Existing programs should be audited periodically to ensure that each component is cost-justifiable in terms of impact on health objectives.

Case Illustration

Using the agreed-on objectives discussed earlier, the planning team for BigHealth's osteoarthritis disease management program identified high leverage in three aspects of care:

- Opportunities for reducing cost of care
  - Reduce the percentage of patients receiving total joint replacement surgery
  - Reduce length of stay for joint replacement surgery
  - Maximize prescribing of more cost-effective pain medications
  - Replace physical therapy services with self-care where appropriate
- Opportunities for reducing joint pain
  - Maximize self-care in the appropriate use of heat, cold, and exercise for managing pain
  - Offer joint replacement to all appropriate candidates
  - Maximize patient compliance with pain medication protocols
- Opportunities for increasing employability
  - Reduce joint pain
  - Adapt the workplace for accessibility to and prevention of arthritis-related physical limitations
  - Increase job satisfaction of persons with osteoarthritis

Upon further review, the team decided to focus its initial disease management efforts on the high-leverage area of joint pain management. Pain reduction is a program goal in its own right, and it contributes significantly to the employability goal. Further, the team felt that more consistent use of conservative pain management techniques, coupled with a joint replacement appropriateness guideline, would result in reduction in the overall costs for the osteoarthritis population.

The team next convened task forces to evaluate the published literature and come to consensus regarding possible best practices and their expected impact on health ROI. Based on the literature review, four specific program interventions were selected for development. The four interventions and their pro forma impact assessments are summarized in table 3-2.

The task forces noted that the cost savings associated with the joint replacement guideline could be realized only if the patient compliance intervention and the self-care pain management intervention were successfully installed. Most of the implementation costs would be incurred in the first

Table 3-2. Osteoarthritis Pro Forma Impact Assessment

Program Components	Expected Impact on			
	Cost of Care	Pain Management	Employability	Cost to Implement
1. Formulary revisions and physician guideline to encourage prescribing less expensive pain medications	−6%	0%	0%	+1%
2. Patient detailing to enhance compliance with pain medication care plans	−1%	+5%	+3%	+4%
3. Educational program to enhance self-care pain management	−2%	+5%	+3%	+5%
4. Appropriateness guideline for joint replacement	−12%	−2%	−1%	+2%
Net Impact, All Components	−21%	+8%	+5%	+12%

year, whereas savings in cost of care and enhanced health outcomes would continue. Because expected costs were within predetermined budget limits, and because the pro forma health ROI promised an acceptable "bang for the buck," BigHealth's top management authorized the planning team to move into the implementation phase of program development.

Program Development

Best practices can have their expected impact on health outcomes only if they are successfully implemented. Successful program development requires the creation of a set of processes that maximize the likelihood of actually achieving the pro forma health return on investment. A sequence of events must take place if a disease management practice is to achieve its outcomes objectives. Table 3-3 presents the "outcomes cascade," which forms the basis for developing a disease management plan that is truly programmatic — explicitly created to optimize health ROI. The left half of the cascade describes the providers' activity sequence, starting with the best practice and leading to an appropriate patient-specific care plan. The right side describes the patient's activity cascade, starting with the care plan and leading to achievement of desired outcomes. Provider steps and patient steps closely parallel each other.

Each step in the outcomes cascade must be planned for and managed. By establishing outcomes measurement criteria for each step in the outcomes cascade, a disease management program can document the immediate

Table 3-3. The Outcomes Cascade

The Provider Cascade	The Patient Cascade
Best practice	Care plan
Knowledge of best practice	Knowledge of care plan
Belief in best practice	Belief in care plan
Ability to perform best practice	Ability to follow care plan
Incentives to perform best practice	Incentives to follow care plan
Self-efficacy regarding best practice	Self-efficacy regarding care plan
Remembering to perform best practice	Remembering to follow care plan
Adherence to best practice	Compliance with care plan
Patient-specific care plan	Desired outcomes

impacts, or "intermediate outcomes," of its interventions. In addition, measuring each step in the cascade can help management identify gaps in the program's ability to achieve health outcomes.

The following list explains considerations for each of the steps in the cascade. Because the steps are so similar for providers and patients, the explanations refer to both groups.

- *Knowledge:* The first consideration in implementing a best practice/intervention is to make sure that *all* affected parties know about it. The effectiveness of dissemination can be assessed by measuring the appropriate intermediate outcome, for example, by asking clinicians whether they are aware of a specific best practice or by quizzing them about the contents of the practice. Likewise, it is possible to ask patients whether they are aware of and understand their care plans.
- *Belief:* Do physicians believe that a best practice is truly "best"? If not, they are unlikely to follow its recommendations. Similarly, patients may not be convinced that their care plans are truly in their best interest. The intermediate outcome of a persuasion effort can be measured by, for instance, asking patients whether they believe that following their care plans is the best way to care for their condition.
- *Ability:* The ability to perform a best practice or intervention may be limited by a number of obstacles: lack of specific skills, inadequate equipment, poor access to supplies, or care settings that do not support performance of the required care activities. A disease management initiative should identify all significant ability-limiting factors, resolve them, and then measure the success of the resolution.

- *Incentives:* Most people will consistently perform a set of activities only if the incentives to do so outweigh the disincentives. Virtually every best practice comes with at least one built-in incentive — it is the right thing to do — and one disincentive — it is harder to do it than not to do it. A disease management initiative must strive to increase incentives for best practice/intervention performance while reducing disincentives.

  Programs should measure the incentives and disincentives to performing specific best practices, as well as their subjective impact on individuals. For example, the time required to perform a best practice is a disincentive. The impact of this disincentive is the perceived inconvenience associated with performing the best practice.

- *Self-efficacy:* To achieve maximum impact, a care plan needs to be "owned" by the patient and other "stakeholders." That is, patients should see themselves as being able to control their own health, using the care plan as a tool in self-management. This sense of self-efficacy applies also to physicians' ownership of the best practices they are expected to follow: They must have a sense that the disease management program's best practices are part of a tool kit that they themselves control in managing patient care.[8] Self-efficacy can be achieved through knowledge, belief, ability, and incentives, combined with a pattern of successful experience in which using the best practice has led to positive health outcomes. Self-efficacy can be measured easily, for example, by asking the arthritis patient, "How confident are you that you can exercise without making your symptoms worse?"[9]

- *Memory:* Clinicians and patients cannot always remember to do the right thing. Obstacles to remembering a best practice or care plan can include its complexity, infrequent need to perform it, the need to perform it while otherwise occupied (for example, at school or work). A variety of memory aids can be incorporated into a disease management program, including case management, variance detailing, and automated decision-support systems. The impact of such aids can be assessed by asking clinicians and patients to estimate how often they forget to perform a specific best practice or care plan component.

- *Adherence/compliance:* The goal of all the prior steps in the outcomes cascade is to ensure that the clinician consistently adheres to the best practice and that the patient consistently complies with the care plan. Individuals can be asked to report their own compliance rates, although this approach is not particularly accurate. More objective methods should be employed where appropriate, for example, a review of pharmaceutical databases to determine whether and when a prescription has been refilled.

- *Desired outcomes:* As previously observed, the pro forma impact assessment sets an estimated upper limit on the potential effect of a best practice on health outcomes. Achieving that potential is determined largely by the disease management program's success in managing the intervening

steps in the outcomes cascade. Table 3-4 summarizes the types of intermediate outcomes that should be measured at each step to evaluate
whether a disease management program is maximizing its impact on
health.

Case Illustration

The third of the four components planned for BigHealth's osteoarthritis
management program (see table 3-2) consisted of patient self-care education. The goals of the initiative would be to reinforce patients' care plans,
to encourage compliance, and to equip patients with successful pain management skills. As planned, the educational component would be developed by
physicians, nurses, rehabilitation specialists, and health educators and would
be implemented as a group program run by nurse practitioners.

In order to maximize the likelihood of successful implementation, the planning team conducted an outcomes cascade review of the proposed education module. The following potential obstacles from both the provider cascade
and the patient cascade (see table 3-3) were identified:

- Provider cascade
  - *Knowledge:* Not all physicians who treat osteoarthritis patients may be
    aware of the educational program and its content.
  - *Memory:* Physicians may forget to refer patients to the educational
    program.
- Patient cascade
  - *Knowledge:* Patients who have not recently seen a BigHealth physician
    may not be aware of the educational program.
  - *Belief:* Patients may not be persuaded that a group educational pro-
    gram is in their best interests.
  - *Self-efficacy:* Patients may not internalize the content of the program,
    thereby reducing ongoing compliance once participation in the formal
    program has concluded.

It was agreed that the program implementation plan should specify interventions that address these potential obstacles. The following intermediate
outcomes were also established and are to be assessed quarterly during
the first year of program implementation:

- Percentage of BigHealth general internists, family practitioners, rheuma-
  tologists, occupational medicine specialists, rehabilitation specialists, and
  orthopedists who are aware of the self-care educational program
- Percentage of patients with an osteoarthritis-related encounter who are
  aware of the self-care educational program, who were referred by their
  physician to the program, and who enrolled in the program

Table 3-4. Intermediate Outcomes to Be Measured for the Outcomes Cascade

Outcomes Cascade Steps	Intermediate Outcome Measures
Best practices/care plans	Pro forma impact assessment: expected outcomes, strength of evidence supporting expectations
Knowledge of best practice/care plans	Self-reported awareness and content knowledge
Belief in best practice/care plans	Self-reported belief that the best practice is in fact "best"
Ability to perform best practice/care plans	Self-reported or independently assessed skills, access to equipment and supplies, supportiveness of care settings
Incentives to perform best practice/care plans	Self-reported or independently assessed incentives and disincentives; self-reported impact of incentives and disincentives
Self-efficacy regarding best practice/care plans	Self-reported self-efficacy
Memory of best practice/care plans	Self-reported frequency of forgetting best practice
Adherence to/compliance with best practice/care plans	Self-reported or objective measures of adherence/compliance

- Percentage of patients with an osteoarthritis-related encounter who believe that the various self-care skills taught in the program are valuable

In addition, patients participating in the educational program were to be assessed prior to enrollment and six months following enrollment using the following indicators of intermediate outcomes:

- Self-reported ability to perform self-care skills taught in the program
- Self-reported self-efficacy regarding their ability to manage their condition
- Self-reported compliance with self-care skills taught in the program
- Pharmacy data regarding refill frequency for prescribed pain medications

• Impact Assessment: Measuring Health Outcomes

Most discussions of health outcomes measurement emphasize methodology: questionnaires and indicators, information systems, risk-adjustment models, and other technical aspects. Although it is important for developers and consumers of disease management to understand the technical functions that must be performed if outcome measures are to be taken seriously, from a strategic perspective, it is more important to specify how the data will be used. This section discusses the core components of an outcomes measurement system, as well as its goals and its uses.

Components of Outcomes Measurement Systems

Outcomes measurement can be described as a system, that is, as a set of interrelated processes. Regardless of the types of outcomes being measured, an outcomes measurement system is successful to the extent that it performs the following core component processes effectively and efficiently:

1. *Define data requirements.* Determine what sorts of outcomes need to be measured and what measurement tools should be used.
2. *Obtain the data.* Define and implement a data-collection protocol.
3. *Manage the data.* Create a database, enter the data collected, and take steps to ensure the quality of the data.
4. *Analyze the data.* Analyze the completeness and quality of the data, determine which method should be used for scoring responses to the outcomes indicator, and perform risk adjustment and outcomes analysis.
5. *Report results.* Prepare a written summary of the results and present it to key stakeholders.

Case Illustration

The disease management team at BigHealth followed these five steps for outcomes measurement of the organization's osteoarthritis program. Table 3-5 shows how the team adapted each step to its specific needs.

Each core component described above requires technical competencies, many of which have been formalized in academic curricula and publications. Management and implementation skills are also essential in making outcomes measurement work. Davies and colleagues have summarized the consensus-based recommendations of several leading health systems regarding organization, project management, financing, and other key issues affecting successful implementation of an outcomes measurement program.[10]

Purposes and Uses of Outcomes Measurement

There are many good reasons to measure the health outcomes of a disease management program:

- *Accountability:* To demonstrate the value of disease management to outside parties, especially payers
- *Continual improvement:* To evaluate the impact of process improvements, to identify opportunities for improvement

Table 3-5. Core Component Processes of Outcomes Measurement

Component	Osteoarthritis Case Example
1. Define data requirements:	
Determine what sorts of outcomes need to be measured.	Pain
Determine what measurement tools should be used	10-point self-reported pain intensity scale
2. Obtain the data	
Define data collection protocol	Mail pain scale to a random sample of individuals 6 months following enrollment in disease management program
Implement data collection protocol	BigHealth outsources questionnaire mailing to a vendor
3. Manage the data	
Create database	BigHealth's information systems department creates a customized PC-based disease management database
Enter data into database	Outsourced data collection vendor enters data and transfers it electronically to BigHealth's disease management database.
Assure quality of data	Perform range checks on data; e.g., correct or delete cases with pain scores greater than 10
4. Analyze the data	
Analyze data quality and completeness	Calculate the response rate to the mailed questionnaire
Determine method for scoring responses to outcome indicator	Define "not in pain" as a score of 3 or less on the pain scale
Perform risk adjustment	Determine the statistical impact of patient age and gender on pain scores
Perform outcome analysis	Calculate risk-adjusted pain scores for the sampled patients
5. Report results	
Prepare written summary of results	Report card presenting the percentage of respondents "not in pain"
Present results to key customers	Mail report cards to all key payers; medical director discusses results separately with each key payer

- *Clinical decision making:* To help clinicians and patients evaluate the expected risks and benefits of alternative treatments
- *Research:* To test hypotheses regarding the effectiveness of treatment in real-world settings
- *Medical record:* To provide a structured format for recording and retrieving encounter-based patient data
- *Management:* To evaluate the degree of success in achieving organizational objectives
- *Incentives:* To reward performance based on achievement of outcomes

Disease management initiatives most often develop outcomes measurement capabilities for accountability and continual improvement. Both of these considerations are discussed in more detail in the following subsections.

Accountability

Payers want evidence that disease management adds value to the care delivery system. Many disease management programs have created their own "report cards" to demonstrate their impact on health outcomes. A good health care report card format is one that conveys information about performance in a way that the consumer can understand and use for purchasing decisions. Well-prepared report cards share certain characteristics:

- *Payer-focused:* Data should be presented on only those patient outcomes that the payer regards as important. Providers may regard other indicators as equally or more important; however, the report card is not created for the providers' benefit. On the other hand, it is appropriate for disease management experts to educate the consumer (payer) about the benefits of excellent care, some of which may include the intermediate outcomes discussed in the preceding section.
- *Brief:* Only a few key outcomes measures should be reported. The report card should briefly describe why the outcome is included, then display the actual results.
- *Simple:* Results should be presented concisely, in a way that can be readily understood by persons with neither the training nor the time to wade through statistical technicalities. Interpretation of results should be intuitive; for example, it is easier to understand the percentage of patients who can walk unassisted than the average score on a multi-item walking scale. Simple tables and graphs work well. Although the methodology underlying the report card is important, it should be relegated to footnotes or an appendix.
- *Comparative:* Payers want the best, and the report card should help them decide whether they are getting it. Where possible, a report card should compare the program's results with some recognized comparative standard.

If no such standard is available, that fact should be noted: Taking the initiative in setting reporting standards is a competitive advantage. Internal comparisons are also useful; that is, comparing the present year's program results with the previous year's.

Continual Improvement

In order to "ace" its own report card, a disease management program needs to concentrate on the outcomes its customers regard as most important. Much can be accomplished by means of outcomes-driven program development, described in the previous section. However, there is always room for improvement — a familiar idea from continuous quality improvement (CQI) initiatives. Core features of successful outcomes-based continual improvement include the following:

- *Outcomes-driven:* In order to improve outcomes, a disease management group must improve and standardize the processes that generate the outcomes. Standardization for its own sake can be worthwhile to clarify patient and payer expectations, to simplify management and evaluation, and to create more accurate estimates of the cost of care. However, the real payoff is not for everyone to do things the same way, but to do them better; that is, to achieve consistently better results.
- *Customer-driven:* It is important that improvement efforts be driven by outcomes that the customer values. Ideally, core customer values are reflected in the outcomes measures incorporated in the report card.
- *Linked to process:* A good outcome is the result of a good process. Measurement activities should be able to confirm that standard care processes lead to good intermediate outcomes, which in turn contribute to good health outcomes. For example, do patients who have participated in a self-care educational program report that they know how to follow their care plan? Do patients who know how to follow their care plan comply with it more often?
- *Attentive to outliers and trends:* Outcomes measures should be able to identify opportunities for improvement. By investigating types of patients or providers who achieve unusually good outcomes, or by looking for upswings in results for a particular time interval, the disease management program may be able to identify new care processes that can be incorporated into the program.

Case Illustration

The BigHealth osteoarthritis management planning team agreed to use the following health outcome measures to evaluate the impact of the overall disease management program:

- Average pain experienced by patients with osteoarthritis-related encounters. The measurement tool of choice was the 10-point pain scale recommended in the U.S. Agency for Health Care Policy and Research (AHCPR) pain management guideline.[11]
- Percentage of working-age osteoarthritis patients who report being neither unemployed nor underemployed because of arthritis-related limitations.

To collect the data, a random sample of osteoarthritis patients will be interviewed by telephone six months following an initial qualifying encounter.

BigHealth top management agreed to incorporate the two health-related outcomes measures into its annual report card, typically sent to all key insurers and employers with which BigHealth does business. Marketing was aware of no other delivery system in the marketplace reporting osteoarthritis health outcomes. Consequently, management felt that simply reporting the results would give BigHealth a competitive advantage regardless of how those results compared with internal or external expectations.

For quality-improvement purposes, the two high-level outcomes indicators incorporated in the annual report card would also be reported quarterly to the osteoarthritis management team. In addition, outcomes measurements were designed for each major component of the overall disease management program. For the self-care educational component, the following health outcomes would be collected by questionnaire from all participants immediately prior to and six months following enrollment:

- Intermediate outcomes related to knowledge, skill, memory, and compliance, specified previously in the outcomes cascade review
- The 10-point pain question from the report card
- The employability questions from the report card
- The "Physical Function" scale from the SF-36, a widely used questionnaire for measuring general health status[12] (The physical function scale measures the impact of physical symptoms on an individual's ability to perform the activities of normal daily living, such as climbing stairs.)
- The "Role–Physical" scale from the SF-36, which measures the extent to which physical problems limit a person's work productivity

Program managers felt that this set of measures would enable them to verify the process–outcome linkages on which the educational program was designed. The process–outcome model used by the team is shown in figure 3-2. Evaluation of trends and outliers helped the program managers identify opportunities for improvement.

• Conclusions and Recommendations

Most disease management initiatives are built sequentially: create the program, sell the program (internally or externally), implement the program,

Figure 3-2.   Osteoarthritis Self-Care Process–Outcome Model

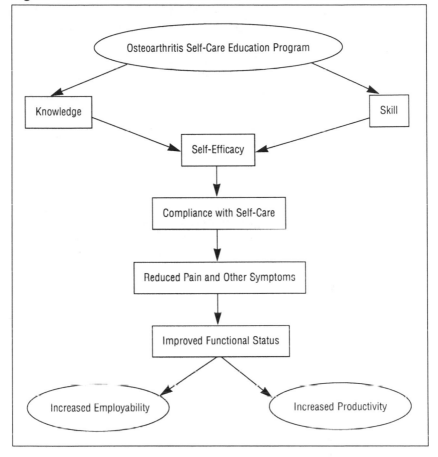

and measure the impact of the program. Since outcomes measurement comes last in the sequence, it often receives the least attention. This chapter proposes that, because the success of a disease management program is judged by its outcomes, all aspects of program development should be driven by an outcomes orientation.

The disease management program should be presold based on its ability to deliver outcomes valued by the consumer. Before building a program, management should determine what the customer wants to buy. In general, customers buy results, not programs.

The disease management program should be designed and implemented so as to achieve maximum outcomes for minimum cost. The outcomes cascade provides a framework for creating program components that can reasonably be expected to improve outcomes. Continual improvement activity is targeted specifically at maximizing outcome performance.

The disease management program should measure outcomes in order to demonstrate that the promised value is a reality. Good report card scores are the natural consequence of a program conceived, designed, and managed with customer-valued outcomes in mind.

This chapter emphasizes and illustrates ways in which disease management can measure and improve health outcomes for populations of patients and plan members. As noted in chapter 1, saving costs has been a main driver for disease management. There is no *inherent* incompatibility between maximizing health and minimizing costs: eliminating inefficiencies can simultaneously reduce costs and improve quality of care; for many health conditions, secondary prevention can be cost-justified by reducing utilization over a fairly short time horizon.

The big question facing disease management is one of emphasis: Are improved health outcomes seen as a means to achieving cost savings, or as ends in their own right? If better health is truly regarded as a goal of disease management, then health systems will find ways to achieve that goal and to demonstrate their successes quantitatively.

References

1. Anders, G. Drug makers help manage patient care. *Wall Street Journal,* May 16, 1995, pp. B1, B7.

2. Brook, R. H., Davies-Avery, A., Greenfield, S., Harris, L. J., Lelah, T., Solomon, N. E., and Ware, J. E. Assessing the quality of medical care using outcome measures: an overview of the method. *Medical Care* 15(Suppl.): Sept. 1977.

3. Lohr, K. N. Outcome measurement: Concepts and questions. *Inquiry* 25:37–50, Spring 1988.

4. Davies, A. R., and Ware, J. E., Jr. *GHAA's Consumer Satisfaction Survey.* 2nd ed. Washington, DC: Group Health Association of America, 1991.

5. *Health Plan Employer Data and Information Set and Users Manual Version 2.0.* Washington, DC: National Committee for Quality Assurance, 1993.

6. Eddy, D. M. *A Manual for Assessing Health Practices and Designing Practice Policies: The Explicit Approach.* Philadelphia: American College of Physicians, 1992.

7. National Asthma Education Program. *Guidelines for the diagnosis and management of asthma.* National Institutes of Health Publication 91-3042. Bethesda: U.S. Department of Health and Human Services, Aug. 1991.

8. Bandura, A. Self-efficacy mechanism in physiological activation and health-promoting behaviors. In: J. Madden IV, editor. *Neurobiology of Learning, Emotion and Affect.* New York City: Raven Press, 1991.

9. Lorig, K., Stewart, A., Ritter, P., Gonzalez, V., Laurent, D., and Lynch, J. *Outcomes Measures for Health Education and Other Health Care Interventions.* Thousand Oaks, CA: Sage, 1996.

10. Davies, A. R., Doyle, M. A. T., Lansky, D., Rutt, W., Stevic, M. O., and Doyle, J. *A Guide to Establishing Programs for Assessing Outcomes in Clinical Settings.* Oakbrook Terrace, IL: Joint Commission on Accreditation of Healthcare Organizations, 1994.

11. Acute Pain Management Guideline Panel. *Acute Pain Management: Operative or Medical Procedures and Trauma. Clinical Practice Guideline.* AHCPR Publication No. 92-0032. Rockville, MD: Agency for Health Care Policy and Research, Feb. 1992.

12. Ware, J. E., Jr. *SF-36 Health Survey: Manual and Interpretation Guide.* Boston: The Health Institute, New England Medical Center, 1993.

Chapter 4

Financial and Actuarial Issues

Richard A. Kipp, FCA, W. Charles Towner, ASA,
and Howard A. Levin, MD

The other chapters in this book define disease management by discussing patient management processes, paradigm shifts, and outcomes management. They also deal to some degree with the financial and economic issues surrounding disease management. This chapter probes deeper into the financial and actuarial issues involved in this new delivery model. In particular, the discussion attempts to give the reader an appreciation of the risks and analytical issues surrounding disease management by defining and identifying the elements of disease management risk and then moving to its quantification. The chapter lays out an approach to analyzing claims history data and specifies a number of studies a financial analyst would want to consider in using these data for disease management product pricing. The calculation of disease management capitation and the use of many of the associated risk-sharing mechanisms, including consideration of the many factors that affect capitation, are touched on. Special attention is given to the importance of understanding the level or degree of medical management present in the disease management system. This is followed with a discussion of financial forecasting and its importance in the planning and overall business risk evaluation process. Finally, the chapter closes with some thoughts on the financial realities of disease management.

The importance of this chapter is rooted in the vital role that reimbursement structure has played and will continue to play in how health care is delivered. Certainly the concepts of risk and capitation discussed in this chapter play a very important role in the success of disease management programs. It should be noted that we will refer to disease management programs and disease management companies in the discussion that follows. Most often they are interchangeable. However, disease management programs can be established by payers for their own exclusive use. We are not as concerned with these because they will not typically involve a carve-out or risk transfer. However, the payer will still be faced with many of the issues discussed here. It is hoped that from the context of the discussion the reader can decide how it applies to each situation.

• Setting the Stage for Altering the Financing of Disease— Identification of Financial Risks

In today's patient management models most of a patient's care is still paid on a fee-for-service basis. Certainly, indemnity insurance carriers and self-paying patients reimburse health care providers via this method. State and federal governments also pay for most of their purchased health care services in this way, and even health maintenance organizations (HMOs) that capitate their primary care providers pay for most of their other nonphysician services on a fee basis. The shift from this historical fee-for-service form of provider reimbursement is beginning to change rapidly as more HMOs capitate both primary care physicians and physician specialists. In addition, a growing number of HMOs are beginning to pay global capitation amounts to provider networks called integrated delivery systems (IDSs).[1] IDSs of one form or another represent one of the fastest-growing organizational structures in the health care delivery system.

This shift in financing is accelerating as the number of people enrolled in HMOs increases and the number of providers being paid via capitation continues to grow. As suggested in other chapters, major changes in reimbursement typically result in major changes in how health care is delivered — enter disease management.

In addition to the shift in how health care is reimbursed, another major force influencing change in the delivery system has been the pharmaceutical industry (see chapter 7). For years pharmaceutical companies appeared to sit on the sidelines, disturbed that their products were not generally seen as the low-cost therapeutic alternatives the companies believed they were. Nonetheless, until the Clinton administration's failed attempt at legislated health care reform highlighted this industry as a contributor to the fast-rising cost of health care, manufacturers seemed content to continue as they were. Today the pharmaceutical industry's desire to change its image is a powerful force that has added momentum to the financing model change. As discussed in chapter 7, pharmaceutical companies, now acting as disease managers, are attempting to proactively integrate themselves into the health care delivery model. They want to change their image from mere suppliers of drugs to players on the center stage of patient management. They are doing this through alliances with managed care companies or through disease management affiliates that sell a management process to their clients (usually managed care organizations [MCOs] such as HMOs).

The types of "products" sold through these alliances vary greatly from educational programs for MCO members to full risk transfer for total patient care for patients of specific disease types (that is, disease state capitation). Disease management as a treatment strategy has considerable appeal on the basis of its focus of clinical and patient management resources on specific health conditions.[2] As suggested in the first two chapters, it is widely believed that disease management programs can achieve significant improvements in quality and efficiency. For health care payers, the appeal of these programs is significantly enhanced by their potential for risk transfer, representing opportunities to carve out the financial risks of some of the more costly segments of a covered population. Although emerging disease management programs have generally not stressed a willingness to accept significant financial risk, it can be assumed that payers are eagerly anticipating the arrival of programs that do. There is certainly a great deal of discussion and activity surrounding disease management within the health care industry, but exactly how successful disease managers will be in achieving their goals of integration and new market development remains to be seen.

Risk

Never has a word been used more often than *risk* in connection with health care than it has these days.[3,4] In its simplest form, risk exists in any situation in which there is a chance, no matter how remote, that something undesired will happen. In insurance terms, it is the possibility that a *loss* (paying for a claim or service delivered) might arise under a policy that has been sold. So for health insurance products or policies it is the possibility of someone using a part of the health care system that is covered under a policy (for example, a stay at an acute care hospital as opposed to over-the-counter drugs, which are not typically covered under a health policy).

For an insurance company, or a provider group accepting capitation, this risk comes into being when the insuring entity agrees to take on responsibility for providing for the payment or provision of a service in exchange for a premium (or a capitation). This is called *risk transfer*. In such a case, the risk is transferred from the individual that has purchased the coverage by paying the premium to the insuring entity.

Given this risk transfer, it makes perfect sense that, once that responsibility has been transferred, the new risk-bearing entity is going to want to take a very active interest in monitoring the good health of the covered individual(s), as well as in providing required services at the lowest reasonable cost, thus reducing its own risk. So, the notion of *risk management* is born. However, risk management[5] is difficult in health insurance because one very quickly encounters the issue of an individual's freedom to pursue treatment as he or she wishes versus the insurer's desire that all clients behave in a prudent, healthy fashion. Risk management is well accepted in workers' compensation and other property casualty insurance products. The use of back braces to prevent back strain on the job is a good example of risk management. Although it is an unacceptable practice in today's environment, requiring people to stop smoking while covered under a specific health policy might be an example of health risk management.

Disease Management Risk

All other things being comparable, the disease management program that assumes the greatest proportion of risk from among its peers will generate the strongest interest from potential contracting partners. For payers, there is a strong incentive to explore and quantify the risk involved in the treatment areas within a disease—finding more cost-effective ways to manage care. From a payer's perspective, the more encompassing the scope of activity included under a risk arrangement, the better. From an actuarial perspective, financial risk for a set of services should only be accepted if the service set is clearly definable and, preferably, if supported by a body of experience data from which expected cost and cost variance can be reliably measured. The ability to accurately quantify risk is dependent on the data used to characterize it.

If an organization is going to take risk on a disease-specific basis, it must have certain information before deciding if the risk is acceptable. Some of these information needs are the answers to the questions shown below:

- For what is the risk being "traded"?
- What are the parameters that define the risk?
- Is the program a carve-out or carve-in?
- How much control can be expected over the risk?
- Are there any limiting factors (for example, benefit provisions)?
- Does the population to be covered have any special characteristics?

Each of these questions is explored briefly in the following subsections.

Risk Trading

As previously mentioned, an insurance company trades premium for risk. In disease management if a risk transfer is involved, as in capitation, the value of the item being traded needs to be determined. If a capitation is being considered, the disease management company should develop its own estimated cost for this product through either a budget or fee-for-service equivalent methodology. Use of a budget methodology is recommended only if the company has several years of experience with the particular disease under a risk contract. Other risk-sharing mechanisms may be used. These are discussed along with capitation later in the chapter. The disease manager's risks arise from three sources: (1) underpricing, (2) random fluctuation, and (3) new business risks.[6]

1. *Underpricing:* Underpricing risk can arise from failing to recognize the many factors that can affect the delivery of care to a group of patients and thereby charging too little for the product. This risk can be

exacerbated in a highly competitive market. Understanding the claim cost risk and the differences in establishing product price for contracts such as capitation vis-à-vis unit pricing such as fee-for-service is essential to success in disease management. This involves knowing something about the expected frequency of various types of service, as well as the relative cost or reimbursement for each type. This will be discussed more fully in the sections that follow.

2. *Random fluctuation:* The essence of this issue is that some events are very difficult to predict. They appear to be occurring randomly. Things like flu epidemics or the sudden appearance of more transplant patients in an at-risk population might be seen as random events from an insurance perspective. When a disease manager takes on a full risk transfer contract such as capitation, those sudden unforeseen occurrences will be the disease manager's responsibility. Handling them becomes a financial management as well as a patient management issue that did not exist in the same way in the fee-for-service world. Some aspects of this type of risk are discussed in later sections of this chapter.

3. *New business:* Disease management represents a new product line for many new disease managers. Some of the reimbursement mechanisms associated with it present special risks (for example, capitation and case rates). Capitation risk was mentioned earlier, there are other risks as well, such as having to account for and track all of the members assigned. Oftentimes HMO benefits have flat copay amounts, which providers are responsible for collecting. Collecting those copays may be a new requirement. Setting up systems for both of these will be important. Additionally, another sometimes significant new business risk for a disease management company is learning how to interact with the insurance industry. Insurance, and in particular managed care, has its own principles and jargon that must be understood by the new risk partners. New skills have to be developed and/or partnered into existing structures for the organization to have a chance for success. Medical management, underwriting, information systems, insurance accounting, and other functions must be brought on-line to lower the risk when entering into this new venture.

Defining Parameters

One of the most critical issues facing both the disease manager and the managed care partner is the problem of scope. How does one identify the point at which a particular patient is the responsibility of the disease manager? As a specific example, assume one wishes to take the full risk for managing asthma patients. Will the disease manager be at risk for the services an asthma patient will need if he or she has an upper respiratory infection? What if the patient develops a cardiac condition?

The real question becomes, Can one easily differentiate between the liability of each party as a payer's claim adjudication system does today? Is there data—such as diagnosis code, procedure code, and so forth— available on something like a claim form to identify cases that are the disease manager's responsibility? If a disease manager is partnered with an MCO to handle anything but the rarest diseases, the answer had better be yes. If not, the deal may not be easily administered—if it can be administered at all.

If the disease manager is taking risk, another way of asking the question might be, Which components (for example, inpatient hospital, physician visits, drugs) should be included? This is discussed further a little later in this chapter.

Carve-out and Carve-in Programs

The term *carve-out* is often used today in association with programs for managing care and, usually, taking risk, where the entire program is segmented in every sense from all other covered services being provided. That is, there is usually a separate provider network and a managing organization with its own contracts and fee arrangements. This organization typically monitors its own performance data. It may even pay its own claims and track its own membership data. It carries out all of the provider network functions (that is, credentialing, disciplining physicians, enrollment, and so on). The term has been used most frequently in connection with managed mental health and substance abuse benefits and outpatient prescription drug programs. In both of these cases payers have easily been able to identify the scope of services of the program and thereby "carve the program out."

The expertise for managing the carve-out program is external to the payer. This represents a constant risk to the carve-out vendor. If the payer becomes dissatisfied with the vendor's service, the payer can replace those services fairly easily. Competitive bids usually find numerous interested suppliers just waiting to take over the prior vendor's role.

A *carve-in* program, on the other hand, is one in which the providers of care are usually the payer's own (at least by contract). The other major difference is that special managed care expertise brought in by the carve-in service vendor is used to educate the payer's provider and is then, in a sense, left with the payer. There can be special ongoing support given by the vendor of these services. Such things as education programs, monitoring reports, and assistance with future provider contracting are all part of the deliverables in this scenario.

The risk taking for each of these may be different. It is far more likely that a carve-out vendor will take full risk than a carve-in vendor. Typically the risk taking in the carve-in scenario is limited to a percentage of the administration fees. Performance measures are established and used to establish the success or failure of the program.

The following are examples of each to help illustrate the differences between them:

- *Example 1: carve-out mental health services:* The Happy Member HMO (HMH) has experienced several years of rising mental health costs. HMH has discussed this cost problem with their contracting mental health providers (psychiatrists, psychologists, and social workers), but no lasting solution has been implemented. Now HMH believes that contracting with a managed health vendor to carve out mental health services is the way to solve the cost problem. HMH issues a request for proposal (RFP) and receives several responses. The RFP requirements include:
  - Provider network development and maintenance
  - Credentialing, provider education, and provider contracting
  - Provider reimbursement
  - Accepting full risk capitation
  - Service scope including all types of service (inpatient, intermediate, and outpatient) for both mental health and substance abuse services
  - Monitoring and reporting
  - Utilization management

  The bid is awarded to a vendor, which results in HMH maintaining its contracts with its own network providers to pay for services outside the scope of services (which are probably few and far between). The vendor contracts with local mental health providers, some of which are the HMH's own contracting providers. The greatest single difference is that the new network is at risk for its services and is being encouraged to behave in a more cost-effective manner through the use of capitation and closely managed utilization.
- *Example 2:* Same HMH scenario except that the solution is to engage a firm that will provide the following services:
  - Provider education
  - Monitoring and reporting improvement
  - Utilization management advice

This firm will not be taking full risk but will put a portion of its administrative charges for its services at risk (for example, 20 percent). Performance criteria will be developed including such financial indicators as overall cost per member per month. The education and training that this firm provides will be for the HMH's current mental health network providers. HMH may also attempt to change the reimbursement method with its network to a full capitation. But there is no contracting relationship between any of the providers and the vendor as there was in example 1. Also, the vendor's risk is limited.

There are parallels to both of these types of programs in disease management, of course. Many people talk in terms of full carve-out for disease management, but this is extremely difficult except for the rarest of diseases. The remaining sections of this chapter do not specifically address the risk issues associated with these programs, although they touch briefly on the intricacies of provider contracting in a disease management environment.

Control

Risk takers usually feel comfortable taking risk in situations where they have some control over the outcome. In the world of health care the controllers of outcomes are primarily the providers of care. The products that providers use and the behavior of patients themselves also can have a major influence on the outcomes achieved. Therefore, a disease manager will want very close contact with providers, probably by contract and possibly as their employer. Further, if the provider is under contract, that contract should have incentives built in to motivate cost-effective behavior. The disease manager will also want the flexibility to first identify and then use the most cost-effective providers and products. This includes the flexibility to use drugs from a nonaffiliated pharmaceutical company.

On a related issue, there has been a great deal of discussion regarding geographic differences in practice patterns among physicians. Effective disease management demands that the most cost-effective alternatives be used at all times along the patient care continuum. Education of patients and providers in the goals of disease management is critical in helping to create the environment necessary to achieve optimal levels of health care management.

The amount of control that can feasibly be applied should become obvious as the program is administered. Process and outcomes measures should be established to monitor the achievement of disease management goals.

Limiting Factors

The payers (MCOs) that most disease managers will be partnering with will have a variety of risk limits built into their insurance policies. These include deductibles; coinsurance amounts; copays; out-of-pocket limitations; exclusions, such as those for preexisting conditions; and annual and lifetime maximums. Such limits create cost sharing between patients and the MCO.

These features need to be considered in determining how much the MCO should pay the disease manager for providing services to its patients. This, of course, assumes that the disease manager in some sense receives all payments made by the MCO for services provided under the disease management contract. If the MCO pays providers directly, the payments are reduced by the appropriate amount to account for patient cost sharing.

Another limiting factor may be a reinsurance policy that the MCO provides or that the disease management company obtains from a reinsurance company. These policies are another form of risk transfer. They are usually sold on either an individual claim or claimant-per-year basis but may also be sold on an aggregate group basis. There will be more discussion of this transfer mechanism in the risk-sharing section below.

Population Characteristics

Insured populations can vary significantly in their use of health services, and a number of factors affect these usage rates. Factors such as age, gender, prior history of disease, and genetics are all important indicators of future use of services. In the insurance world, governmental programs are usually segmented from commercial business, and individually sold policies are looked at separately from large- and small-employer groups. Uninsured people also have unique health care utilization characteristics.

When the disease manager prices a contract, especially a capitation contract, he or she essentially determines the value to be placed on differences in these and other factors from one block of business to another. In some cases, a deal may be determined to be too risky to accept. The insurance world calls this determination *process underwriting*. It involves both analytical skill and good judgment. It does not seem to be practiced often by disease managers and is rarely discussed in these terms, but its essential nature should become clear as the chapter progresses.

• Quantification Issues

In discussing risk and how to measure it, an initial goal is the development of common descriptive statistics such as the mean and variance of the cost-per-covered-member for some specified period of time — usually a year or month (where a member is anyone covered by a health care contract — the employee and the dependents). To derive the mean cost per member per year for a group of covered members, information is needed regarding the dollars spent on services used. Also, it is necessary to have information as to how many people *could have* used a service.

The notion of "could have" is key to the notion of risk and its measurement, especially in connection with disease-specific risk. People get sick and need health care services in what appears to be a random fashion to an outside observer like an insurance company. The fact is that some diseases are more readily controlled or prevented than others. The occurrence of some diseases is far from a random process, especially those of a genetic nature. To take risk for any type of disease, it is important to have some sense of how often it occurs in the at-risk population. Comparisons of current disease prevalence and incidence rates for an at-risk population to expected rates for the population's demographic characteristics are helpful in projecting patient volume.

In order to estimate the costs of providing disease-specific treatment, a base of treatment experience data is necessary. Assuming that a database of experience specific to the disease management program has not yet been sufficiently accumulated, these experience data represent an unmanaged population (at least in terms of specific disease management). Using this base, costs can be derived and later adjusted to reflect clinical modifications and patient management effects. These types of data are available in insurance company or HMO claims histories, but they are not accessible to the public. So unless a disease manager is also the payer of claims, he or she must acquire data from some other source (see below).

Disease Management Risk Measurement

The nature of the treatment-cost risk for particular diseases under a disease management program is somewhat unique in comparison to risk for more diversified health conditions; it calls for a different approach to utilizing experience data to quantify it. The patient base is homogeneous with respect to the illness. This is a departure from other risk arrangements, such as physician primary care or specialty capitation, which have a much more diverse collection of patients with a multitude of ailments generating the demand for care. Under these arrangements, there is no particular subgroup within the population that drives the costs for the group — other than the people who happen to be sick at a specific point in time — and this group is more or less in flux.

Under a disease management program, the patient base is the subgroup of patients having the disease. This subgroup has new additions from time to time as well as exiting patients, but represents a much more constant set of patients than the subgroup of generic sick people who generate costs under a generic physician specialty capitation. Thus, under a disease management program, the primary treatment-cost risk determinant is the nature of the patient group. Because of this, the emphasis in analyzing experience data should be on per-patient costs and their variation within the patient group. This requires modifying existing methods of measuring risk.

Existing Methodologies and Their Shortcomings

For those acquainted with how costs are estimated for sets of medical services, such as in the development of case rates, global rates, capitation rates, and so on, a familiar process comes to mind:

* Define the services to be included, translated into the coding scheme used in hospitals' and facilities' claims and billing — such as the Physician's

Current Procedural Terminology (CPT), the Health Care Financing Administration's Common Procedure Coding System (HCPCS) codes for physicians and other professionals, diagnosis-related groups (DRGs), and ambulatory patient groups (APGs) for facilities.
- Determine the reimbursement level for each service.
- Derive the frequency of expected occurrence for each service, usually obtained from a data source representing the total volume of services for a defined population for a specified period of time.
- Multiply the reimbursement amount by the expected frequency for each service and sum these amounts to determine total cost.

A natural extension of this methodology for estimating costs under a disease-specific scope of services would be to narrow the focus of the process to a particular disease. This would translate into modifying the data source used to derive the frequencies so it would contain only the services performed on patients with the particular disease, normally defined in terms of an International Classification of Disease (ICD-9) code. In theory, this would appear to be a sound methodology. In practice, however, it has a number of deficiencies.

Probably the main reason this methodology comes up short is the difference in the approach to and the role of the experience data required for determining disease management risk. Whereas the method discussed previously focuses on the most basic unit of health care delivery—the discrete service—the focus of disease management programs is the patient and the more comprehensive units of treatment, such as encounters or episodes. A panel of asthma experts could gather together with CPT code and ICD-9 manuals and develop a comprehensive and detailed specification of what constitutes asthma treatment. Whatever the set of coding specifications used to gather the activity from the experience data for measuring risk, significant numbers of services would be omitted due to the simple fact that different providers would code the diagnosis differently for the same patient during the same encounter. The gathering of activity to measure risk for disease management should be done by identifying the patients first, then collecting the activity. Decisions on whether an encounter is generated by the disease would determine whether the services performed during the encounter should go into the risk measurement or not, thereby including services that would have been missed by the previously described process.

There are more important flaws in this service-oriented methodology than omitting services that should be included in at-risk amounts. The orientation itself is fundamentally out of sync with the disease management approach. By focusing on services as the important units of risk, it fails to produce the types of patient-based information that are of much greater use in characterizing and ultimately quantifying the risk involved in the treatment of a specific disease. The important unit of risk in disease management is the patient, and the evaluation of risk should be made from this basis.

A Patient-Based Approach

For the purposes of this discussion, let us assume an ideal data source is available with which to measure full risk, that is, all aspects of the treatment of a disease. This source covers several years, representing the claims activity of a large, stable population with known demographic characteristics. Such sources are not plentiful, but they do exist.

Just what are these patient-based types of information, and how do they characterize the risk in disease-specific treatment? The initial shift from a service-oriented approach to a patient-centered one consists of constructing larger units of health care delivery from discrete services. These units are typically inpatient admissions, emergency room encounters, outpatient encounters, office visits, and home health care. From these units, even more comprehensive collections called *episodes* can be constructed, representing particular disease stages or courses of treatment.[7] A more detailed discussion of the nature of these episodes follows later in this chapter. An important point to emphasize is that in the formation of encounters and episodes, the underlying composition of these larger units in terms of discrete services is recorded. The usefulness of a discrete-service characterization of disease treatment is not abandoned, just superseded.

After these larger units have been constructed, per-patient summaries are developed. The most basic type is cost per patient. There are many ways of looking at these per-patient costs, with several being particularly informative:

- *Distributions of aggregate per-patient cost, that is, by-percentile measurements of yearly treatment costs per patient.* This allows determination of what proportion of total patients account for a given proportion of total costs. It also helps in considering outlier points and analyzing reinsurance possibilities.
- *Distributions of per-patient utilization and costs by encounter and episode type.* Focusing on ranges of per-patient costs by these categories allows for the following characterizations:
  - Severity levels can be estimated.[8-10] Although aggregate costs can be a crude measure of severity, occurrence thresholds of particular encounter types are often a more reliable indicator. A common indicator of severity for asthma patients is the incidence of inpatient admissions or emergency room encounters. Severity-level information is important for two reasons.
    - Cost differences between severity categories can be dramatic. A potential contracting population may have a significant enough difference

in severity mix from the baseline in the experience data to warrant an adjustment to the baseline costs.

–Cost variances within severity categories may indicate that a particular severity level has costs that are more predictable, which could suggest a possible segregation of the risk arrangement by severity category.

— Episode types are indicative of particular disease stages or courses of treatment. The utility of cost and utilization information by episode parallels some of the points made above in connection with severity levels. Cost differences between stages and courses of treatment, and variance within these episodes, can have implications similar to those for severity levels. In addition, by-episode cost and utilization summaries can be useful in three ways.

–For diseases with well-defined disease stage progression, identification of per-patient cost ranges by stage can be useful in projecting future costs, based on the current mix of stages in a patient population and the subsequent stages through which they may be expected to pass. A given patient population may represent a quantity of risk that may change significantly over time.

–In the opening remarks of this section, the importance of including cost allowances for currently untreated patients in the overall estimate of costs for a population was noted. Categorization of a separate episode type for treatment connected with the initial diagnosis for a disease would allow for a more precise estimate of costs for these untreated patients. On the other hand, some disease management programs may assume that a patient enrolled in the program would have already been definitively diagnosed and the costs associated with the initial diagnosis would not be included in the scope of risk. In either case, it is useful to treat the initial diagnosis as a distinct episode with quantified costs.

–Certain types of care may be appropriate for a specific stage of a disease but may not be the kind of treatment that requires the resources or expertise of specialized disease management providers. These categories of care could be returned to a primary care provider and omitted from the scope of disease management risk. An example of this type of care would be purely palliative treatment. Knowing the cost distribution of this type of care would aid in determining whether or not to retain it in the scope of risk.

— There is an opportunity to measure savings opportunities under disease management. By building per-patient distributions of costs and utilization by severity levels and encounter and episode types, while retaining the underlying service composition information, both of the larger units and their component services are encapsulated. This allows modeling of savings potential through modification of the utilization frequency of particular services or the larger encounters/episodes,

replacing them with alternatives or eliminating them altogether. These modifications could be based on targets established by treatment protocols or expected patient-management effects.
— Trend measurement by severity/encounter/episode categories has the potential to zero in on the primary trend drivers. These drivers could be the overuse of a particular service or encounter. A new course of treatment using an expensive new technology might be identified. In any case, once identified, action could be taken.
• *Distribution of costs by comorbid conditions.* Comorbid conditions may not be directly related to the disease in question, but do impact the overall health of the patient and, in so doing, may warrant some degree of inclusion into the risk arrangement. Again, information as to the range of costs for these conditions could be valuable in deciding what to consider.

Cost-per-patient information is probably the most important product of a patient-oriented analysis of experience data for the purpose of quantifying risk under disease management. If reliable cost-per-patient measures are the cornerstone units of disease management risk, disease prevalence and incidence rates are the most important parameters in summarizing these units. As stated in the previous section, different populations in different areas can exhibit widely varying disease incidence rates. Then, there are populations that may be similar in terms of incidence rates but, for whatever reason, have different current prevalence rates. In either case, capitation rates have to reflect these differences. Populations showing large variations in incidence rates may be too unreliable to accept full population-based risk. In such cases, a contact capitation may be the best alternative. Contact capitation involves taking on risk only for those patients who have met the criteria for inclusion in the risk pool, which, in a disease management program, would be patients with the disease. The risk associated with the variability of incidence and prevalence rates is removed.

These are some of the more important characterizations of risk under a disease management program. Most of these items require a source close to the ideal described. This is not to say that workable estimates of risk can only be derived from such sources. Separate sources representing the same type of care may be aggregated by adjusting the utilization characteristics of each source to simulate a common population. However, a source close to the ideal is preferable.

• Using Data

Given the preceding descriptions of some of the data characterizations that can be made and their usefulness in quantifying risk, this section suggests an outline for the process of using ideal experience data for this purpose.

Analyzing Experience Data

The overall goal of this process is to describe as fully as possible all aspects of the disease that can be observed through the window of health insurance claims history. This description includes the following elements:

- Summaries of utilization and cost of treatment over both the covered population and the diagnosed patient base by discrete service and encounter types (basic groupings of services, such as inpatient admissions, office visits, and so on)
- A definition of meaningful episodes of disease manifestation and/or treatment courses, including initial diagnosis
- Episode profiling, that is, summaries of the utilization, mix, and cost of the encounters and drugs/equipment comprising the episodes of disease manifestation and/or treatment course
- Identification of patient strata by disease severity and/or progressive state
- Incidence rates of new cases and prevalence rates by patient strata
- Patient profiling, that is, distributions of frequencies and costs of discrete services, encounters, and episodes by patient strata
- Identification of comorbidities and summarization of service cost and utilization for treatment of these comorbid conditions

Most of these characterizations are necessary for defining and quantifying the scope of the risk that might be assumed for treating the disease. Some, such as episode profiling, are useful in comparing prevailing modes of treatment both to each other and to disease management protocols, with a view to estimating savings under disease management programs.

Forming the Claims History

The first step in analyzing experience data consists of gathering the claims history generated by patients with the disease. Basically, this process consists of identifying the patients with the disease and collecting their claims. However, certain aspects of the disease and the specificity of the existing ICD-9 coding determine at what chronological point in the body of available claims data the gathering of the data for inclusion in the analysis should begin. This concern with determining a starting point for collecting the claims data is necessary in order to establish points of disease onset and subsequent stages.

Some diseases have ICD-9 coding that may indicate the initial diagnosis or progressive stage of the disease. Others may have onset and disease-stage points that are characterized by specific services or drug regimens. Others may have neither. For these diseases, it is necessary to have a period of claims history for observation preceding the period to be used for actual claims gathering. This period of observation is used to identify the patients in the gathering period who are ongoing in status and those who are initially diagnosed.

Building and Classifying Encounters

Once the necessity for an observation period has been decided and the starting point for claims collecting has been determined, all claims activity for the identified patients is gathered. The next step is building the basic encounters from the discrete, line-item-level services. The basic encounter types are:

- Inpatient admissions
- Emergency room encounters
- Outpatient encounters at:
  - Physician offices
  - Outpatient facilities
- Home-based care

As the encounters are constructed, information on the discrete services comprising them is recorded, including information as to provider type, service type, and diagnosis. The diagnostic information is especially important to be able to classify the encounters as having been generated by the disease in question or by a comorbid or unrelated illness or condition.

Interpreting the diagnostic information for the purpose of encounter classification is problematic. There are two main issues to resolve in connection with this diagnostic classification. The first is manifested primarily with inpatient and emergency room encounters, with which a multitude of charges can exist. Some are facility charges and some are professional charges. There is frequently disagreement between the facility diagnosis and the diagnoses specified by the various physicians involved. There can also be differences in diagnoses among the physicians.

Sometimes the presence of differing diagnoses within an encounter is readily interpreted, such as a psychiatric consult for an admitted asthmatic suffering depression or other isolated services for specific incidental treatment. Other cases are not so clear-cut, such as hospital charges for a respiratory diagnosis and physician charges with predominantly asthma diagnoses. To avoid a painstaking encounter-by-encounter analysis, general classification rules must be developed with clinical input based on a grid of the observed mix of diagnostic coding by provider type.

The second issue involves a judgment as to what treatment related to a disease should be included under a risk contract. Some treatments not coded under the ICD-9s for the disease are nonetheless closely related to the disease or may be manifestations due to the disease. Again, clinical input is needed for these judgments. Using asthma as an example, a decision could be made to classify certain respiratory admissions (such as pneumonia) under the asthma treatment classification using the logic that normally such conditions do not warrant admission — although for asthmatics they do.

In light of this discussion, attempts at constructing average costs per patient per month should not be made until these service inclusion issues are resolved.

The formation of encounters is the first step in organizing collections of discrete services into more meaningful parcels of care. Characterizing disease treatment by the frequency and cost of these encounters allows for an initial classification of patients into severity levels, with a higher incidence of admissions or emergency room encounters generally indicating a higher severity. It also facilitates comparisons to proposed treatment protocols and an estimation, by way of modeling a reduction or shifting of encounters in accordance with protocol standards, of savings potential under the proposed protocols.

Forming Episodes

For some diseases, an additional level of treatment grouping may be useful as a way of viewing the care given over a particular course of treatment or disease stage.[11] Episodes are a means of collecting the encounter activity and drug utilization over a period of uniform treatment or for the duration of a recognizable disease stage. Examples of episodes include the following:

- Periods corresponding to specific drug regimens
- Periods of particular therapies, such as a course of radiation or chemotherapy for cancer
- A stage of a progressive disease, such as AIDS

Clinical input is needed to determine which meaningful episodes may exist for a given disease and how they should be defined in terms of health claims information.

The formation of episodes has several potential uses, several of which were mentioned in the previous section on measuring risk. Beyond their use in quantifying risk, episodes representing particular therapies/courses of treatment/drug regimens can be compared on a cost and resource-use basis. The periods following these episodes can be analyzed for the purpose of developing and comparing efficacy measures in terms of the observed frequency and cost of postepisode care.

In a manner similar to that discussed for encounters, the use of treatment episodes may be another way of comparing prevailing courses of care to proposed protocols. In light of specific treatment episodes either recommended or discouraged by proposed protocols, changes in the relative mix of these treatment courses can be modeled and potential savings estimated.

For progressive diseases, the segregation of costs by episodes representing disease stages may indicate significant cost differences between the stages. For these diseases, a subdivision of the risk by disease stage may present a more palatable alternative to assuming total risk.

At this point in the analysis, it should be possible to develop some meaningful criteria for classifying patients by severity and/or disease stage. Once these strata are defined, a process of patient profiling can be undertaken to develop distributions of encounter/episode costs and frequencies by patient strata and in aggregate. As mentioned previously, such characterizations are useful in quantifying disease management risk.

Comorbidity Analysis

At this point the disease manager has constructed encounters and possibly grouped encounters generated by the disease in question into episodes. He or she also has summarized the frequency and cost of these service groupings over patient strata. What can be done with those encounters generated by other illnesses or conditions? Viewing summaries of this comorbid activity by patient strata could be informative. Other possibilities include summarizing the activity for periods preceding or following particular episodes.

These analyses may or may not yield anything useful. They may suggest comorbidity conditions that a risk-taking entity may want to explicitly exclude. On the other hand, they may indicate conditions that would be clinically consistent with the expertise of physician specialists and financially favorable to include in a risk arrangement.

An analysis of the experience data, such as the one already outlined, should produce the information needed to better understand the nature of the treatment risk for a disease. From this understanding, a scope of risk can be established and defined. The body of treatment activity corresponding to this definition can be extracted from the experience data and used to derive the statistics needed to quantify the risk.

Descriptive Statistics

Now that the treatment activity under the disease-scope definition has been isolated, the average cost for the included disease care on a per-member-per-year (PMPY) or per-member-per-month (PMPM) basis can be derived. This is done by summing all dollars for the included care and dividing by average members per year or by member months (which is a count of the number of members having coverage for each month of coverage during the year):

Average PMPM cost = Dollar amount ÷ Member months

The variance of the PMPM cost is also important. With this knowledge, a determination can be made as to how stable the costs for a disease are and how large a population is needed to ensure that the estimated average PMPM is a reasonable estimator of the true value of that statistic. A distribution of yearly per-member costs, such as the one shown in table 4-1, illustrates how variance is estimated.

Actuarial Cost Model

The cost of health care services has two components: utilization of services and service reimbursement amounts. For example, the PMPM for hospital inpatient costs is equivalent to:

Number of days × Average charge per day ÷ Number of member months.

It is useful to view PMPM costs and their utilization and reimbursement components by types of care (inpatient hospital, outpatient hospital, surgical, and so on). Such a breakout of costs is called an *actuarial cost model,* a flexible tool for modeling the effects of utilization changes (possibly accomplished through patient management or treatment changes) and reimbursement-level modifications. An example of an actuarial model is given later in this chapter.

Table 4-1. Illustrative Distribution of Costs by Dollar Amount for Asthma in an Unmanaged System

Amount of Claims ($)	Percentage of Members	Average Amount of Claims ($)
$0	95.0	0
$0–$249	3.0	175
$250–$499	1.15	375
$500–$999	.45	750
$1,000–$1,999	.25	1,500
$2,000–$4,999	.10	3,500
$5,000+	.05	7,500

Mean per member per year: $23.94
Mean per member per month: $2.00
Standard deviation: $224.71
Sample size for 95% confidence ±5% of mean: 135,000

Other aggregations of cost and its components that can be incorporated into an actuarial cost model include:

- Geographic area or region
- Age and gender
- Employer group
- Industry

Aggregations by these categories produce characterizations of costs in terms of the parameters of the population from which they were derived. By adjusting the mixes of these parameters, diverse populations can be modeled.

Further aggregations, such as the following, can be especially useful in a disease management context:

- Severity level
- Episode type
- Provider (for closed panels of providers such as IDSs)

Constructing these aggregations can highlight the cost characteristics of patient or provider subgroups and allows for more specific modeling of treatment alternatives.

Use of an actuarial cost model allows flexible modeling of many aspects of disease management. More sophisticated studies can be incorporated to understand the impact of disease management intervention on clinical outcomes.

Trends

Another aspect of the data analysis is the consistency and predictability of the cost over a period of years. To begin to get a sense of this, the analyst can collect data for a time series and look at the changes in the mean cost per member over time. This might be expected to follow some pattern like the medical consumer price index (CPI) or local medical charge increases. If not, the analyst must look deeper, slicing the data for each year into the many pieces already described. With this process, observations about year-to-year changes can be made.

Modeling Potential Cost Savings

The analyses described can make the significance of the savings potential easier to understand. When using an actuarial cost model, changes in expected utilization due to a managed system can be viewed and used to reconfigure the costs. This provides insight into the opportunity for savings. For asthma these savings would have the cost characteristics shown in table 4-2.

The analyst must be careful to include in any model an accounting for diseased people in a population who previously went untreated. In an analysis

Table 4-2. Sources of Asthma Savings

Type of Savings	Cost Characteristics
Reduced admissions	High
Reduced length of stay	Moderate to high
Reduced emergency room admissions	Moderate
Reduced physician visits	Low to moderate
Increased drug therapy	Slight cost increase*

*Some argue that the reduction of noncompliance with drug therapy actually cuts down on drug costs by eliminating wasted product.

of asthma, these people would probably be untreated mild asthmatics who do not realize they have asthma or have been misdiagnosed. If the patient/member education envisioned for disease management actually works, these untreated members should be identified and brought into the system for treatment. This could represent an initial increase in cost, but the long-term benefits in reduced stress to the member and reduced lost time to the employer may more than offset the additional short-term expenses. Consideration of these effects is beyond the scope of this chapter, but could certainly be of significant interest to employer groups.

Table 4-3 shows a very simple model for calculating the overall impact on medical claim cost of implementing a disease management program. It indicates that while the number of people treated increased by 10 percent (5 percent to 5.5 percent), the medical claims cost per patient was reduced by 50 percent, thus resulting in a net 45 percent savings overall.

Other diseases, such as AIDS and cancer, present much greater risk to the disease manager due to the large number of undetected, untreated cases that may be present in a population at any given time. In the case of cancer, early detection could enhance the chance for a cure. That is not the case with AIDS. Until a cure is found, the greatest gain is that early detection may help to halt the spread of the disease. In any case the more complex the disease process, the more complicated the modification to the model shown in table 4-3.

• Methods of Financing and Risk Sharing

Capitation and fee-for-service were discussed briefly earlier in the chapter. These and other methods of financing, as well as the risks associated with each method, are displayed in table 4-4.

Fee-for-service, the method with the lowest level of risk transferred, is becoming rarer all the time. The global fee usually involves only professional

Table 4-3.   Asthma Claims Savings Model

	Prior to Disease Management Program		With Disease Management Program		
	No. of Patients Treated	Cost per Patient	No. of Patients Treated	Cost per Patient	Cost Reduction per Patient
Current patients	5	$635.00	5.5	$320.00	(50%)
Nonpatients*	95	0	94.5	0	
Total members	100	$ 31.75	100.0	$ 17.60	(45%)

*Nonpatients include nonasthmatics as well as untreated asthmatics. The additional cost of disease management administrative functions is *not* included.

Table 4-4.   Risk Associated with Various Financing Methods

Common Methods of Financing*	Nature of Mechanism	Level of Risk Transferred	Nature of Risk Transferred
Fee-for-service	Fee for procedure	Lowest	Time to perform service
Global fee	Fee for multiple procedures	Low to medium	Shift in intensity of services required
Case rate	Payment for total care of patients for an episode (usually short time horizon)	Medium	Shift in intensity of services required
Capitation	Payment made per member regardless of services rendered	Highest	Frequency of cases and cost/intensity of a case

*Per diems paid to hospitals for a day's care are a special category within fee-for-service. Diagnosis-related groups are a special category within case rates.

services delivered as a group and priced as a package. The case rate generally involves facility and professional charges, but many times excludes drugs and other extras. Contact capitation, which is similar to a case rate but with an open-ended time horizon, has particular applicability in a disease management context and is discussed with capitation.

Capitation is one of the primary methods of financing used in managed care today. There are several risk-sharing mechanisms that may be used in combination with capitation. The general characteristics of each are discussed in the following sections.

Capitation

The method of financing at the provider level that is getting the most attention these days is capitation, which is defined by the following characteristics:

- Dollar amount paid in advance for any and all services that *may be* provided
- Usually paid to a provider or provider organization
- Typically on a regularly scheduled basis and most often monthly
- Paid for each person or policy that is eligible to receive a service

Capitation is most often calculated on a fee-for-service equivalent basis, as shown in table 4-5, but can also be developed through a detailed budget analysis. The cost model shown in the table is for all health care costs, but the same method of calculation would be used for a specific disease. The model shown does not allow for patient cost sharing which must be accounted for in setting the disease budget amount. Also, many other factors may affect the cost and utilization levels expected for a given population of people.

The calculated PMPM value, a fundamental part of the capitation, would be paid to the disease manager on a scheduled basis for every enrolled

Table 4-5. Example of an Actuarial Cost Model for Beneficiaries under Age 65 in an Unmanaged System

Type of Service	Annual Admits per 1,000	Average Length of Stay	Annual Utilization per 1,000	Average Cost per Service	Per Member Monthly Claim Cost
Hospital					
Inpatient	89	5.75	510	$1,800	$76.50
Outpatient			700	310	18.08
Physician					
Surgeries			480	580	23.20
Office visits			2,600	50	10.83
Radiology			800	120	8.00
Pathology			2,100	40	7.00
Other			3,200	90	24.00
Other					
Prescription drugs			4,300	40	14.33
Miscellaneous other			220	250	4.58
Total			14,910		$186.52

member. It is usually thought of as a full risk transfer mechanism. However, the disease manager may not have the capacity to accept full risk.

A particularly onerous component of total risk under a disease-specific, full risk arrangement, is disease prevalence/incidence rate risk. These two rates combine to determine how many patients with a particular disease are present in a given population. An implicit expected number of people receiving treatment for a disease is assumed in any PMPM estimate. Variance from this assumption in the actual experience, assuming that per-patient costs do not change, translate directly to the PMPM estimate. For example, if the number of asthma patients increases from the assumed 5 percent to 6 percent of the population, the expected PMPM will increase by a corresponding 20 percent.

Incidence rates for diseases may or may not be particularly stable. Even when they are stable, prevalence rates, representing the number of patients present in a given population, can be erratic. Groups of covered lives can undergo patient mix changes due to changes in health plans, additions of new groups, and so on.

If the nature of the prevalence/incidence risk is too volatile for a given population for any reason, a reasonable alternative to a full capitation may be contact capitation. A *contact capitation* is a per-patient amount paid on a periodic basis (monthly or yearly) as of the time contact is first made between the patient and the disease management providers for treatment or diagnosis of the disease. Risk is assumed only for the treatment of patients, not for the number of patients.

Aside from contact capitation, a number of other methods can be employed alone or in conjunction with capitation to share the risk among the various parties involved in the delivery and financing of care. The most often used — withholds, risk corridors, pooling by degree of control, stop loss, and incentives — are discussed in the following sections.

Withholds

These are dollars held in abeyance until actual fee-for-service results (or fee-for-service equivalents) are known for the period in question. The percentage can vary by type of provider. It is usually 15 percent to 20 percent, but can be as low as 5 percent and as high as 30 percent. Withholding a portion of funds is a process most often applied to a capitation payment, but has also been used with fee-for-service payments. In either case, an incentive is created for the disease manager, or its providers, to pay attention to overall costs so the withholds will be returned.

For example, if a disease manager negotiated a $.50 capitation PMPM and had a 20 percent withhold, the actual monthly payment would be $.10 less, or $.40. The $.10 would be held until the year ended, and a settlement calculation would be performed. This calculation would compare the actual to expected experience for services not being paid by capitation, say $1.50 PMPM for referrals such as inpatient and specialty physician costs. If the experience were $1.50 or less, the withhold would be returned. If the experience were more than $1.50, a portion of the withhold would be retained to offset the loss. If the loss exceeded $.10, the entire withhold would be retained.

In the preceding example, $.50 (or $.40) is paid on a pure capitation basis and $1.50 of expected cost is paid on a fee-for-service basis. Alternatively, the full $2.00 could be used only as a fee-for-service equivalent target (pseudocapitation) for settlement purposes and all services could be paid for on a fee-for-service basis less the withhold. At the end of the year, the settlement would be done in a similar fashion.

Each method has its advantages. In either case, the downside risk is limited to the withhold. The upside gain is most when the services at full risk are the greatest. However, part of the deal may involve upside limitations. These would be established in a similar fashion through the year-end settlement. Both alternatives (labeled as cases I and II) are recapped in table 4-6.

Risk Corridors

Risk corridors are a way of limiting gains and losses. First a target claim cost per member is established. The risk corridor is usually expressed as a symmetric percentage above and below the target.

If the target is $2.00 with a ±10 percent risk corridor, the disease manager's risk would be full within $.20 of $2.00. So, if the actual expenses are less than $2.20, the disease manager pays them. If the expenses are below $1.80, the disease manager gets to keep an additional $.20 PMPM ($1.80 − $2.00) but may have to refund money to the payer if the $2.00 was paid in advance as a pseudocapitation.

Actually, the $2.00 can be paid on a fee-for-service basis or a capitation basis. In both cases, a settlement must be done at the end of the year to determine if money is owed by either contracting party.

The risk corridor can be used in combination with the withhold. If it is, the withhold often defines the greatest possible loss and the greatest gain

Table 4-6. Sample Settlements: Withhold Mechanism

Case	Capitation	Target Fee-for-Service	Withhold	Downside Risk*	Potential Return*
I	$.50	$1.50	$.10	$.10	$.10
II	—	$2.00	$.10	$.10	$.50

*Additional gains would arise only if the actual cost for the capitated services was less than the capitation payments. In the fee-for-service payment model there would be a return upon settlement.

is set at an equal amount. However, there are many variations on this theme, including establishing a carry-forward mechanism for gains and losses. One common variation is to set a capitation for services of primary responsibility. For an HMO using a standard contracting approach, it would be office visits for primary care physicians. For asthma, it might be the pulmonologists' services. All other services that are paid as fee-for-service are set up into pools (that is, hospital pool, referred physician pool, and pharmacy). Experience is monitored monthly, and settlements on the pools are done annually. The settlement compares actual experience to expected targets for each pool. The gains or losses on each pool are shared between the risk-taking partners based on a formula (for example, 50/50). The provider's or disease manager's share is usually capped at some multiple of the withhold amount. The risk sharing in the following example is 50/50 with a capping device. Using the earlier $2.00 case, the arrangement might look like this:

Capitation $.50
Withhold   20% ($.10)
Hospital risk fund target $.75
Physician and other medical risk fund target $.10
Pharmacy $.65
Risk share   50/50 with gain up to 3× withhold
Losses carried forward/gains paid after withhold threshold of 1× is achieved

If actual claims come in below target, the distribution of funds is made as shown in table 4-7. In this case the withhold ($.10) is returned in full. The $.05 gain is carried forward until the following year's settlement. It is then used to offset losses, and a profit distribution is made the following year if the gain in the total risk pool exceeds $.05. Remember, a protective threshold of $.10 is being established in the carry-forward account. This is a reserve of about 7 percent of the value of the fee-for-service target.

It is easy to see how this all gets very complicated and can easily be made more so.

Pools by Degree of Control

The risk-sharing agreement can recognize all of the participants in the care's delivery. If it does, it may be desirable to establish shares based on the level of control each participant has over the services being rendered.

Using the $2.00 PMPM example with $.50 capitation, participants might choose to split the fee-for-service funds into risk shares as shown in table 4-8. The partners in this model are an HMO, a hospital, a group of disease management physicians, and the disease manager/pharmaceutical company. This arrangement involves first establishing how gains and losses are to be capped (if at all). A settlement is done at the end of the year on each fund

Table 4-7. Sample Financial Settlement: Risk Corridor

Fund	Actual Claims ($)	Target ($)	Difference ($)	Risk (%)	Provider (Gains)/ Loss ($)	Distribution
Hospital	.60	.75	(.15)			
Physician	.15	.10	.05			
Pharmacy	.65	.65	0			
Total	$1.45	$1.50	($.10)	50	(.05)	0

Table 4-8. Sample Risk Shares Varying by Partner

		% Partner Risk Shares			
Component	PMPM	HMO	Hospital	Physicians	DM/ Pharmacy
Hospital inpatient	$.50	30	30	20	20
Hospital outpatient (including E/R)	$.25	30	30	20	20
Total facility	$.75				
Physician service/ other medical	$.10	30		70	
Pharmacy (drugs)	$.65	30		20	50
Total	$1.50				

Note: DM = disease manager; E/R = emergency room services.

(component), not in total as in the risk-corridor example. Shares of gains or losses are divided based on the percentage share scheme shown in the table.

Risk corridors can be used, and withholds can be layered in as well. The shares and the corridor should all be decided on in view of the risk-based capital available.

Stop Loss

Another way of limiting or sharing risk is to purchase a stop-loss policy or provision from either a reinsurance company or the partnering payer. There are essentially two types of stop loss with a couple of modifying features. The most common form of stop loss in the provider market is *individual,* or *specific, stop loss.* This limits the primary risk taker's risk to a predetermined limit (attachment point). Often this is $50,000 or more, but for some specialties and diseases, lower amounts are used.

Going back to the claim amount distribution in table 4-1, this would normally be used to establish the probability of claims by dollar amount. From this distribution, claims over $5,000 occur only .05 percent of the time. If a disease manager wants to be sure that it can never be more than $5,000, a stop-loss policy may be appropriate. The charge for such a policy would be the percentage of the claim dollars represented by the excess over $5,000. From the sample distribution, the average cost of claims over $5,000 is $7,500, which equates to $2,500 per claim over $5,000. This amount is multiplied by the probability of a claim that size to estimate the cost for this protection: $2,500 \times .0005 = \$1.25$ per member per year, or $.10 per month, or roughly 5 percent of the overall expected claims.

Now a reinsurance company will not charge the $.10. It also will have to load in its expenses and profit margins, which could easily double the cost. So a great deal of thought should go into the decision of whether to purchase reinsurance from a reinsurance carrier. The decision is one that should reflect the level of control the disease manager will have on the cost of large cases, the amount of capital that is available to offset that type of risk, and the other risk-sharing features that have been incorporated into the contract. Lastly, the manager should consider how much of the risk is really only *capacity risk* (the risk of working harder for less) before making the decision to pay for reinsurance.

The second type of stop loss is called *aggregate stop loss*. This is usually sold as a percentage of the expected claims amount per member per month. Values such as 120 percent, 150 percent, and 200 percent are often used.

At 120 percent the disease manager's risk would be limited to the cost up to 120 percent of the agreed-on target. If $2.00 is used as the target, the risk exposure is an additional $.40 (20 percent of $2.00). This type of insurance is priced using a probability distribution that reflects the manager's ability to predict the overall cost of claims. Typically, this is called an *actual to expected distribution.*

It should also be noted that aggregate stop loss is often sold in tandem with individual stop loss, and many times reinsurers will use coinsurance and liability caps to further complicate the analysis. A common construct for an individual stop loss contract is to begin to pay at some attachment point (for example, $50,000) but to pay only a percentage of the cost (such as 80 percent) to some limit (for example, $1,000,000), at which point the liability reverts back to the disease manager.

Incentives

In addition to the risk-sharing methods already described, a disease manager may be interested in adding an incentive mechanism to the contract. Such mechanisms are usually designed in such a way as to motivate provider behavior. Usually, the desired behavior has a financial element to it, but lately incentive programs have also included a quality element. The National Committee for Quality Assurance's (NCQA's) Health Plan Employer Data and Information Set (HEDIS) performance measures are commonly used for these elements. For disease management, outcomes are often used in the design of incentive/compensation systems. The best systems are simple and use a limited number of significant measures, for example, inpatient admissions and emergency room usage for asthmatics.

Strategies to Avoid Undue Risk

It is obvious that all of the risk-sharing mechanisms described, except pure capitation, can be used to reduce disease management risk (other than from the payer's perspective). However, there are several other methods of side-stepping risk that are worth mentioning.

Phase-In Risk

If the long-range goal is to accept full risk but the start-up risks are a barrier to entry into the market, the disease manager can phase in to full risk over a period of years. This sort of scheme is shown in table 4-9. In this example the transfer of risk begins with full risk in the corridor around ±5 percent. The next 4 percent (5 percent to 9 percent) are split 75/25 between the transfer-risk bearer (for example, the disease manager) and the payer (an HMO). The next 3 percent corridor is split 50/50 and the next 2 percent is split 25/75. In the first year there is no risk over 14 percent.

A settlement under this method, where the target was $2.00 PMPM and the actual results were $1.50 is shown in table 4-10. In this case if the disease manager was paid $2.00 PMPM in advance via capitation, $.30 PMPM would have to be returned to the payer. The full "savings" are $.50. The disease manager is entitled to $.20 of the $.50, given the risk-sharing mechanism. This is the maximum amount of savings the disease manager will retain with this arrangement in the first year. If the actual PMPM was $2.50 and the disease manager was paid $2.00 PMPM, the payer would have to pay the disease manager an additional $.30 PMPM based on the settlement process. This would represent a $.20 loss to the disease manager. To reduce the amount of money the disease manager must return, a withhold can be held in abeyance until settlement time.

This example depicts a situation in which the disease manager is paid an amount as pseudocapitation (that is, the disease manager is not at full risk but is paid on a monthly per capita basis). This is often the way disease management capitation is discussed, but phasing in risk is awkward in this situation. Far more common in the HMO world is a situation in which a provider (for example, a primary care physician) is paid a capitation for the services it performs directly. Targets are set for services performed by other providers, but for which the capitated provider is also at risk (such as referral services). A withhold is taken on the capitated amount, and the risk percentage is applied to the savings or losses on the other fund as described earlier.

In the disease management world an analogous situation can be drawn. Full capitation with a withhold is paid for the pharmacy costs and/or the physician component of the disease dollars. All other dollars paid to other providers (presumably on a fee-for-service basis) are set up in a risk fund to which appropriate risk percentages are applied. A settlement under this type of arrangement looks like table 4-11. The total amount the disease manager is at risk for here is $.15. The withhold was $.10; therefore, the disease manager owes another $.05 at settlement time. If the disease manager had been at full risk, $.25 would have been lost instead of $.15 as in this scenario.

Exclusion of Outlier Conditions

This may be hard for the disease manager to argue, but the highly complicated conditions within the disease category can be left out of the risk

Table 4-9. Sample Risk Phase-In Mechanism

Corridor %	First Year	Second Year	Third Year
First ±5%	Full risk	Full risk	Full risk
Next ±5%–9%	75% risk	Full risk	Full risk
Next ±9%–12%	50% risk	75% risk	Full risk
Next ±12%–14%	25% risk	50% risk	75% risk
More than ±14%	No risk	25% risk	25% risk

Table 4-10. Sample First-Year Settlement: Phase-In Approach 1

		Corridor Thresholds					
	Target	5%	5%–9%	9%–12%	12%–14%	14%+	Actual Experience PMPM
	$2.00	$1.90	$1.82–$1.90	$1.76–$1.82	$1.72–$1.76	$1.72	$1.50
% risk		100%	75%	50%	25%	0%	
Maximum PMPM corridor		.10	.08	.06	.04	0	
Maximum share		.10	.06	.03	.01		

Table 4-11. Sample First-Year Settlement: Phase-In Approach 2

		Corridor Thresholds					
	Target	5%	5%–9%	9%–12%	12%–14%	14%+	Actual Experience PMPM
	$1.50	$1.575	$1.575–$1.635	$1.635–$1.68	$1.68–$1.71	$1.71	$1.75
% risk		100%	75%	50%	25%	0%	
Maximum PMPM corridor		.075	.06	.045	.03	0	
Maximum share		.075	.045	.0225	.0075		

contract. In this case they are paid for on a fee-for-service basis, but probably at a discount. An example of such an arrangement might be heart transplants in a coronary artery disease contract.

Dynamic Utilization Thresholds

Given that the data for calculating disease management capitation are at best unproven, a model could be created that allows for modifications of a capitation if a greater number of services are demanded of the system than could have reasonably been expected from the data that were analyzed. This assumes that a substantial analysis of opportunity was conducted using the payer's own data. Clearly, the less correlation between the data used to set capitation assumptions and the population at risk, the more reason there is to use a mechanism to adjust the original capitation using actual experience.

Every capitation model for disease management ought to consider the possibility of an influx of previously untreated patients resulting from a greater prevalence of disease than the incidence of treatment would indicate. However, if the true prevalence in a population cannot be known and disease management screening devices uncover new risk for treatment, an adjustment may be warranted.

Recognition of Case Severity

This issue is worth a chapter unto itself. If the data elements are available for use in a severity classification system, one should be considered. There are a number of severity classification systems under investigation today, some of which were recently compared by Iezzoni and colleagues.[12] Also, the Society of Actuaries has just concluded a study contrasting several risk-adjusting mechanisms.[13] Some of these mechanisms are quite sophisticated, whereas others are very simple. One simple way of recognizing case severity is to make outlier payments for cases that exceed predetermined limits. This type of mechanism is used by the federal government in making its DRG payments to hospitals for Medicare beneficiaries.

However it is done, a severity/risk-adjusting process can help recognize unusual costs for high-risk patients.

Membership Thresholds for Capitation

One of the most troubling things about payers that want to capitate everything is the total lack of appreciation of the statistical issues around capitation. A capitation or PMPM claim cost amount is an estimator of the average expected cost PMPM for a population of people. That amount is used to contract with small groups of providers for very narrow sets of services that can vary dramatically in amount used from patient to patient.

A claim distribution such as the one shown in table 4-1 can be used to help set a membership threshold for capitating a given set of services. No *full risk* capitation contract should be entered into unless the population being managed is of sufficient size.[14,15]

The example in table 4-1 shows that the mean PMPY amount for asthma was $23.94. The standard deviation was approximately $225. The formula for sample size (n) is a function of z (the standard normal deviate for the desired level of confidence, such as 95 percent), the standard deviation, and d (the degree of precision required). Given parameters of a mean = $23.94, d = ±5 percent of the mean, and a confidence level of 95 percent (z = 1.96), the required sample size is:

$$n = \left(\frac{z\,(\sigma)}{d} \right)^2 \quad or \quad n = \left(\frac{1.96\,(224.7)}{1.197} \right)^2 = 135,372$$

This means that given the claim size distribution and its implied variance, a population of at least 135,000 members is needed to be 95 percent confident that the PMPM estimate found from analyzing a payer's data is within 5 percent of the true PMPM value.

The values for z and d can be varied, which essentially allows the disease manager to vary confidence in the estimate of the true population PMPM (capitation). The distribution specified in table 4-1 does not have a particularly large variance. In fact, it is easy to imagine other diseases with very diverse claim sizes ranging well up into the tens of thousands of dollars. These types of diseases require even larger population bases. The results of analysis like this should be used to indicate when risk sharing of some sort is appropriate. It should be obvious that it is essential to understand the nature of a given disease state's fluctuations in claim size prior to entering into any type of substantial risk sharing, such as capitation.

Clearly, an effective case management component of the disease management system is very important to minimize the overall risk to the disease manager. This raises the point of disease management's impact on financial results.

• Medical Management's Impact on Disease Management Financial Results

Without any doubt whatsoever the single most important aspect of disease management is the efficient, effective medical management of the patients. Before a disease manager has a track record for managing patients that can be analyzed and fully understood, various steps can be taken to begin to understand how well the system is likely to perform.

This involves a combination of statistical data analyses, patient chart audits, therapeutic compliance surveys of patients and providers, and outcome studies. Each of these is discussed briefly in the following subsections.

To be successful, the disease manager must use skills including epidemiology, medicine, management, finance, statistics, and data analysis. A thorough understanding of the incidence, prevalence, treatment, and outcomes of specific illnesses is required.

Components of Program Development

As detailed in chapter 2, a disease management program designed to achieve cost reductions and outcome improvements requires the following:

- Basic medical knowledge of disease treatment and outcomes
- Identification of markers to track patients with the illness
- Data analysts to develop profiles
- Implementation staff to promote changes that include physician education specialists, case managers, patient education specialists, and financial assistance in developing incentives

The effectiveness of treatment alternatives and how they potentially can affect outcomes become the basis of successful action. The process of care for different levels of severity of the illness must be laid out and methods determined to categorize the population to determine the cost of various treatment plans and outcomes. Some of this information comes from the medical literature, and some is created in the disease management process. The basis of all disease management is the known medical knowledge concerning the illness, and assessing this information effectively is often an intense and expensive process. Once it is established, the maintenance of any system relies on a thorough and regular review and update based on any changes in scientific knowledge. The disease manager should not underestimate the expense of this process in more complex disease management strategies. When a specific protocol has been developed to handle an episode of illness and has passed appropriate review by the medical specialist, medical management's responsibility is to move current medical practice toward the new standard and to track changes in outcomes and costs.

The next challenge is to track the diagnosis, process, and outcomes of an illness using efficient measurement techniques. Ideally it would not require chart review or additional tracking sheets for the patient and physician. Initially, markers are found for this information in available data sets such as claims data. The use of electronic records greatly simplifies the disease manager's role by having all information easily available. The current challenge for the disease manager at this stage is to use the available data in sophisticated ways to easily develop disease management profiles for large numbers of people.

Once the desired patterns of care have been decided on and there is a clear understanding of current patterns and their costs, the next step is to develop methods to move the existing patterns toward the desired one. The tools available to medical management include physician and patient education, financial and other incentives, and case management assistance. Physician education may include supplying physicians with copies of articles from the medical literature, seminars, tapes, and other communications. Working with actuaries and financial specialists, incentives can be constructed to further encourage change. Feedback of performance to the physician also is important. Self-care is a powerful tool to use with patients. In an age in which people desperately want some ability to take control, providing tools through pamphlets, newsletters, videotapes, and CD-ROM can make the patient a crucial link in the promotion a new treatment modality. For example, with asthma, recognition of the need for treatment, appropriate use of drugs, and appropriate use of the emergency room can be essential to improve outcomes and reduce costs.

If feedback to physicians includes outcomes of care showing improvement in patients, that alone is a powerful motivator. However, if there are added incentives that financially reward the physicians, the total effect is extremely powerful in effecting changes in practice patterns.

The end result of medical management should be similar to a total quality management outcome, which is to reduce variation in process by encouraging the use of the best practice.

Statistical Data Analyses

Various uses of data for understanding disease-specific cost and utilization measures were discussed earlier. This section is concerned with the use of those same data to establish the practice patterns for the providers in the disease management network. This usually involves the specification of a benchmark or standards and the comparison of utilization levels of groups of the providers' patients against those standards.

Profiling Systems

Over a dozen systems sold today purport to give one the ability to rank and compare, or in some way analyze, physician practice patterns. Without identifying them or commenting on their capabilities, suffice it to say that they all have pros and cons and different features that can be helpful in identifying aberrant physician practice patterns. The one thing that all of them have in common is the limited ability to truly identify good or bad physician practice. In most cases, these systems are not intended for such use. Rather, they are intended to be used as educational tools first to find physicians who seem to practice differently from a norm, then to organize data for that physician's patients into meaningful categories, which facilitates the physician's education in cost-effective medical management. The systems can be very powerful tools for education, but extreme caution must be exercised when using them to try to identify "good" and "bad" physicians. This is due to a lack of sufficient physician patient samples to allow statistically credible estimates of cost per patient or the number of services performed per patient.

Earlier discussion mentioned the population threshold size needed to capitate a provider group for a specific set of services. Imagine how many data (how many patients' worth of data) might be needed for a single physician before the payer could be sure of accurately describing the physician's practice pattern for a given type of service. This is a problem. Usually, in group or staff model programs, no single payer has a sufficient amount of a physician's practice to be able to do such a thing. This is what makes an all-payer data source attractive. Such files already exist for inpatient discharges and have been used to do some interesting profiling of hospitals.

Inpatient Hospital Practice Patterns

Milliman & Robertson, Inc. (M&R), has published a system for monitoring and evaluating inpatient care.[16] Within these guidelines the reader first observes a construct called Optimal Recovery Guidelines (ORGs), a sample of which is shown in figure 4-1. These ORGs are for uncomplicated cases and as such do not pretend to specify care for the most difficult-to-manage patients. They have been widely accepted and are used to determine, on a statistical basis, how efficient the lengths of stay are for a given hospital. To accomplish this, the ORG lengths of stay are needed in a data set and

Figure 4-1.   A Sample of Milliman & Robertson Health Care Management Guidelines

---

Optimal Recovery Guidelines: M-60 Asthma
(ICD-9: 493.01, 493.11, 493.21, 493.91)

Day 1:   Admitted to the ICU for respiratory failure (CO_2 retention) or to regular floor care for failure to respond to hours of outpatient or emergency room treatment, including parenteral steroids, beta-agonists by inhalation, injection or oral administration, and parenteral oral theophylline. ABGs, chest x-ray, flow rates, CBC, chemistries, theophylline level, parenteral hydration and medication, inhalation treatments, culture as indicated, possible oxygen, possible bronchoscopy or ventilation.

Day 2:   Patient has not required ventilation and is breathing comfortably. ABGs or oximetry satisfactory. Convert to oral medication, including large doses of systemic corticosteroids, and appropriate doses of beta-agonists and theophylline. Discharge, possibly with home care to include respiratory therapy, nursing visit for assessment, or continued parenteral treatments as appropriate, if oximetry and flow rates are stable.

Goal Length of Stay: 1 Day

Source: Doyle, R. *Health Care Management Guidelines.* Vol. I. *Inpatient and Surgical Care.* Seattle, WA: Milliman & Robertson, Sept. 1995 (2nd printing).

detailed discharge data with diagnosis and procedure codes present are required.

Another approach to the same type of analysis has recently been developed.[17] This is called the length of stay (LOS) efficiency index, a process that compares discharge lengths of stay to standards that have been developed using statistical analysis with clinical review. The standards incorporated in this model were developed by analyzing uncomplicated cases as determined by the 3M All Patient Refined (APR)–DRG grouper Version 12 for 12 states' all-payer discharge data sets. This independent method of analysis yields a set of discharges similar to the "optimal" used by the M&R Healthcare Management Guidelines in the ORG and can be used to statistically evaluate performance. A summary of a comparison done on the Florida discharge data set is shown in table 4-12.

This analysis indicates that HMOs in Florida in 1993 and 1994 were slightly better managers of care than non-HMO payers but both were relatively high in comparison to most efficient practices. This is shown for the entire state but can also be done at the provider level.

These studies can be used to identify the opportunity for savings and to identify providers that seem to be practicing at the most efficient levels. The data can also be viewed at a more detailed diagnosis/procedure code level, which is more refined than the DRG level.

Patient Chart Audits

In *Calculated Risk,* Doyle and Axene refer to a process that uses patient chart data to determine the "degree of health care management."[18] This notion is an important one to payers in a given market because it can be the difference between financial success or failure. Basically a sample of patient charts are pulled and the cases are reviewed in light of the ORGs contained in the M&R Healthcare Management Guidelines (HMGs). This process reveals not only the presence, but also the causes, of inefficiencies — from this practice pattern changes can be instituted. This type of analysis can be used as a complement to provider profiling and inpatient discharge analysis to help determine the current level of managed care and where improvements can be made. For disease managers these analyses should be directed to the diseases under their risk arrangement and the providers in the networks they are using.

Therapeutic Compliance Survey for Patients and Providers

These surveys are self-report–type surveys conducted to help establish, where no other data exist, whether the patients and their providers are using the most cost-effective alternatives in an appropriate fashion. Data obtained in this fashion should be compared to the analysis of the episodic claims data described earlier. We will not describe the details of what might be contained in a survey of this type except to say that, from a financial perspective, data are obtained that then can be used to paint a more complete picture of how service is being delivered to patients with specific diseases. This can then be used to reward provider behavior or to target areas in need of education.

Outcomes Studies

Nothing may be more important to the disease manager and the utilization managers of payers than the monitoring of outcomes. This has long been a missing piece of the delivery system data. Disease managers in search of a market need to tout their achievements in delivering the best outcomes. Critics of managed care have speculated for years that MCOs are so watchful of cost they must be delivering less quality.

The topic of how to measure clinical outcomes is covered in chapter 3. The relationship between medical outcomes and the finances of the disease manager and the payers is obvious. In fact, risk sharing and incentives can be fashioned around the achievement of acceptable clinical outcomes. Today these systems rely on simple criteria like readmission rates and lengths of stay. As mentioned, a simple design for a system for asthma would be one that measures the number of emergency room encounters and inpatient

Richard A. Kipp, W. Charles Towner, and Howard A. Levin

Table 4-12. Comparison of Florida HMO, Non-HMO, and Best Practice Inpatient LOS

MDC	Description of MDC	HMO 1993	HMO 1994	Non-HMO 1993	Non-HMO 1994	Case Mix-Adjusted Model LOS HMO 1993	HMO 1994	Non-HMO 1993	Non-HMO 1994	HMO 1993	HMO 1994	Non-HMO 1993	Non-HMO 1994
1	Nervous system	2.44	2.44	2.42	2.44	3.77	3.45	3.75	3.61	1.54	1.41	1.55	1.48
2	Eye	1.08	1.08	1.08	1.08	1.15	1.30	1.60	1.50	1.07	1.20	1.48	1.39
3	Ear, nose, mouth, and throat	1.25	1.22	1.18	1.17	1.78	1.89	1.78	1.71	1.43	1.55	1.52	1.47
4	Respiratory system	2.84	3.06	2.81	2.78	3.89	4.09	3.65	3.67	1.37	1.34	1.30	1.32
5	Circulatory system	2.07	1.99	2.04	2.08	3.28	2.98	3.37	3.11	1.59	1.49	1.65	1.50
6	Digestive system	2.07	2.10	2.04	2.07	2.71	2.58	2.71	2.63	1.31	1.23	1.33	1.27
7	Hepatobiliary system and pancreas	1.54	1.50	1.50	1.46	2.56	2.51	2.73	2.53	1.66	1.67	1.82	1.73
8	Musculoskeletal system and connective tissue	2.63	2.81	2.40	2.50	4.08	4.02	3.83	3.57	1.55	1.43	1.60	1.43
9	Skin, subcutaneous tissue, and breast	1.85	1.92	1.76	1.83	2.51	2.58	2.45	2.42	1.36	1.34	1.39	1.33
10	Endocrine, nutritional, and metabolic	1.82	1.76	1.84	1.86	2.61	2.33	2.58	2.49	1.43	1.32	1.40	1.34
11	Kidney and urinary tract	2.68	3.18	2.88	2.97	3.34	3.78	3.59	3.52	1.25	1.19	1.25	1.18
12	Male reproductive system	1.78	1.97	1.95	2.22	3.45	3.24	3.63	3.51	1.94	1.65	1.86	1.58

13	Female reproductive system	2.07	2.09	2.07	2.07	3.02	2.79	3.04	2.81	1.46	1.33	1.47	1.36
14	Pregnancy, childbirth, and the puerperium	1.45	1.43	1.43	1.41	2.03	1.77	2.10	18.4	1.40	1.24	1.47	1.31
16	Blood, blood-forming organs, and immune system	4.15	4.18	4.19	4.18	4.00	5.30	4.87	4.48	0.96	1.27	1.16	1.07
17	Poorly differentiated neoplasms	2.70	2.63	2.69	2.62	4.10	3.38	3.23	3.05	1.52	1.28	1.20	1.17
18	Infectious and parasitic diseases	2.96	3.01	2.95	3.00	3.50	3.70	3.91	3.34	1.18	1.23	1.32	1.11
21	Injury and poisoning	1.49	1.48	1.47	1.44	2.23	1.82	2.09	2.10	1.49	1.23	1.42	1.46
23	Factors influencing health status	1.05	1.05	1.05	1.05	2.00	1.33	1.88	1.20	1.90	1.27	1.78	1.14
24	Multiple significant trauma	6.18	5.86	5.80	6.03	7.43	6.47	8.72	8.18	1.20	1.10	1.50	1.36
	Total	1.77	1.78	1.80	1.81	2.57	2.37	2.70	2.49	1.45	1.33	1.50	1.38

admissions. Low numbers of these events is a good proxy indicator for good management of asthmatics. Coupled with a patient assessment survey, these outcomes would indicate the care being delivered was high quality and cost-effective.

Financial Impact

Any model constructed to calculate a capitation or case rate on a disease-specific basis allows for reflection of a number of factors. One of the most important is the change that can be expected in utilization due to changes in medical management. The variables affected are both cost and use by component of care. Models should be run to test the sensitivity of the calculations to changes in the assumptions affecting both variables. Once that testing is complete the scenario(s) with the greatest likelihood are selected and used to form the basis of risk taking.

• Other Factors Affecting Expected Health Costs

As mentioned in the last section, there are a number of factors that can have an impact on capitation calculations; some are more obvious than others. The factors include:

- Overhead expenses and profit target
- Demographics (such as age, sex, marital status)
- Geographic location
- Health status
- Insurance status
- Benefit level
- Managed care level
- Providers in the network
- Level of quality delivered
- Scope of services covered (such as types of service, out-of-network)
- Economic conditions (for example, inflation, unemployment)
- Payer payment level expectation (that is, Medicare, HMO, insurance company [or companies])
- Stop-loss level
- General cost and use of service patterns
- Payer marketing and underwriting practices
- Access of technology
- Severity of illness
- Substitution pattern

Most of these factors have already been discussed, or they are obvious from their description, but some of the more subtle factors need a bit more explanation.

- *Overhead expense and profit target:* A forecast of the detailed administrative expenses necessary to run the disease management organization and a competitive analysis are keys to the knowledge one needs to appropriately price a product.
- *Insurance status and benefit level:* These two factors are closely related. The first has to do with whether someone is insured or not and whether they are paying for the coverage themselves. The second deals with the richness of the benefit package. That is whether there are significant barriers to service, such as a large deductible or coinsurance. As a rule, people who have insurance use more services, and people who pay for it themselves — as opposed to getting it through an employer — tend to use it more often. People with no barriers to the system, like a deductible, behave totally differently than people who share care costs with providers and insurers.
- *Providers in the network:* It is important to know who the provider partners are and how they will act in a managed care environment. Physicians who manage their patients well typically refer patients less often and tend to use more conservative approaches to treating disease, such as "watchful waiting" in potential surgical cases. When setting the assumptions in any calculation model, one must have some knowledge of what to expect in terms of cost and utilization patterns for the network providers and how this compares to other providers practicing in the area. This knowledge should include the desired level of quality with regard to outcomes.
- *Payer payment level expectation:* The federal government is a large buyer of health care services. It sets the price it is willing to pay and contractors need to know this. Many large HMOs behave in the same way. Negotiations can be tough because many times the market sets the rates.
- *Payer marketing and underwriting practices:* This is one of the trickiest factors to identify but can be extremely important when risk is being transferred. Payers all have differing levels of sophistication with regard to their marketing techniques and their ability to attract favorable risk populations (people who are not very sick). Having a notion about how well or badly a payer handles risk selection can have a great deal to do with the level at which the capitation rate should be set. The worse the risk manager, the higher the rate may need to be.
- *Substitution pattern:* This simply refers to the approach for using the local health care infrastructure. Where available, is home care used? How often? Are drug therapies used where appropriate? How often is magnetic resonance imaging used instead of standard filming techniques? Answers to these questions give the actuary an idea on how to set the utilization assumptions by component of care.

• Risk-Taker Forecasting and Business Plans

Any organization that is about to undertake a new line of business or start a brand-new business should go through a formal strategic-planning process.

This includes (1) developing a vision or mission, (2) doing an environmental analysis to understand the market and how it is changing, and (3) performing an internal assessment to determine its capabilities and how to improve on them. In the disease management world, partnering to bring together all of the necessary skill sets is a strategy used by many disease managers. Once steps 1 through 3 have been completed, a detailed business plan and supporting financial forecast should be prepared.

Of interest here is the final forecast and development of the risk-based capital requirements. Both of these topics are very complex, and a full discussion is beyond the scope of this chapter. However, this section presents the basic concepts.

Financial Forecasting

Earlier sections covered methods of financing and risk sharing that could be used to develop risk-transferring contracts between providers, disease managers, and payers. These risk-sharing mechanisms presume that the product is known—that is, whether it is a specific disease capitation product or an administrative service contract (ASC) with simple performance risk or some other construct.

With capitation the risk taker is directly at risk for some portion, and perhaps all, of the claims expense. With ASC contracts the risk is usually limited to percentages of the administrative fees paid to perform the disease management function.

A disease manager can potentially sell products with characteristics of each of these methods of transferring risk. Therefore, the forecaster needs to know the types of products and the nature and extent of the risk that is being transferred for each. The main elements of the forecast are revenue and expenses. These are of significantly different magnitude in full-risk transfer versus the performance-risk model. An illustrative forecast model is shown in table 4-13.

This forecast is presented as if an insurance company were evaluating it. Claims are on a full incurred basis (paid claims plus an accrual for outstanding claims). The idea of incurred claims is an important notion. A disease manager must understand that the employer contracts between the employer groups and the payers are on an incurred basis. If a service is rendered to a covered employee or dependent while that contract is in effect, it is the liability of the payer. More than likely the disease management contract will be written in a similar fashion, passing along the incurred risk. The notion of an "outstanding" claim (or one that has not yet been paid) is also an important point. At the end of each reporting month, an insurance company estimates the amount for claims that have been incurred by covered members but that have not yet been paid at the time the report month ends. So, for example, if a patient enters the hospital on December 31 and

Table 4-13. Sample Five-Year Financial Forecast

	Year 1	Year 2	Year 3	Year 4	Year 5
Revenue:					
Capitation	$1,000	$1,200	$1,500	$1,400	$1,300
Case rate	500	700	900	800	700
Administrative service contracts	2,000	2,500	3,000	3,500	4,000
Reinsurance recoveries	150	250	300	250	200
Incentives/withhold	300	400	200	400	100
Investments	150	200	250	200	150
Other	25	30	35	40	45
Total	$4,125	$5,280	$6,185	$6,590	$6,495
Expenses:					
Actual claims and cap components	$800	$1,100	$1,600	$1,700	$1,800
Case rate contracts	400	800	950	1,000	1,000
Operating expenses	1,600	2,000	2,400	3,000	3,500
Reinsurance premium	150	300	350	300	400
Total	$2,950	$4,200	$5,300	$6,000	$6,700
Gain/(Loss)	$1,175	$1,080	$885	$590	($205)
Surplus	$1,175	$2,255	$3,140	$9,140	$8,935
# member months	2,000	2,500	2,900	3,100	3,000
# cases	100	125	145	155	150
# employee months	800	1,000	1,160	1,240	1,200

is discharged January 5, the liability for that expense is assigned to December. The fact is the hospital may submit the claim for payment on January 10 (along with many others). It may take the payer a week or two to process and pay the claim (sometimes a lot longer). Therefore, at the time the December financial statement is prepared, the payer might not have accounted for that claim but must estimate its value as part of the incurred but not reported (IBNR).

In the forecast, most of one's attention is focused on developing the assumptions to complete the year 1 projections. The out-years 2 through 5 are usually developed using factor increases and decreases to values developed for the first year.

Behind each element of the forecast, there is another level of detail. For instance, the capitation in the revenue section might be developed by multiplying the number of estimated member months by the average capitation rate for each disease product sold during the first year. At another level, the capitation rates may be looked at by payer contractors. If differences exist from payer to payer (reflecting the factors discussed in the last three sections), this must be accounted for in developing the total capitated amount.

Each contract sold may vary just because its effective date is later in the year. So an identical product sold in January for $2.00 may be sold for $2.10 in December. The projection of each element of the forecast is developed in a very detailed fashion, making financial forecasting one of the most challenging tasks the disease manager faces.

The operating expense budget is probably the easiest to complete. This usually involves identifying the people needed to perform various tasks and estimating their wages and other benefits along with the expenses associated with purchasing systems support, equipment, buildings, lights, heat, phones, travel, and so on. The complicating factor here for the disease manager is to estimate direct expenses versus contracted expenses for purchasing partnered services. For instance, if the disease manager needs utilization management expertise and would rather partner than develop it, the cost of that contract must be estimated. This usually requires a separate bidding process to obtain quotes for the partnered service components.

The preparation of a good forecast is a tedious, time-consuming, and clearly essential task. Once the model budget is prepared and factored into the overall forecast model, scenarios should be run to reflect a range of potential financial outcomes. This is done by altering the assumptions used to develop the elements (revenue by type and expenses by type) of the forecast.

The results of the forecast scenarios begin to paint a picture about the potential gains and losses over time. This leads directly to a picture of the start-up and ongoing capital requirements for the disease manager.

Risk-Based Capital

The National Association of Insurance Commissioners (NAIC) uses the term *risk-based capital* to describe the amount of money an insurance company should have on hand to back the risk involved in delivering on promises to its policyholders or members to pay their claims. The NAIC has prescribed formulas to calculate the amount of risk-based capital an insurance company needs to have on hand to pay for unforeseen events and to avoid interference by the state insurance department in its affairs. At this point in time risk-based capital requirements for provider-sponsored insurance entities have not been universally adopted by the states. However, some states do have rules regarding capital maintenance and reporting requirements to their insurance departments. All risk-taking disease managers should look into what the states require in each of their markets. Now this all sounds very onerous, but it actually may prevent some catastrophes in risk taking. Organizations that are not financially fit to participate in and manage risk should not do so.

The contingencies that risk-based capital accounts for are primarily claim cost related. There are several contingencies that must be considered when contemplating a company's ongoing capital needs. They are fluctuations in the following:

- Claim cost risk (inflation and use trends)
- Asset value (book versus market value)
- Market conditions
- Operating expenses (budget versus actual expense variances)
- Susceptibility to random catastrophic events
- Rapid changes in technology

Claim Cost Risk

The many facets of disease management claim cost estimation have already been discussed in a fair amount of detail. Having an understanding of the variability of the cost of patients in specific disease categories helps in developing possible risk-taking scenarios. From these data (in combination with the other factors) a calculation of the required capital can be made.

Asset Value

Book versus market asset values can differ substantially depending on the type of investment instruments held by the company. To analyze this issue, the investment portfolios are reviewed to determine the risk level (that is, mix of equities, bonds, real estate, cash, and other assets). Judgments can be made as to the probability of fluctuation of various magnitudes for each type of investment.

Market Conditions

The market for disease management products is very new. However, the market for other capitated specialty products has been around for a while and is very competitive. Because the payer's market for employer group products pressures overall prices for health care, one should assume that market prices for disease management products are very competitive. This holds down margins except for the best managers. The tighter the margins, the more surplus one may need to weather a stormy business cycle.

Operating Expenses

Most organizations prepare budgets with the best intentions. Most also monitor their budget throughout the year fairly closely to help assure that the budget is adhered to. However, unforeseen events take place or new business requirements present themselves that lead to unintended expenditures. The accumulated risk-based capital would also be used to fund these unexpected events.

Susceptibility to Random Catastrophic Events

Disease managers typically have a narrow scope of services under their control. However, if they are responsible for a patient type (for example, asthmatics) under all conditions, they may be more susceptible to a catastrophic event such as a flu epidemic or a sudden increase in environmentally caused asthma. New strains of infectious disease present the latest threat to patients of all kinds. Writing a contract with a payer that recognizes and accounts for random unforeseen events of this sort is the best form of protection. Stop loss that applies to cost on an aggregate basis can be purchased. This protects a fledgling enterprise from this type of risk.

Rapid Changes in Technology

Of all the contingencies mentioned here, this has to be the most familiar of all. Technological changes are occurring at a rapid pace for a broad spectrum of patients, from diagnostic tools to drug therapies and beyond. This risk is real but controllable for the disease manager. New therapies can be experimented with and initiated when their benefits are proven and return on investment is assured. Nonetheless, for disease managers that do not tightly control the use of new technologies, the specter of high-cost substitute procedures looms large. The impact of these contingencies is difficult to anticipate, but it is clearly an important consideration in developing the overall magnitude of risk-based capital.

From the preceding discussion, one can see that a forecasting process is key to developing both a road map of expectation for return on investments and an idea about the amount of capital necessary to run this new business. The sharpest businesspeople use forecasting to assist them in determining whether to embark on these new ventures.

• Specific Issues Related to Asthma Management

Discussion of asthma has been sprinkled throughout this chapter. Asthma is one of the simpler diseases to identify for analysis purposes. It is reasonably easy to establish distinct levels of the scope of service:

- Simple asthma (by diagnosis codes)
- Asthma and directly related pulmonary problems
- Asthmatics (for all services)

Episodes are linked to exacerbations. Severity is indicated by the cost to manage, which is heavily related to the need for inpatient or emergency room care.

This disease is a fairly common one, and it is one that has been widely studied. The methods and treatments an asthmatic should use have been written about frequently.[19] The cost on a PMPM basis in typical under-65 populations probably ranges from just under $1.00 for a narrow-scope product to around $3.00 for a broader-scope product.

What then is the attraction for disease managers? Why do they believe their approach will interest a payer? If the most common cost is close to $1.00, and the disease manager believes it can be cut by 50 percent, $.50 PMPM is saved. Part of this is shared. The payers may realize $.25 of the savings. This is normally not enough to attract a payer's attention. A reduction of this magnitude, while appreciated, could cause significant contracting problems for the payers' primary care physicians as depicted in figure 4-2. The interfering circles of influence show the many possible capitated providers involved in treating asthmatics today and how an asthma management program needs to be integrated with all of these relationships — a task not so easily done.

Figure 4-2. Interfering Circles of Influence

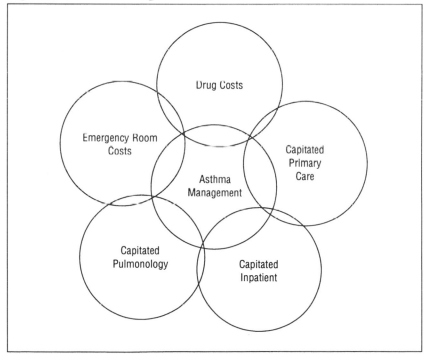

Therefore, one could argue that although asthma is a good demonstration disease for managers to use to sell the effectiveness of their services, it is not the program to sustain them. Niches need to be developed that clearly add value to payers' delivery mechanisms before they will take on risk transfer for specific diseases. There is too much potential for the creation of ill will among the many partners a payer already has.

Other problems also exist for disease managers. The disease manager must realize that once a saving is created, there is enormous pressure to encroach on the disease manager's share of that savings in future contract periods. This is due to the pressure employers are putting on payers to lower their prices (see figure 4-3). This contracting spiral portends trouble for disease managers in the out-years, especially when margins are small.

• The Likely Future of Disease Management

To readers who have made it to this point, the discussion should have provided some insights into disease management risk and its measurement. But more than that, this chapter should promote a more open discussion of the financial issues facing the disease management industry. Risk transfer

Figure 4-3. Payer Contracting Cycle

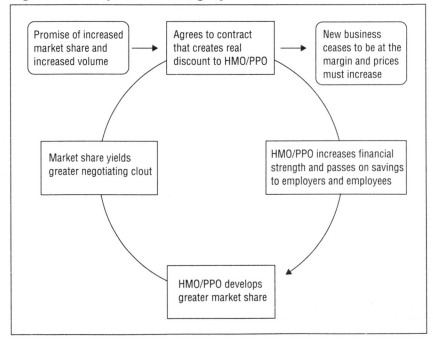

and the incentives it creates can be a powerful force in the health care industry, but using it inappropriately may cause many more problems than it could ever be worth. Careful consideration of sound data is the only path for the risk taker to follow.

Disease management cost modeling must account for the many factors that can affect the cost and use of medical services. Overall savings must account for the medical costs as well as operating costs for disease managers. Alternative financial futures must be reviewed to determine ongoing capital needs and, more importantly, to determine the feasibility of achieving present financial goals.

It is the authors' feeling, from a medical management point of view, that disease management will be the patient management approach that carries the health care industry into the next century, in spite of the lack of clarity on exactly how disease managers (as separate companies) will fit into the paradigm. Chapter 12 addresses the obstacles to the success of disease management and reviews the evolution of disease management into total population-based health management.

Some experts believe that adding value is the key, but all believe that information and its management is crucial to success. There will be no place for smoke and mirrors. Managers that help treat rare chronic conditions will be of interest. Managers that help with the big three—heart disease, cancer, and diabetes—will be sought after also. Disease managers that demonstrate that outcomes and not product sales of pharmaceuticals are paramount will prevail.

Payers that can solve the difficult partnering problems that disease management can pose will be the first to achieve the next major-level reduction in health care cost. And, of course, any payer or disease manager that can instill a sense of individual responsibility in its members for taking care of their own health (that is, health management) will achieve the greatest long-term savings.

References

1. Pagnani, E., editor. *The Grand Alliance: Vertical Integration Strategies for Physician and Health Systems.* Washington, DC: The Advisory Board, 1993.

2. MacKinnon, N. J., Flagstad, M. S., Peterson, C. R., and Mesch-Beatty, K. Disease management program for asthma: baseline management of resource use. *American Journal of Health System Pharmacists* 53(5):535–41, Mar. 1, 1995.

3. Rosenbloom, J. S. *A Case Study in Risk Management.* Englewood Cliffs, NJ: Prentice Hall, 1972.

4. Follmann, J., Jr. *Medical Care and Health Insurance.* Homewood, IL: Irwin, 1963.

5. Rosenbloom.

6. Pyenson, B., editor. *Calculated Risk: A Providers Guide to Assessing and Controlling the Financial Risk of Managed Care.* Chicago: American Hospital Publishing, 1995.

7. Wingert, T. D., Kralewski, J. E., Lindquist, T. J., and Knutson, D. J. Constructing episodes of care from encounter and claims data: some methodological issues. *Inquiry* 32:430–43, Winter 1995–96.

8. Iezzoni, L., Shwartz, M., Ash, A. S., Hughes, J. S., Daley, J., and Mackiernan, Y. D. Severity measurement methods and judging hospital death rates for pneumonia. *Medical Care* 34(1):11–28, Jan. 1996.

9. Thomas, J. W., and Ashcraft, M. L. F. Measuring severity of illness: six severity systems and their ability to explain cost variations. *Inquiry* 28:39–55, Spring 1991.

10. Dunne, D., Rosenblatt, A., Taira, D. A., Latimer, E., Bertko, J., Stoiber, T., Braun, P., and Busch, S. *A Comparative Analysis of Methods of Health Risk Assessment Final Report,* a research study sponsored by the Society of Actuaries, Chicago, Oct. 1995.

11. Wingert and others.

12. Iezzoni and others.

13. Dunne and others.

14. Snedecor, G., and Cochran, W. *Statistical Methods.* Ames: The Iowa State University Press, 1978.

15. Cochran, W. *Sampling Techniques.* 3rd ed. New York City: John Wiley and Sons, 1977.

16. Doyle, R. *Health Care Management Guidelines.* Vol. I. *Inpatient and Surgical Care.* Seattle, WA: Milliman & Robertson, Sept. 1995 (2nd printing).

17. Cookson, J. An analysis of the efficiency of HMO inpatient length of stay in Florida. Unpublished paper written at Milliman and Robertson, Radnor, PA, 1996.

18. Pyenson.

19. MacKinnon and others.

Chapter 5

Disease State Considerations

Charles E. Barr, MD, MPH, Daniel L. Bouwman, MD, MPH, and Frank Lobeck, PharmD

Selecting specific diseases or care episodes for application of disease management techniques involves weighing at least three important factors: impact, interventions, and value.

The *impact* of a disease state can be described in terms of economic costs (for example, payments, productivity); humanistic costs (such as fatalities, functional changes, suffering, quality-adjusted life years); and scope (for example, incidence, prevalence, care encounters). The availability of effective *interventions* is another important consideration. Evaluating interventions involves comparison of treatment options, identification of potential barriers to treatment delivery, and assessment of interventions designed to overcome these barriers. For example, one of the reasons for the selection of asthma by many disease management organizations is the belief that available interventions will prove effective in reducing the total cost of the disease in the (relatively) short term. Finally, the potential *values* of specific disease management programs are estimated in terms of economics, quality of care, patient satisfaction, and provider satisfaction. Evaluating programs in terms of impact, interventions, and values can aid in the selection and prioritization of disease management programs.

This chapter examines these three considerations in the selection of disease states for disease management and provides a case example of one of the more "popular" diseases being selected by many organizations for implementation — diabetes.

We would like to thank the following people who helped us write this chapter: Judith A. Kepler, PharmD, for her editorial assistance and guidance in preparation of the manuscript; William Spalding for his assistance with MarketScan[SM] data analysis; and Sheri Staak for her overall support throughout the project.

• Impact

Disease impacts diverse aspects of life, and these effects can be experienced from a variety of perspectives. Impact may stem from advances in technology, publication of new research, or newly published consensus statements or guidelines. For example, the Diabetes Control and Complication Trial (DCCT) confirmed that attempting to maintain near-normal blood glucose concentrations decreases the development and progression of microvascular diabetic complications (for example, retinopathy, nephropathy, neuropathy).[1] Because of the potential humanistic and economic impact of reducing microvascular complications, programs designed to efficiently implement the DCCT finding are worthy of careful consideration.

Identifying Impact

Various evidence-based guidelines, consensus statements, and opinion guidelines are available and can be used as a basis for disease management programs. Government agencies, such as the National Institutes of Health (NIH) and the Agency for Health Care Policy and Research (AHCPR), publish consensus statements and guidelines that are useful in assessing disease management programs. In addition, professional organizations, including the American College of Obstetricians and Gynecologists (ACOG), the American College of Physicians (ACP), and the American Society of Health-System Pharmacists (ASHP), develop and publish guidelines and technical guides for their respective members. Chapter 6 addresses the development and use of clinical practice guidelines.

Disease management programs that utilize newly released consensus statements or guidelines have the potential to hasten incorporation of new standards into patient care, thereby impacting the cost and quality of that care. There are also established consensus statements or guidelines with low perceived rates of implementation, such as diabetes, asthma, hyperlipidemia, prenatal care, immunization, and use of corticosteroids in preterm labor. These areas represent opportunities in which a disease management program can impact quality of care by driving care processes into compliance with statements and guidelines. *Healthy People 2000* and the Health Plan Employer Data and Information Set (HEDIS) "report cards" are being used to compare care among care providers.[2] These report cards are visible and have impact from the health plan's perspective because they may affect decisions by purchasers of care and should be considered when selecting disease states for program development.

The identification of potential impact of a program may come from other subjective sources. Conditions with high humanistic impact, such as HIV infection, may warrant program development even when there is a low prevalence in a specific population. Some employers require implementation of disease management programs for specific conditions in their plans. Adverse drug reaction monitoring may identify areas where improvements can be made, and news of malpractice suits may stimulate consideration of programs to address areas with high legal risks. Although all these subjective considerations are important, it is essential that objective impact measures be reviewed.

Evaluating Impact

Objective health and disease impacts are generally described and measured in terms of financial payments; number of patients affected (incidence and prevalence); frequency of care episodes; and human costs, such as functional or emotional status. A number of resources can be employed to aid in the estimation of these impacts. Various branches of the government, including the Health Care Financing Administration (HCFA), the Public Health Service (PHS), the Veterans Administration (VA), and the National Center for Health Statistics (NCHS), have data related to health economics. Data from these sources are occasionally summarized in other government documents, such as the *Healthy People 2000* report. Although government data can be extremely valuable in accessing the nationwide impact of disease, the populations summarized may not be entirely reflective of those served by specific organizations that wish to implement disease management programs.

The published literature is another source of information for disease impact. Systematic review of the literature can identify relevant studies on incidence, prevalence, disease costs in subpopulations, indirect costs, and human costs. Although more narrowly focused than government databases, published studies may contain greater depth and specificity of information. The published literature can also be used to evaluate various perspectives, such as those of the patient, payer, provider, employer, and society. The limitations of this type of information include age of data (related to the duration of the research and publication process), narrow scope, and use of populations differing from those to be affected by proposed programs.

Evaluation of "normative" claims databases may be also be useful. Available proprietary databases contain medical claims data, prescription claims data, or both from specific health care plans or groups of plans. Other databases are assembled from sampling subpopulations and then projecting the data to larger populations. In any case, a normative database containing data from patients comparable to the target population in terms of geography, occupation, age, gender, and risk factors should be selected. Severity adjusting should be employed, when appropriate, so the database matches the target population as closely as possible. Examples of impact evaluation developed from a normative database, MarketScan[SM], are presented in figures 5-1, 5-2, and 5-3. The MarketScan[SM] database contains claims payment data from several large, self-insured employers and is representative of employed adults and their dependents. Similar databases are also available for Medicaid, Medicare, and federal employee groups (see table 5-1).

Inpatient conditions associated with the highest *aggregate* payments in the MarketScan℠ database are related to reproduction, cardiovascular conditions, psychiatric conditions, and back and neck disorders, as indicated in figure 5-1. In the outpatient setting, the largest aggregate payments were made for procedures related to pulmonary, gastrointestinal, psychiatric, back or neck disorders, and hypertension. If this database were reflective of a program's population, back and neck conditions would merit careful evaluation because there are high aggregate payments for both inpatient and outpatient care of these disorders.

Conditions associated with the highest *per-episode/admission* inpatient payments in the database are noted in figure 5-2. In this database, the most costly care is probably provided by a relatively low number of highly specialized caregivers. Because of high per-care expenses, the small number of providers involved, and the potential for high return in both economic and humanistic terms, it may be possible to justify expensive interventions for these disease states. For example, plan-sponsored multiday seminars on new

Figure 5-1. Care Episodes with Highest Aggregate Payments

Inpatient	*Outpatient*
• Uncomplicated vaginal delivery	• Respiratory symptoms
• Psychosis	• Abdominal and pelvic symptoms
• Coronary bypass	• Neurosis
• Uterine procedures	• Back and disk disorders
• Percutaneous cardiac procedures	• Hypertension
• Cesarean section	
• Back and neck disorders	

Source: Prepared from the MarketScan℠ database using DataProbe™: The Medstat™ Group, Ann Arbor, MI, 1995.

Figure 5-2. Inpatient Care with High per-Episode Payments

Inpatient Episode

• Burns
• Transplants (liver, heart, kidney, bone marrow)
• Cardiac valve procedures
• Cardiac bypass
• Prematurity or respiratory distress syndrome

Source: Prepared from the MarketScan℠ database using DataProbe™: The Medstat™ Group, Ann Arbor, MI, 1995.

Figure 5-3. Most Frequent Billing Episodes

Inpatient	*Outpatient*
• Vaginal delivery	• Allergic rhinitis
• Psychosis	• Essential hypertension
• Uterine and adnexa procedures	• Back disorders
• Cesarean section	• Respiratory symptoms
• Chest pain	• Dislocation
• Alcohol and drug abuse related	• Abdominal and pelvic symptoms
• Back and neck procedures	• Neurotic disorders
	• Diabetes mellitus
	• Lipid disorders

Source: Prepared from the MarketScan℠ database using DataProbe™: The Medstat™ Group, Ann Arbor, MI, 1995.

Table 5-1. Differences in Medicaid Claims Paid, by Intervention Group

Intervention	Pharmacy Costs ($)	Physician Costs ($)	Lab Costs ($)	Hospital Costs ($)	Total Costs ($)
Reminder	54.71*	(22.38)	9.64	(18.46)	23.51
Unit-of-use	74.09*	(19.51)	(6.73)	(22.91)	22.94
Both	124.86*	(66.79)*	(18.05)*	(107.69)*	(67.67)*

*p < 0.05 as compared to control.

surgical procedures may be warranted for all surgeons billing for valve or bypass procedures. Extensive evaluation, care mapping, and continuous improvement programs may also be justified in high-payment or high-volume conditions.

Another criterion for disease management programs is the number of people impacted. Figure 5-3 summarizes the *most frequent billing episodes* from the MarketScan℠ database in both inpatient and outpatient settings. Programs that have high impact on large numbers of people with frequent health care encounters can be targeted from this type of data. As in the first example of conditions with high aggregate payments, the data suggest that back disorders may be worth further attention as they appear in both inpatient and outpatient lists.

Normative databases are useful in preparing a preliminary assessment of the impact of diseases in a particular type of population without performing costly, plan-specific data acquisition and integration projects. These databases are also useful in settings where limited claims data are available, such as in staff-model HMOs. However, normative databases are limited by potential differences between the database population and the population where the programs will be implemented.

Whenever possible, data analysis should be performed on the database of the specific patient population in which interventions are being considered. This increases the accuracy of impact and value estimations. Although a large part of health care occurs in the outpatient environment, outpatient data are often limited and difficult to obtain because of the fragmentation of health care services. Inpatient data, although much more readily available, are also often fragmented into several types of databases. Rapid advances in information technology and the gradual integration of health care services are beginning to make the collection and evaluation of large amounts of outpatient claims data possible. For example, provider profiling against local or normative peer groups and geographic mapping may help identify specific areas in which opportunities for improvement exist, even if care for the population as a whole appears within guidelines. There are also many other ways of evaluating plan data to determine impact on the population or subpopulations within health care plans.

Databases typically describe impact from a plan provider perspective. Merging databases with clinical, employment, and/or quality-of-life information can allow for analysis of impact from other perspectives. Regardless of which variables and measurement tools are employed, impact is an important factor to weigh when considering potential disease management programs.

• Interventions

Once potential disease states and health conditions with high impact are identified, possible interventions should be cataloged and evaluated. Disease management involves the efficient implementation of effective interventions to improve care. It is important to identify and understand the following factors before choosing interventions and designing a disease management program:

- Current processes of care over the entire course of the disease
- Current practice patterns
- Barriers to management of the disease
- Benefits of treatment and other interventions
- Previous successful and unsuccessful implementations of interventions

Care Process and Practice Patterns

For most diseases, the process of care includes prevention, screening, diagnosis, treatment, treatment of complications, rehabilitation, and secondary prevention. In developing disease management programs, the best practices or protocols for the selected disease must be identified (see chapter 6). A panel of local or national thought leaders should be consulted to modify practices to meet the needs of the specific patient population. Consideration also should be given to the practices of various caregivers, including primary care physicians, physician specialists, pharmacists, nurses, dietitians, behavioral specialists, and allied health professionals. In addition, it is important to realize that disease management takes place in various settings, including clinics, hospitals, nursing homes, rehabilitation facilities, homes, school, and the workplace.

Barriers

Once the care process is understood, an inventory of potential barriers to delivery of the desired care is conducted. There are three basic classes of barriers: system barriers, provider barriers, and patient barriers.

System barriers are often related to access, reimbursement, and processes. Examples of system barriers include:

- Benefit plans that do not cover reagent strips for self-monitoring of blood glucose (a barrier to tight control of blood glucose in diabetic patients)
- Misdirected formulary programs that result in shifts to more expensive therapies, delays in treatment, increases in hospitalization rates, or use of inappropriate agents (barrier to quality and cost-effectiveness of care)
- Lack of reimbursement for health care education, therapy monitoring, diet planning, or exercise design by allied health professionals (barrier to self-implementation of treatment)
- Lack of appropriate community-based resources to provide possible outpatient procedures (barrier to lower-cost, alternative sites of care)
- Lack of quiet, private counseling areas in pharmacies (barrier to effective patient education)

These examples show a variety of points in the care process where system barriers may arise, but there are certainly many more possibilities.

Provider barriers are obstacles that impede the implementation of best practices. The overwhelming amount of new medical information generated on a daily basis is a provider-based barrier to acquisition and integration of new knowledge and changes in practice behavior. There are several effective vehicles for providing provider education to overcome the information overload. Decision-support tools may supplement provider education in applying new findings to specific patients. When considering provider barriers to implementation of effective treatment changes, physicians are often targeted because they direct many of the health care resources. However, opportunities for enhancement of care exist throughout the health care system; the needs and barriers presented by nurses, pharmacists, dietitians, and other allied health care providers all merit attention.

Time is another common provider barrier. Physicians' time to manage patients may be limited by the large number of patients they are required to see. The shift from hospital care to office care has resulted in not only larger numbers of patients in physicians' offices, but in patients who are more acutely ill. Floor nurses in hospitals may not have time to provide optimal professional services because of clerical and administrative duties. A lack of trained technical support staff may force pharmacists to perform routine dispensing tasks rather than counsel patients about the proper use of medications.

Patients also face health care information overload. A large variety of information is available from printed media, talk shows, on-line resources, and well-intentioned friends and loved ones. The information is often miscommunicated or conflicting and can lead to information paralysis. Benefits designs may also cause patient barriers in terms of financial disincentives or "hassle" factors. All of these factors can lead to noncompliance with recommended care. *Patient barriers* often are discussed in terms of compliance with or adherence to treatment plans. There is vast medical literature related to this topic, and an in-depth discussion of compliance is beyond the scope of this chapter. However, in designing disease management programs, it is important to have a firm grasp of general concepts related to noncompliance and specific details related to compliance in the disease state being evaluated.

Although identification of barriers based on a review of the medical literature is essential, analysis of plan- or site-specific data can help identify very specific barriers to treatment implementation. Administration of corticosteroids to women during preterm labor can be used to illustrate this point. A recent NIH consensus statement recommends administration of a short course of inexpensive corticosteroids during labor when the estimated gestational age is between 24 and 34 weeks and delivery is expected within seven days.[3] Although decreased infant morbidity and mortality resulting from such treatment was first documented in 1972, only 13 percent of eligible women receive this treatment. A plan-specific comparison of time of hospital admission for women in preterm labor not receiving corticosteroids and time of delivery may help identify the actual barrier. A short interval between admission and delivery suggests that patients do not recognize when they are in labor and do not present soon enough, or that there are barriers to being admitted. A long interval between admission and delivery for women in preterm labor not receiving corticosteroids suggests a physician-based barrier and inadequate processes for assuring proper treatment. Armed with an analysis specific to the plan, interventions that focus on the actual barriers can be developed and implemented with greater confidence.

Intervention Selection

Once the care process and treatment barriers for a particular disease or health state are understood, interventions to improve care and outcomes can be evaluated in proper context. Many types of intervention tools can be used in disease management programs. Education of both patients and health care providers is usually an important part of disease management. Consideration should be given to the cultural and educational mix of patients and the types of providers involved in the program. Other interventions include data collection and analysis systems, facilitation of process or system change, and development and implementation of decision-support tools for policy, administrative, and clinical decision makers. An in-depth discussion of the availability and assessment of interventions is beyond the scope of this chapter. However, assessment of potential interventions provides information essential to the determination of value for specific interventions and programs employing them.

After a number of interventions have been identified, the success of these interventions needs to be evaluated. An important method of assessing potential success is to review previous performance through review of published and unpublished program assessments. Programs that have overcome system, provider, or patient barriers in specific, high-impact potential disease states warrant careful scrutiny. Plan-specific data analysis can be used to identify cohorts of patients similar to those involved in previously successful intervention programs. By selecting like cohorts, intervention studies hopefully can be recreated with similar outcomes.

It is, perhaps, even more important to identify programs that did not achieve measurable outcomes. For example, a recent study evaluated the effect of patient medication education videotapes on compliance to a lipid-lowering drug, a calcium channel blocker, a beta-blocker, and transdermal estrogen.[4] More than 80 percent of patients reported both viewing the tapes and finding them "useful" or "somewhat useful." However, there was no difference in apparent compliance between patients who received a videotape and a matched control group. Results of this study should be considered when evaluating potential use of patient drug education videotapes in improving medication compliance. On the other hand, if the education itself is the desired outcome, such videotapes might be a cost-effective way of providing basic information. This report represents something of a rarity; there are fewer reports of unsuccessful interventions than successful ones, and negative studies tend not to be published. As such, the lack of a literature evaluation of an intervention does not mean it has not been tried and found wanting.

Interventions can be focused to maximize success. In this process, specific cohorts of patients or providers that closely resemble those in successful intervention research programs are identified. Several interventions can be applied to different cohorts of the same population, thereby decreasing the cost of the interventions (applied to fewer people) and increasing success (applied to those with known response rates).

• Value

Several types of values can be attached to intervention programs. Health outcomes, as discussed in detail in chapter 3, are the ultimate values driving disease management programs. Outcome measurements may include mortality and morbidity (hospital admissions, return-care episodes); health status (such as that measured using the SF-36 Health Survey and similar health status or quality-of-life tools); or achievement of predetermined clinical goals.[5] For example, outcome value for a lipid disorder disease management program may be measured as change in individual or population mean cholesterol concentration, or change in quality-of-life measurements, cardiovascular morbidity, and overall mortality.

Less specific, but often easier to document, are values based on completion of processes. Process indicators have value as surrogates for clinical outcome values. Evaluation of the number of diabetic patients receiving eye examinations to screen for diabetes would be a process indicator. In this case, the process indicator has value in that it is part of the HEDIS report card. Soft values, such as public relations and patient satisfaction, also merit consideration. Although it is difficult to measure specific clinical or humanistic outcomes for some interventions, there may be measurable value in terms of increased patient knowledge and sense of empowerment.

Economic value is also an important consideration in choosing disease management programs. Economic values should be determined from a variety of perspectives, including those of patients, providers, employers and/or payers, and society. Both short- and long-term economics should be considered, although data are generally lacking in regard to the long-term economic benefits of most health care practices.

Use of economic modeling techniques, as discussed in chapter 4, may enhance the estimation of value. Normative databases can be used in developing models and providing estimates of value in various populations. If the disease management planning team has access to databases from the actual populations for which the programs are to be implemented, more sophisticated value modeling can be conducted. Plan-specific data can be used as a baseline to enhance estimates and for modeling in various cohorts of the target population. This allows for delivery of more focused intervention programs.

The potential values of specific programs can be determined by weighing the cost of implementation with the return. If interventions with known success records are employed, the value of the program can be quantified.

With knowledge of the number of patients to whom an intervention will be delivered, the cost of the intervention, and the known or estimated return from the intervention, rough estimates of program value can be made. By determining program value from a variety of perspectives for a number of programs, opportunities for enhancement of care in a population can be prioritized.

• Case Example of a Diabetes Disease Management Program

In the following case example, diabetes is used to demonstrate the three major considerations already discussed, that is, impact, interventions, and value. The example is meant to follow the analysis that a disease management development team might conduct in determining whether a disease is a reasonable candidate for development of a disease management program. It is also meant to demonstrate the difficulty of quantifying disease appropriateness for program development when both the clinical *and* economic outcomes must be considered.

Impact Considerations

As suggested earlier, the first step in assessing which diseases should be candidates for disease management development is to quantify the impact of the disease. In this case, published literature was used for the analysis.

Diabetes is a multifaceted disease with potential consequences to the patient; the patient's family, employer, and health care providers; and society. Patients are faced with many potential complications. Diabetic nephropathy develops in 35 percent of patients with insulin-dependent diabetes mellitus (IDDM).[6,7] Retinopathy develops in 75 percent to 97 percent of patients within 15 years of onset of IDDM.[8,9] In patients with non–insulin-dependent diabetes mellitus (NIDDM), 80 percent of those who are insulin-treated and 55 percent of those who are non–insulin-treated develop retinopathy within 15 years of onset of diabetes.[10] Cardiovascular disease was noted among 58 percent of diabetics and 26 percent of nondiabetics.[11] The incidence of peripheral vascular disease in one community was 25.1 and 2.6 per 1,000 person-years in diabetic versus nondiabetic subjects, respectively. Patients with diabetes have a 4.4 to 5.1 times higher incidence of stroke than nondiabetic patients.[12] Approximately 30 percent to 70 percent of patients with diabetes mellitus experience neuropathy.[13] The incidence of foot ulcers in people with diabetes is 2 percent to 3 percent per year, and osteomyelitis and cellulitis of the feet are 12 to 14 times more prevalent in patients with diabetes.[14] People with diabetes have a 16 times higher incidence of lower-limb amputation, and 50 percent of all lower-limb amputations in the United States are performed on diabetics.[15] Approximately 15 percent of diabetics have amputations.[16] Diabetic gastroparesis (nausea, diarrhea, vomiting, and abdominal distention) is an episodic condition occurring in 20 percent to 30 percent of patients with diabetes mellitus.[17]

In addition, diabetes accounted for 144,000 premature deaths, a loss of 1,445,000 years of productive life, and total disability for 951,000 people in 1986.[18] In the 54–65-years age group, 49 percent and 68 percent of diabetic and nondiabetic persons, respectively, were in the work force approximately 10 years later.[19] Swedish citizens under 65 with diabetes had twice the rate of early retirement and twice as many hospital days as nondiabetics. People using insulin used twice the number of sick days as other people. In the United States, overall, diabetics had $7,000 per year lower productivity than nondiabetic people.[20]

Health care expenditures for confirmed diabetics in the United States in 1992 were $11,157 per patient, compared to $2,604 per nondiabetic patient.[21] Expenditures for drugs and medical devices were $1,056 per patient with confirmed diabetes and $232 for nondiabetic patients.

Most diabetic patients do not face the economic burden of the disease alone; 86.5 percent of people under 65 and 98.8 percent of patients over 65 have at least some health insurance.[22,23] Government programs include 96 percent of older patients and 26.4 percent of younger patients. Private health insurance is held by 69.3 percent of people with diabetes.[24,25]

It was estimated in 1995 that 3.1 percent of Americans had diagnosed diabetes. There were roughly 7.8 million diagnosed cases of diabetes in the United States, and an additional estimated 7 million undiagnosed cases.[26] Over 90 percent of the cases were classified as NIDDM. Insulin was used by roughly 43 percent of diabetics and oral agents by roughly 49 percent; 2 percent to 10 percent used both an oral agent and insulin.[27] The total annual economic burden of diabetes in 1992 was estimated to be $85.7 billion to $91.8 billion, approximately $45.2 billion in direct costs and $46.4 billion in indirect costs.[28]

Based on this literature analysis, diabetes clearly deserves a closer look as the subject of a potential disease management program. The next step would normally be to define the impact on a specific population through evaluation of normative databases from representative populations and actual plan-specific data analysis. However, for illustrative purposes, it will be assumed that the plan and plan population so closely emulates the literature in epidemiology and costs that the data can be extrapolated directly to a 100,000-member plan; 3.1 percent (3,100) of members have diagnosed diabetes.

Further extrapolation of disease impact from a broad-based impact analysis to a specific population can be achieved by identifying a best clinical practice or guideline and defining current practices in a population. This "gap analysis" is used to help identify potential interventions and, later, to assess program value. Diabetes therapy involves diet, exercise, and often insulin or oral medication. Practices consistent with American Diabetes Association (ADA) guidelines should improve control of blood glucose, reduce or delay development of diabetes complications, and reduce consumption of medical resources.[29] The goal for glycemic control in diabetic patients is a fasting blood glucose concentration of less than 120 mg/dL, bedtime glucose of 100 to 140 mg/dL, and HbA;ilc of less than 7 percent. Guidelines also call for patient education, regular eye and foot exams, and proper foot care.

Interventions and Value Considerations

For this hypothetical case example it is assumed that, similar to previous descriptions, 51 percent of eligible patients had not had eye exams (31 percent to 35 percent stated they were never told to get an exam), and 55.7 percent had not had foot exams in the previous two years.[30-32] It also is assumed that intensive insulin therapy is being prescribed to half the patients requiring insulin and that 50 percent of non–insulin-using patients with NIDDM have less than full compliance to oral drug therapy. Within the framework of these baselines, potential interventions (opportunities) can be identified and evaluated.

Determination of interventions and the eventual assessment of their value is best facilitated by review of the landmark 1993 Diabetes Control and Complications Trial. This study by the NIH followed the care of 1,441 people with IDDM. The results indicated that traditional methods of treating diabetics may not be effective and that more aggressive blood sugar monitoring is indicated. Based on a review of the literature and with the DCCT study as guidance, five interventions were selected for evaluation in this case example. In most cases, there are many more possible ways to package and deliver interventions to address system barriers (system and process change), patient barriers (education and behavior change), and provider barriers (education and behavior change).

Intervention 1: Intensive Glucose Control

The DCCT trial employed four- to five-times-daily blood glucose monitoring and three- to four-times-daily glucose concentration-guided injections of insulin.[33] With this regimen, 44 percent of patients achieved at least one HbA;ilc of 6.05 percent or less, and the mean glucose concentration was 155 ± 30 mg/dL compared to 231 ± 55 mg/dL in patients assigned to conventional treatment. In the DCCT study, intensive therapy reduced occurrence of retinopathy, in patients with no baseline retinopathy, by 76 percent.

In patients with preexisting retinopathy, intensive therapy slowed progression by 54 percent and occurrence of proliferative retinopathy by 47 percent.[34] Intensive therapy also reduced the risk for development of nephropathy: There were 39 percent fewer cases of microalbuminuria and

54 percent fewer cases of albuminuria in intensive-treatment patients. The occurrence of clinical neuropathy was reduced by 60 percent. However, there was also a two to three times greater risk for hypoglycemia in the intensive-treatment group.

The cost of intensive therapy of diabetes, as delivered in the DCCT trial, is significant. Diabetes-related medications, supplies, and office visits were $1,700 per year for patients treated with conventional insulin therapy (control group). For patients treated with intensive therapy, the yearly diabetes-related drug, supply, and office costs were $4,000 for patients using multiple daily insulin injections and $5,800 for patients using insulin pumps.[35] Because no economic analysis has been reported on non-diabetes-related health care costs, the value of intensive therapy is expressed as significant reduction in complications over several years for an incremental cost of $2,300 to $4,100 per year.

Although no prospective studies have shown that aggressive control of blood glucose prevents the development of complications in patients with NIDDM, there is strong circumstantial evidence that control is related to complications. This evidence is based on studies relating past control to current health status (outcome). Note that ADA guidelines call for tight control of NIDDM.

Case example population—cost of intervention 1

Assumptions:

- Membership includes 3,100 diabetics, 51 percent on insulin.
- Fifty percent of those on insulin (790) do not employ multiple blood sugar assessments and multiple injections, and 50 percent of those (395) accept an offer for intensive treatment.
- Sixty-nine percent of program patients (273) elect multiple injections and 31 percent (122) elect insulin pumps.
- Costs reported by the DCCT are used.

   Incremental, first-year cost (treatment initiation plus incremental difference in cost) of intensive therapy (over conventional therapy) for multiple daily injections is:

Multiple injections, 273 ($2,824 + $2,300) = $1.40 million
Insulin pump therapy, 122 ($4,100 + $2,903) = $0.85 million
Total first-year incremental costs = $2.25 million

Intervention 2: Ophthalmic Screening

Based on economic modeling, the current rate of compliance with annual ophthalmic screening in U.S. diabetic patients yields a cost savings of $247.9

million per year and 53,986 per person-years of sight.[36] If 100 percent compliance with guidelines were achieved, cost savings would be $472 million and 94,304 person years of sight.[37] However, patients given a single leaflet on the importance of eye care for patients with diabetes did not have eye exams any more frequently than a matched group of patients that did not receive the materials.[38]

Case example population — cost of intervention 2

Studies on economic savings are from a federal government perspective. A single mailing of educational materials is unlikely to achieve any benefit; therefore, cost would likely outweigh benefit. The disease management design team either needs to research the literature concerning eye screenings or pilot a program(s) in this area.

Intervention 3: Clinical Practice Guideline Education/Usage

In an interim assessment of nine urban public health diabetes programs, several process improvements were achieved when practice guidelines were implemented with provider education.[39] Rates for eye exams went from 8 percent to 26 percent, and rates for foot exams from 18 percent to 44 percent. Blindness decreased from 9.5 to 2.7 per 1,000 patients during a four-year period, and 77 percent with hypertension had blood pressures lower than 160/99. However, there was no change in weight or glucose control compared to the baseline.

Case example population — cost of intervention 3

Implementation of clinical practice guidelines throughout a medical plan is difficult and depends heavily on the plan structure (see chapter 6). Successful guideline development usually employs local development of the protocol to gain provider acceptance of results. The major costs will be hundreds of hours of staff time for the protocol development process, introduction of the program with oral or written education, and monitoring of progress. Consultants or partnerships with vendors might be available to "jump-start" the program in this area. Careful analysis of the direct and indirect costs of these arrangements are warranted.

The study described was conducted with employed physicians. If the example population is served by employed physicians or a relatively small population of physicians in a limited geographic area, this approach is worth further evaluation. It is more difficult to extrapolate the study to other plan types.

Once again, the quantification of the impact of this type of intervention is very difficult to measure. The disease management development team may want to arrange for a pilot of the proposed intervention.

Intervention 4: Patient Compliance

A survey found high satisfaction among patients who subscribed to a free monthly newsletter.[40] The highest level of satisfaction was noted among patients who were older, had lower incomes, had more diabetic complications, and had lower baseline knowledge about diabetes.

> *Case example population—cost of intervention 4*
>
> The study evaluating the newsletter was able to document patient satisfaction with the newsletter, but did not document change in any behavioral, clinical, or economic outcomes. As such, the newsletter cost should be weighed against the value of patient satisfaction.

Intervention 5: Medication Possession Ratio

Medication possession ratio (number of tablets received divided by number of tablets needed for full compliance) was greater in patients receiving a mailed refill reminder 10 days before a refill was due (.73), unit-of-use packaging (0.71), or a combination (.87), as compared to a control group.[41] As detailed in table 5-1, patients receiving mailed reminders and unit-of-use packaging together had less per-capita health care utilization.[42]

> *Case example population—cost of intervention 5*
>
> For the unit-of-use dispensing and reminder program, the potential savings is $102,790 ($67.67 per each of the 1,519 [49 percent] of patients on an oral agent, but not on insulin). However, it is not clear from the study report whether costs for the packaging and reminder system were factored into the cost determination. If packaging and reminders could be contracted for $5.63 per month or less, the economic benefits might outweigh the risks. It also might be possible to reduce the costs without reducing the benefits by focusing the interventions only on those with refill patterns that suggest noncompliance.

• Conclusion

There are tremendous opportunities for enhancing the quality and cost of health care through implementation of disease or health management programs. One of the challenges is deciding where to start. Many sources of information can be employed to aid in making these decisions, including previous institutional or expert experience, published literature, and normative databases. The most important source of information is the population to be served. Well-designed analysis of available demographic, claims, clinical, employment, functional, and quality-of-life information is invaluable. With these sources of information, selection of disease or health states for disease (or care) management programs and selection of specific programs within disease or health categories can be directed by assessment of potential impact, evaluation of available interventions, and estimation of program value.

References

1. The Diabetes Control and Complications Trial Research Group. The effect of intensive treatment of diabetes on the development and progression of long-term complications in insulin-dependent diabetes mellitus. *The New England Journal of Medicine* 329(14):977–86, Sept. 30, 1993.

2. U.S. Department of Health and Human Services, Public Health Service. *Healthy People 2000: National Health Promotion and Disease Prevention Objectives.* DHHS Publication No. (PHS) 91-50213, 1991.

3. NIH Consensus Development Panel on the Effect of Corticosteroids for Fetal Maturation on Perinatal Outcomes. Effect of corticosteroids for fetal maturation on perinatal outcomes. *JAMA* 273(5):413–18, Feb. 1, 1995.

4. Powell K. M., and Edgren, B. Failure of educational videotapes to improve medications compliance in a health maintenance organization. *American Journal of Health-Systems Pharmacists* 52:2196–99, Oct. 15, 1995.

5. Ware, J. E. *SF-36 Health Survey: Manual and Interpretation Guide.* Boston: The Health Institute, 1993.

6. Francisco, G. F., and Brooks, P. J. Diabetes Mellitus. In: J. T. DiPiro, R. L. Talbert, P. E. Hayes, G. C. Yee, G. R. Matzke, and L. M. Posey, editors. *Pharmacotherapy: A Pathophysiologic Approach.* 2nd ed. New York City: Elsevier, 1992, pp. 1121–45.

7. Gilbert, R. E., Tsalamandris, C., Bach, L. A., Panagiotopoulos, S., O'Brien, R. C., Allen, T. J., Goodall, I., and others. Long term glycemic control and the rate of progression of early diabetic kidney disease. *Kidney International* 44(4): 855–59, Oct. 1993.

8. Francisco and Brooks.

9. Harris, M. I. Summary. In: M. I. Harris, C. C. Cowie, M. P. Stern, E. Beyko, G. E. Reiber, and P. H. Bennett, editors. *Diabetes in America.* 2nd ed. National Diabetes Data Group, 1995. NIH publication no. 95-1468:1–13.

10. Harris.

11. Glauber, H., and Brown, J. Impact of cardiovascular disease on health care utilization in a defined diabetic population. *Journal of Clinical Epidemiology* 47(10):1133–42, 1994.

12. Stegmayr, B., and Asplund, K. Diabetes as a risk factor for stroke. A population perspective. *Diabetologia* 38:1061–68, 1995.

13. Francisco and Brooks.

14. Harris.

15. Lesse, B. Diabetes mellitus and the St. Vincent declaration: the economic impli-
    cations. *Pharmacoeconomics* 7(4): 292–307, 1995.

16. Shenaq, S. M., Klebuc, M. J. A., and Vargo, D. How to help diabetic patients
    avoid amputations: prevention and management of foot ulcers. *Postgraduate
    Medicine* 96(5):177–92, Oct. 1994.

17. Francisco and Brooks.

18. Huse, D. M., Oster, G., Killen, A. R., Lacey, M. J., and Colditz, G. A. The eco-
    nomic costs of non-insulin-dependent diabetes mellitus. *JAMA* 262(19):2708–13,
    Nov. 17, 1989.

19. Harris.

20. Olsson, J., Persson, U., Tollin, C., Nilsson, S., and Melander, A. Comparison
    of excess costs of care and production losses because of morbidity in diabetic
    patients. *Diabetes Care* 17(11):1257–63, Nov. 1994.

21. Rubin, R. J., Altmann, W. M., and Mendelson, D. N. Health care expenditures
    for people with diabetes mellitus, 1992. *Journal of Clinical Endocrinology and
    Metabolism* 78(4):809A–809F, Apr. 1994.

22. Harris.

23. Harris, M. I., Cowie, C. C., and Eastman, R. Health-insurance coverage for
    adults with diabetes in the U.S. population. *Diabetes Care* 17(6):585–91, June 1994.

24. Harris.

25. Harris, Cowie, and Eastman.

26. Harris.

27. Harris.

28. Harris.

29. Raskin, P., editor. *Medical Management of Non-Insulin-Dependent Diabetes.*
    3rd ed. Alexandria, VA: American Diabetes Association, 1994.

30. Agardh, E., Agardh, C. D., and Hansson-Lundblad, C. The five-year incidence
    of blindness after introducing a screening programme for early detection of treat-
    able diabetic retinopathy. *Diabetic Medicine* 10(6):555–59, June 1993.

31. Moss, S. E., Klein, R., and Klein, B. E. Factors associated with having eye exami-
    nations in persons with diabetes. *Archives of Family Medicine* 4(6):529–34, 1995.

32. Wylie-Rosett, J., Walker, E. A., Shamoon, H., Engel, S., Basch, C., and Zybert,
    P. Assessment of documented foot examinations for patients with diabetes in
    inner-city primary care clinics. *Archives of Family Medicine* 4(1):46–50, 1995.

33. The Diabetes Control and Complications Trial Research Group.

34. The Diabetes Control and Complications Trial Research Group.

35. The Diabetes Control and Complications Trial Research Group. Resource utili-
    zation and costs of care in the diabetes control and complications trial. *Dia-
    betes Care* 18:1468–78, Nov. 1995.

36. Javitt, J. C., Aiello, L. P., Chiang, Y., Ferris, F. L. III, Canner, J. K., and Green-field, S. Preventive eye care in people with diabetes is cost-saving to the federal government. Implications for health-care reform. *Diabetes Care* 17(8):909–17, Aug. 1994.

37. Javitt and others.

38. Newcomb, P. A., Klein, R., and Massoth, K. M. Education to increase ophthal-mologic care in older onset diabetes patients; indications from the Wisconsin Epidemiologic Study of Diabetic Retinopathy. *Journal of Diabetes Complications* 6(4):211–17, 1992.

39. Baker, S. B., Vallbona, C., Pavlik, V., Fasser, C. E., Armbruster, M., McCray, R., and Baker, R. L. A diabetes control program in a public health care setting. *Public Health Reports* 108(5):595–605, 1993.

40. Anderson, R. M., Fitzgerald, J. T., Funnell, M. M., Barr, P. A., Stepien, C. J., Hiss, R. G., and Armbruster, B. A. Evaluation of an activated patient diabetes education newsletter. *The Diabetes Educator* 20(1):29–34, 1994.

41. Skaer, T. L., Sclar, D. A., Markowski, D. J., and Won, J. K. Effect of value-added utilities on prescription refill compliance and Medicaid health care expenditures—a study of patients with non-insulin-dependent diabetes melli-tus. *Journal of Clinical Pharmacy and Therapeutics* 18(4):295–99, 1993.

42. Skaer and others.

Chapter 6

Clinical Practice Guidelines: Foundation for Effective Disease Management

John T. Kelly, MD, PhD, and David B. Bernard, MD, FACP

Health care professionals, purchasers, consumers, and others have raised significant concerns about the quality, utilization, and costs of health care services during the current period of enormous change in the American health care system.[1-4] Researchers have identified substantial variations in clinical practice; overuse, underuse, and inappropriate use of health care services; and significant differences in the costs of health care.[5] Numerous important efforts to improve health care have been initiated. One of the most visible efforts to address concerns about the quality, utilization, and costs of health care services has been the development, dissemination, and implementation of clinical practice guidelines as tools to improve clinical decision making.[6-8] These practice guidelines provide a useful foundation for effective disease management activities.

Supporters of practice guidelines include numerous national organizations, such as the American Medical Association (AMA), the American Hospital Association (AHA), the Joint Commission on Accreditation of Healthcare Organizations (JCAHO), the National Committee for Quality Assurance (NCQA), the Agency for Health Care Policy and Research (AHCPR), the Institute of Medicine, the Health Care Financing Administration (HCFA), the Physician Payment Review Commission, and the U.S. General Accounting Office.[9-14] For example, the AMA, which refers to practice guidelines as *practice parameters,* has stated: "Practice parameters enable physicians to: (1) obtain the advice of recognized clinical experts, (2) stay abreast of the latest clinical research, and (3) assess the clinical significance of often conflicting research findings."[15] Numerous health care professionals and health care delivery systems, including many managed care organizations, employ and encourage the use of practice guidelines.

This chapter discusses the benefits and challenges associated with the use of practice guidelines and the role of practice guidelines in disease management activities. It also provides two case examples of the use of practice guidelines in disease management and emphasizes that scientifically sound, clinically relevant practice guidelines provide a useful foundation for effective disease management activities.

• Diversity of Clinical Practice Guidelines

Numerous practice guidelines are available; almost 2,000 have been developed by over 70 national organizations.[16] Many other practice guidelines have been developed at the regional and local levels, whether by adaptation from national guidelines or independently.[17-19]

Practice guidelines address a wide array of clinical issues. Some provide comprehensive recommendations for the diagnosis and management of a specific clinical condition, such as angina, asthma, or diabetes. Others provide recommendations for a less comprehensive set of issues, such as the indications for the use of a specific diagnostic test or therapeutic intervention. The practice guidelines listed in figure 6-1 were developed by the American College of Physicians (ACP) and illustrate the variety of clinical issues that available practice guidelines address. The ACP practice guidelines vary considerably in the scope and content of their recommendations.

Figure 6-1.   Selected Practice Guidelines by the American College of Physicians

- Cardiac rehabilitation services
- Common screening tests
- Diagnostic evaluation of carotid arteries
- Diagnostic uses of the activated partial thromboplastin time and prothrombin time
- Eating disorders: anorexia nervosa and bulimia
- Evaluation of patients after recent acute myocardial infarction
- Glycosylated hemoglobin assays in the management and diagnosis of diabetes mellitus
- Hormone therapy to prevent disease and prolong life in postmenopausal women
- How to study the gallbladder
- Implantable and external infusion pumps for the treatment of thromboembolic disease in outpatients
- Indications for arterial blood gas analysis
- Management of gallstones
- Management of hypertension after ambulatory blood pressure monitoring
- Parenteral nutrition in patients receiving cancer chemotherapy
- Screening low-risk, asymptomatic adults for cardiac risk factors
- Screening for diabetes mellitus in apparently healthy, asymptomatic adults
- Screening for hypertension
- Selected methods for the management of diabetes mellitus
- Serum enzyme assays in the diagnosis of acute myocardial infarction
- Thrombolysis for evolving myocardial infarction

Source: Summarized, with permission, from *Directory of Practice Parameters*. Chicago: American Medical Association, 1995.

Each of these practice guidelines, used singly or in combination with others, may provide useful information for important aspects of disease management.

• Benefits of Using Clinical Practice Guidelines

Various studies have demonstrated the benefits of practice guidelines in improving the quality, utilization, and outcomes of clinical practice.[20-30] Practice guidelines provide a foundation for professional education,[31-34] as well as for clinical pathways, algorithms, protocols, clinical order sets, and other tools used in patient management.[35-38] They also facilitate the development of review criteria and other performance measures used to evaluate clinical practice.[39] The following is a list of several other important benefits associated with the use of practice guidelines:

- Authoritative source of information on important clinical issues
- Comprehensive evaluation of relevant scientific literature
- Source of reliable expert opinions
- Clarification of significant clinical controversies
- Specific, practical recommendations for patient management
- Evaluation of economic consequences of alternative patient management strategies
- Identification of specific patients who will benefit from the use of specific clinical recommendations
- Useful basis for effective disease management activities

One of the most valuable benefits of practice guidelines is the compilation and analysis of relevant scientific literature. Comprehensive literature reviews facilitate identification of areas for which reliable scientific information is available (or unavailable). For example, the Agency for Health Care Policy and Research practice guidelines on topics such as acute lower back pain problems in adults, acute pain management, benign prostatic hyperplasia, cataracts in adults, depression, heart failure, poststroke rehabilitation, pressure ulcers in adults, sickle cell disease, unstable angina, and urinary incontinence in adults provide extensive literature reviews that include detailed information on the strength and weakness of the evidence from various research studies.

Practice guidelines also provide access to the recommendations of recognized experts in specific clinical areas. Such information allows identification of areas of consensus and controversy, facilitates determination of clinical areas in which disease management activities might be effective, and provides useful information to guide clinical practice.

• Challenges in Using Clinical Practice Guidelines

Many complex issues surround the development, dissemination, and implementation of practice guidelines. Some of the challenges involved include the following:

- The unreceptive attitude of many health care professionals toward practice guidelines
- Limited published literature regarding successful implementation
- Uncertainty about optimal processes with which to develop practice guidelines
- The large number of available practice guidelines, including multiple guidelines addressing similar clinical issues
- Incomplete justification for specific patient management recommendations
- Inadequate evaluation of scientific literature
- Inappropriate use of expert opinion
- Recommendations that are out of date
- Conflicting recommendations in available practice guidelines
- Incomplete recommendations on important patient management issues
- Failure to address the full continuum of care (for example, prevention, diagnosis, treatment)
- Inadequate evaluation of the economic consequences of alternate patient management strategies
- Recommendations that are not easy to implement in patient management
- The need to modify recommendations prior to use
- Difficulty in identifying specific patients who will benefit from specific recommendations
- Difficulty in using practice guidelines to develop practical clinical management tools (for example, clinical pathways, order sets)
- Delivery system barriers to effective use of recommendations
- Concerns about legal implications of practice guidelines
- Difficulty in evaluating the results of implementation of recommendations

Issues such as how to evaluate the scientific literature, the role of expert opinion, and the reliability of specific clinical recommendations are important in developing practice guidelines, whereas assessment of the scientific soundness of specific clinical recommendations is an important priority in evaluating existing practice guidelines.[40,41] Although some groups consider economic information in developing the recommendations in their practice guidelines or provide information regarding the economic consequences of those recommendations, this is not the standard. Implementation of recommendations is often hampered by the absence of reliable information regarding the cost of alternate clinical management strategies. Issues such as the relative benefits of alternate types of publications and other methods of communicating information, and identification of how to incorporate recommendations into patient management tools arise in the dissemination of practice guidelines.[42-44]

A significant challenge is presented by practice guidelines that provide recommendations for some, but not all, of the important issues that must be addressed to facilitate comprehensive disease management. Although recommendations that focus on a narrow set of issues may be valuable, users need to rely on other practice guidelines or other information sources to develop more comprehensive strategies for effective disease management.

Another challenge is the availability of practice guidelines with conflicting recommendations, or disagreement with the results of scientific research completed after the practice guidelines were developed. For example, various professional organizations have developed recommendations for strategies to facilitate disease prevention (such as mammography or measurement of cholesterol levels); however, the recommendations often differ on important issues such as which screening tests to perform and their frequency.[45] Locally developed practice guidelines may include clinical recommendations that differ from those made by national practice guidelines. Such conflicts may create confusion and controversy and undermine support for the use of specific guidelines.[46]

Professional liability issues related to practice guidelines have received considerable attention because the impact of guidelines in this area is controversial.[47-49] Evidence on whether practice guidelines are being used as exculpatory evidence (to exonerate a defendant physician) or as inculpatory evidence (to implicate a defendant physician) is not decisive. In a study of 259 malpractice claims from two insurance companies, of the 259 claims, guidelines were involved in 17 cases: 4 used guidelines as exculpatory, and 12 used them as inculpatory (1 was undetermined).[50] In the second part of the same study, a survey of 980 malpractice attorneys reported that once a suit was initiated, practice guidelines were likely to be used for inculpatory purposes. However, Maine passed the Medical Liability Demonstration Act in 1990, which provided that physicians can use the fact that they adhered to practice guidelines as an affirmative defense in a claim of professional neglect.[51] The law has not been tested in court to date. It is unresolved whether practice guidelines will increase or decrease professional liability litigation; nevertheless, these considerations do not present a significant impediment to the successful development and use of practice guidelines.

To address some of these challenges, health care professionals should implement a systematic process to review the reliability of the recommendations in practice guidelines, and, as necessary, modify specific recommendations. Both the Institute of Medicine and the AMA have suggested approaches for such evaluation.[52,53] The probability of successful practice guideline use may be increased by modeling practice guideline activities after successful efforts already implemented by other health care organizations; the AMA and the AHA have compiled extensive information on the successful implementation of practice guidelines.[54,55] Dissemination of such positive information should encourage receptive practitioner attitudes toward practice guidelines.

• Incorporating Clinical Practice Guidelines into Disease Management Activities

Effective disease management is a complex activity that requires a wide variety of capabilities, including information management, provider education, patient identification, case management, and clinical practice. Expert scientific and clinical knowledge regarding optimal management of all major aspects of patient care is needed. Practice guidelines based on reliable scientific information and expert clinical judgment are valuable tools to facilitate disease management. The nine steps discussed in the following subsections have been modified from steps originally proposed by the AMA for implementing practice guidelines and are relevant to the incorporation of practice guidelines in disease management activities.[56] Following the discussion of these steps, two hypothetical case examples are used to demonstrate some of the more important process issues.

Step 1: Issue Identification

The first step in using practice guidelines in disease management involves the identification of specific clinical areas of interest to be managed. Potential clinical issues include comprehensive management of a disease or condition (for example, prevention, diagnosis, and treatment) or management of an important aspect of a disease or condition (such as outpatient management of patients with advanced diseases). Identification of clinical areas for disease management may be based on many different factors, including:

- Availability of relevant, high-quality practice guidelines
- Successful implementation of such practice guidelines in specific clinical areas by other organizations
- Concerns over quality, utilization, outcomes, or cost-management issues
- Significant and unexplained variations in current practice patterns
- Clinical services involving substantial expenditures
- Improvements in clinical management methods that are expected to provide significant benefits
- Requirements of managed care, payer, accreditation, or other influential organizations

Reliable practice guidelines that have been successfully implemented by other organizations, with demonstrated benefits in quality, utilization, outcomes, or cost management, provide a useful foundation for determining specific clinical areas for disease management activities.

Step 2: Issue Refinement

Once clinical issues of potential interest are identified, it is essential to refine and focus this list to select those issues that meet the objectives of the disease management initiative. Many of the considerations identified in step 1 are relevant to refining and prioritizing the list of issues for disease management. The availability of relevant, high-quality practice guidelines and information about successful implementation in specific clinical areas by other organizations can be useful. For example, published reports identifying effective use of practice guidelines in disease management provide a model that can be imitated in other disease management activities.

Step 3: Identification of Relevant Practice Guidelines

With the large number of practice guidelines already available and the ongoing development of new ones, it is useful to follow a systematic strategy to identify those that are potentially relevant to the planned disease management initiative. Practice guidelines developed by national organizations provide useful information, and the AMA's *Directory of Practice Parameters,* which is published annually, provides a comprehensive list of these practice guidelines. *Practice Parameters Update,* published quarterly by the AMA, provides information about new practice guidelines and recent modifications in existing practice guidelines developed by national organizations. Both publications also identify practice guidelines that have been withdrawn or replaced. Practice guidelines developed by regional or local organizations can also provide useful information.

Many articles that discuss the implementation of practice guidelines have been published, and the National Library of Medicine is a valuable source of information about publications related to this topic. Such publications often include information about regional or local practice guidelines that have been derived from those developed by national organizations, practice guidelines that have been produced independent of national models, the benefits and challenges of using practice guidelines, and practical advice regarding how to use practice guidelines.

Step 4: Evaluation of Practice Guidelines

Once the clinical issues to be addressed through disease management activities are determined and the practice guidelines relevant to these issues are identified, the practice guidelines and their recommendations should be evaluated fully. The Institute of Medicine and the AMA have suggested approaches for this evaluation. Among the issues to be considered are the following:

- The reputation of the sponsoring organization
- What processes were used to review the scientific literature
- What processes were employed to obtain expert opinion
- Links between the results of the scientific literature review and expert opinion with practice guideline recommendations
- The date the recommendations in the practice guideline were developed
- The presence of conflicting recommendations in other reliable information sources
- Benefits and challenges to implementing the practice guideline recommendations

Many practice guidelines include information to facilitate such evaluation. Although this process can be complicated, preliminary evaluation of available practice guidelines may be sufficient to determine their relevance for specific disease management activities.

Step 5: Selection and Modification of Practice Guidelines

Health care professionals whose practice will be affected by the recommendations in practice guidelines should be involved in the review and selection of the practice guidelines to be used in disease management. Successful local implementation of practice guidelines benefits from substantial local review and, as appropriate, local modification of the original practice guidelines. Practitioners are more likely to modify their behavior if they have been involved in developing the practice guidelines and have a sense of ownership.[57] Recommendations in the selected practice guidelines may be suitable for use without change, but their length, format, or language may be modified to facilitate dissemination or implementation. For example, the recommendations may be condensed or rewritten to facilitate their use. Alternatively, the recommendations may be modified to accommodate relevant scientific or clinical information. Research findings published after the completion of the practice guideline may necessitate modification of some or all of the recommendations.

The recommendations in specific practice guidelines may be modified to accommodate factors specific to the health care delivery system, such as patient population, health care services available, health care benefits, or professional preference. For example, certain recommendations may provide greater clinical benefit than others; recommended services may not be available within a particular geographic locale or may not be included in relevant health benefits packages; or specific alternative practices may be deemed preferable to the recommendations because of professional preference or financial considerations. Additionally, selected practice guidelines may not provide clear recommendations on important clinical issues, such as a challenging or controversial issue that the disease management activity seeks to address. In such circumstances, modifications or additions to the recommendations may be essential for effective disease management.

It is also important to recognize that given the existence of approximately 2,000 clinical practice guidelines by a diverse group of organizations including the AHCPR, Centers for Disease Control (CDC), specialty societies, managed care organizations, and local institutions, the potential for conflicting recommendations is high. At the present time there is no clearinghouse for identifying and resolving differences among practice guidelines. This creates problems in the selection and implementation process.

Step 6: Dissemination of Practice Guidelines

After relevant practice guidelines have been selected and modified as necessary, they should be disseminated to the health care professionals who are expected to use them in disease management efforts. Effective dissemination strategies include:

- Preparing practice guidelines in formats relevant to the needs of the specific users
- Facilitating ready access to the various formats of the practice guidelines
- Distributing information about the practice guidelines through routine communications mechanisms (for example, correspondence, seminars)
- Addressing concerns among health care professionals regarding the use of practice guidelines
- Using respected "opinion leaders" to provide support for practice guideline use
- Distributing published information about successful implementation of practice guidelines in other settings

Condensed versions of practice guidelines, which provide recommendations for patient management without full discussion of the scientific rationale behind the recommendations, may be adequate to meet the needs of certain health care providers. Effective dissemination should assist health care professionals in obtaining the adopted practice guidelines and promote a receptive attitude toward their use among physicians and other health care professionals. Dissemination should also clarify the expected benefits associated with the use of these practice guidelines and indicate how they enhance disease management objectives.

Step 7: Implementation of Practice Guidelines

The availability of scientifically sound, clinically relevant recommendations for disease management may be sufficient to encourage their adoption and implementation. Additional strategies to promote implementation of the recommendations include using the adopted practice guidelines to accomplish the following:

- Develop practical products to assist patient management (for example, algorithms, protocols, clinical pathways, clinical order sets, health care provider reminder systems)
- Guide utilization, quality, and outcomes management activities (for example, design of health benefits, incentive systems, preauthorization of services, case management)
- Design information systems to identify specific patients who will benefit from the use of specific recommendations
- Manage incentives for health care professionals and consumers to use practice guidelines
- Remove health system barriers to the use of specific recommendations

These strategies incorporate recommendations into disease management mechanisms that influence and assist clinical management. For example, developing clinical order sets and clinical pathways that reflect practice guideline recommendations helps clinicians to manage patients in accordance with those recommendations. Collection and dissemination of information regarding compliance with specific recommendations (for example, screening mammography, diabetic eye examinations) encourages health care professionals to follow them. Effective implementation of these strategies fosters implementation of practice guidelines.

Step 8: Evaluation of the Impact of Practice Guidelines

Evaluating the impact of adopted practice guidelines and the various patient management tools derived from them is essential. The practice guidelines provide a basis for data collection and analysis, a foundation for review criteria and other performance measures used to assess clinical practice, and a framework for practice profiles and other reports generated to provide information about clinical practice.[58] Strategies to evaluate the impact of practice guidelines include:

- Evaluation of practice guideline use by health care professionals
- Measurement of the degree of compliance with practice guideline recommendations
- Evaluation of the clinical consequences of practice guideline use (for example, quality of care, resource utilization, outcomes)

- Measurement of the economic consequences of practice guideline use (for example, direct costs to the health care delivery system, indirect costs to enrollee or employer)
- Assessment of the consequences (clinical and economic) of the use of various patient management tools derived from the practice guidelines
- Identification of barriers to effective practice guideline use
- Assessment of the attitudes among health care professionals toward practice guidelines
- Assessment of the attitudes among patients and consumers toward practice guidelines
- Evaluation of the role of practice guidelines in facilitating the objectives of disease management

These strategies should provide reliable information with which to evaluate the impact of practice guidelines, identify the benefits and challenges associated with their use, and provide a basis for information dissemination to health care professionals to facilitate practice improvement. Demonstration of the benefits of practice guideline use in facilitating disease management (such as improvements in clinical outcomes, patient satisfaction, utilization of services, and costs of patient management) should enhance support for such activities. For example, periodic reports that demonstrate improved compliance with practice guideline recommendations (such as improved screening for breast and cervical cancer and improved management of patients with asthma and renal disease) and the benefits of such compliance (such as reduced frequency of advanced cancer, reduced costs in the management of patients with asthma or renal disease) should encourage support among health care professionals for specific disease management activities. One example of a successful practice guideline relates to the use of prophylactic antibiotics before elective thoracic surgery at the LDS Hospital in Salt Lake City.[59] Improved compliance with the practice guideline lowered the postoperative infection rate to 0.4 percent from a preguideline rate of 1.8 percent. Such data provide strong incentive to physicians to follow the practice guideline recommendations.

Step 9: Periodic Review and Modification of Practice Guidelines

With the rapid evolution of new scientific and clinical information, periodic review of adopted practice guidelines, the patient management tools derived from them, and the disease management activities based on them is essential. Information obtained through the evaluation described in step 8 provides useful material to facilitate ongoing improvements in both the practice guidelines and the patient management tools. Effective strategies to review and modify adopted practice guidelines include:

- Establishing a schedule (for example, annual, semiannual) to review adopted practice guidelines
- Developing an effective system to monitor the publication of new or modified practice guidelines that may be relevant
- Monitoring publications that provide useful information about practice guideline implementation
- Ensuring that information about the results of implementation of the practice guidelines are used in the review and modification of the practice guidelines
- When practice guidelines are modified, using strategies similar to those employed in their initial development, dissemination, and implementation

For example, a national organization's release of new practice guidelines for the management of diabetes should encourage review and, as necessary, modification of practice guidelines adopted for specific disease management activities. Such efforts should ensure that practice guidelines are current and consistent with disease management objectives and that disease management activities are based on current scientific information.

• Case Examples: Use of Practice Guidelines in Disease Management Activities

The use of practice guidelines in disease management activities is illustrated by a description of the efforts of two hypothetical disease management programs. Case 1 focuses on how one committee uses practice guidelines to identify patients who would benefit from a disease management program for asthma. Case 2 examines how the appropriate selection of practice guidelines for each stage of progressive renal disease can improve disease management at all points on the continuum of care.

Case 1: Identification of Patients to Participate in Disease Management

A committee comprising physicians, nurses, pharmacists, and other health care professionals is assigned responsibility for developing disease management activities. The committee is also responsible for the review and adoption of practice guidelines to facilitate disease management activities. The committee follows the nine-step process described in the last section to identify opportunities for more effective and efficient disease management.

Aware of a wide variety of successful initiatives to improve the management of patients with asthma, the committee decides to focus on this disease. Important tasks for the committee include identification of asthmatic patients, determination of the asthmatics who might benefit from modification in their clinical management, and identification of the health care providers whose management of patients with asthma might be improved.

To facilitate the committee's efforts, analyses of available data are undertaken. Useful data sources for the evaluation of clinical practice related to asthma include computerized administrative information (for example, encounter and claims data) about patients, their diagnoses, and the services they have received. Additional data sources include medical record data.[60]

The committee uses computerized administrative data as an efficient preliminary way to identify asthmatics. Through analysis of data on patient encounters and claims, patients are presumed to be asthmatics if a primary or secondary diagnosis of asthma occurs during one or more of their health care encounters or in one or more of their claims. Alternatively, through analysis of data on the use of pharmaceuticals, patients may be identified as asthmatics if they take specific pharmaceuticals associated with the management of asthma (for example, isoproterenol, theophylline). Some patients may be identified through both encounter and pharmaceutical data, whereas other patients may be identified from only one source. For example, patients who are taking medications for asthma but who did not receive medical care specifically related to the management of that disease may appear in a database related to the use of pharmaceuticals but not appear in an administrative database related to encounters or claims.

Use of analytical rules to manage computerized administrative data, such as identification of all patients with ICD-9 code 493 ("asthma") or all patients receiving pharmaceuticals related to the management of asthma, permits preliminary identification of asthmatics, characterization of the services these asthmatics received, identification of the severity of their condition, and assessment of opportunities for improved patient management.

The committee analyzes encounter or claims data regarding the frequency of outpatient visits, emergency department visits, and inpatient hospital stays among asthmatics.* It then uses pharmaceutical data to identify which medications and combinations of medications are used to manage asthmatics, which regimens are prescribed (for example, dosages, frequency), and what patterns patients follow in filling their prescriptions (compliance). Data may be analyzed in various ways, such as by site of service, health care provider, or patient. The data may be risk adjusted or modified in other ways to facilitate analysis, and data from multiple sources may be combined to permit more sophisticated analyses.

The committee also analyzes information regarding the costs of these services. Through these efforts, it profiles patients with asthma and evaluates health care providers who manage asthmatics. Issues of interest include

---

*Data for inpatient and outpatient services may be combined to calculate episodes of care.

variations in patterns of care, utilization of specific health care services, use of pharmaceuticals, and costs of care. The committee is especially interested in the identification of patients and health care providers who will benefit from targeted interventions such as education, modification in practice patterns, or case management. Conclusions made through analysis of administrative data may be verified or modified, as necessary, through evaluation of medical records.

To identify practice guidelines relevant to the management of asthma, the committee reviews the AMA's *Directory of Practice Parameters* and *Practice Parameters Update*. It identifies 11 practice guidelines sponsored by five different national organizations—the American Academy of Allergy and Immunology, the American Academy of Pediatrics, the AMA, the American Thoracic Society, and the National Heart, Lung, and Blood Institute. As shown in table 6-1, these practice guidelines address a broad array of issues regarding the diagnosis and management of asthma. The committee also obtains selected practice guidelines on asthma and asthmatic patient management tools developed by various regional and local organizations, such as managed care organizations, health care delivery systems, hospitals, and group practices.

Table 6-1.   Selected Examples of Practice Guidelines on Asthma

Practice Guideline	Sponsoring Organization
Drugs used in bronchial disorders	American Medical Association
Exercise and the asthmatic child	American Academy of Pediatrics
Guidelines for the diagnosis and management of asthma	National Heart, Lung, and Blood Institute
Guidelines for the evaluation of impairment and disability in patients with asthma	American Thoracic Society
Management of asthma during pregnancy	National Heart, Lung, and Blood Institute
Metered-dose inhalers for young athletes with exercise-induced asthma	American Academy of Pediatrics
Office management of acute exacerbations of asthma in children	American Academy of Pediatrics
Practice parameters for diagnosis and treatment of bronchial asthma	American Academy of Allergy and Immunology
Progress at the interface of inflammation and asthma	American Thoracic Society
Use of antihistamines in patients with asthma	American Academy of Allergy and Immunology
Use of inhaled medications in school by students with asthma	American Academy of Allergy and Immunology

Source: Summarized, with permission, from *Directory of Practice Parameters*. Chicago: American Medical Association, 1995.

The committee identifies the clinical issues of greatest interest, evaluates the available practice guidelines, selects those that are most relevant, modifies them as necessary, disseminates them to the health care professionals who will use them, and develops patient management tools to facilitate improved management of asthmatics. For example, to reduce the frequency of avoidable hospitalizations among patients with severe asthma, the committee develops a list of asthmatic patients at greatest risk of hospitalization and establishes a case management program for them. The committee also develops recommendations regarding how specific pharmaceuticals, such as metered-dose inhalers or corticosteroids, should be used; how patients with asthma should be monitored (for example, use of peak flow meters); when patients should contact their physicians; and how patients should be managed in emergency departments.

After the adoption, dissemination, and implementation of the asthma practice guidelines, a data system is maintained to provide information on current and evolving practice patterns for managing patients with asthma. The committee provides input on the system's design and management to ensure that the data collected and reports available for analysis are relevant. Health care providers can use the reports to evaluate their performance relative to the practice guideline recommendations and develop strategies to modify their practice as necessary. The reports enable the committee to monitor the success of the disease management program and to identify opportunities for improvement in clinical decision making and patient management. The committee can also use the reports to review the adopted practice guidelines and modify the recommendations as necessary. Modifications in the practice guidelines may be made when opportunities for more effective and efficient management of asthma are identified, when improved practice guidelines become available, and when medical knowledge advances.

Case 2: Selection of Practice Guidelines for Specific Stages of a Disease

Effective disease management programs require development and implementation of clinical strategies tailored to a particular disease or condition. The natural history of a disease should be taken into account to ensure that disease management activities are appropriate for and relevant to the various disease stages for individual patients. The management of patients with progressive renal disease illustrates how practice guidelines can be useful in disease management, and how different practice guidelines are relevant for different stages of the disease.

Once the population at risk for progressive renal disease is defined and identified, the first step is to design early screening and disease-prevention strategies. Hypertension and diabetes mellitus are important conditions that account for the majority of patients who subsequently develop chronic renal failure or receive renal replacement therapy. Various practice guidelines for managing hypertension provide recommendations designed to reduce the frequency of progressive hypertensive renal injury. The National Kidney Foundation has developed practice guidelines for the screening and management of microalbuminuria in patients with diabetes mellitus to delay the development of diabetic renal disease.[61,62] These practice guidelines provide useful information for disease management activities to facilitate identification of risk factors for and prevention of renal disease.

Another aspect of disease management is to identify patients who have developed renal disease and design appropriate treatment strategies. Abundant evidence exists that the natural history of chronic renal disease is relentless progression to end-stage renal failure. Most patients with chronic renal failure lose residual renal function in a predictable fashion. Various studies have identified factors that play a role in the progressive destruction of renal tissue. Interventions designed to monitor renal function and minimize the influence of destructive factors should be instituted.

Available practice guidelines, such as those in table 6-2, provide recommendations regarding the management of various aspects of chronic renal disease. Early in the course of the disease (with renal function over 30 percent of normal), practice guidelines describe how to manage factors responsible for progressive renal injury (such as hypertension, diabetes, hyperlipidemia, proteinuria, excessive dietary protein and phosphorus) and provide recommendations as to how to minimize renal damage that may be caused by the use of nephrotoxic drugs (for example, aminoglycosides), volume depletion, and other factors. Later in the course of the disease (with renal function below 30 percent of normal), important electrolyte, metabolic,

Table 6-2. Selected Examples of Practice Guidelines for Progressive Renal Disease

Practice Guideline	Sponsoring Organization
Adequacy of hemodialysis	Renal Physicians Association
Analgesic-associated kidney disease	National Institutes of Health
Diabetic renal disease	National Kidney Foundation
Laboratory tests in end-stage disease patients undergoing dialysis	Agency for Health Care Policy and Renal Research
Management of staghorn calculi	American Urological Association
Morbidity and mortality of dialysis	National Institutes of Health
Percutaneous nephrostomy	American College of Radiology
Prevention and treatment of kidney stones	National Institutes of Health

Source: Summarized, with permission, from *Directory of Practice Parameters*. Chicago: American Medical Association, 1995.

and clinical abnormalities must be identified and managed if a patient is to be maintained in optimal status prior to the onset of end-stage renal disease. Available practice guidelines provide recommendations for case managers, health care providers, patients, and family members to facilitate the management of these abnormalities and of superimposed complications (for example, infections) that might necessitate emergency care or hospitalization.

Once end-stage renal disease occurs, available therapeutic options include chronic dialysis and renal transplantation. There are practice guidelines to assist health care providers and patients in identifying which of these interventions is appropriate and when it should be provided. Practice guidelines for patients on long-term dialysis and patients with a renal transplant identify complication prevention and management strategies that, if implemented effectively, may enable patients to function optimally.

The use of relevant practice guidelines appropriate for the management of each stage of renal disease improves the probability that optimal management of these complex patients will occur during every phase of the disease, thereby resulting in improved clinical outcomes, greater patient satisfaction, and more efficient utilization of health care services.

• Conclusions

Successful disease management strategies to improve the quality, utilization, outcomes, and efficiency of health care services must take into account relevant scientific information and clinical experience, identify optimal ways to manage groups of patients and individual patients, and achieve acceptance by health care providers and patients. Properly developed practice guidelines and patient management tools derived from them — modified as necessary to meet organization-specific, patient-specific, and condition-specific needs — are important mechanisms to facilitate the goals of disease management. Practice guidelines provide a useful scientific foundation for disease management activities. Moreover, patient management tools derived from these practice guidelines provide an effective mechanism to facilitate implementation of practice guideline recommendations. Numerous challenges exist in the development of practice guidelines, their adaptation in the development of patient management tools, and their use in the management of individual patients and as a foundation for the evaluation and modification of clinical practice. Nevertheless, practice guidelines are valuable tools to guide the design, implementation, and monitoring of effective disease management activities.

If practice guidelines are to emerge as a constructive tool that will improve quality of care and facilitate efficient use of resources, health care providers should promote the following goals:

- Better access to information on regional and local practice guidelines and patient management tools derived from practice guidelines
- Reliable data and practical data management tools to enable effective evaluation of ways to use practice guidelines to improve clinical practice
- Expanded research on effective and efficient ways to use practice guidelines in disease management
- Evaluation of the influence of health care delivery systems on the implementation of practice guideline recommendations

References

1. Kelly, J. T., and Kelly, J. M. Comparing quality in managed care and fee-for-service delivery systems. *American Journal of Managed Care* 1:129–31, 1995.

2. Epstein, A. Performance reports on quality—prototypes, problems, and prospects. *The New England Journal of Medicine* 333(1):57–61, July 6, 1995.

3. Kassirer, J. P. The quality of care and the quality of measuring it. *The New England Journal of Medicine* 329:1263–64, 1993.

4. Kassirer, J. P. The use and abuse of practice profiles. *The New England Journal of Medicine* 330:634–36, 1994.

5. Kelly, J. T., and Kellie, S. E. Appropriateness of medical care: findings, strategies. *Archives of Pathology and Laboratory Medicine* 114:1119–21, 1990.

6. Woolf, S. H. Practice guidelines: a new reality in medicine; I: recent developments. *Archives of Internal Medicine* 150:1811–18, 1990.

7. Woolf, S. H. Practice guidelines: a new reality in medicine; II: methods of developing guidelines. *Archives of Internal Medicine* 152(5):946–52, May 1992.

8. Woolf, S. H. Practice guidelines: a new reality in medicine; III: impact on patient care. *Archives of Internal Medicine* 153:2646–55, 1993.

9. Kelly, J. T., and Toepp, M. C. Practice parameters: development, evaluation, dissemination, and implementation. *Quality Review Bulletin* 18:405–9, 1992.

10. Kelly, J. T. Role of clinical practice guidelines and clinical profiling in facilitating optimal laboratory use. *Clinical Chemistry* 41:1234–36, 1995.

11. Shapiro, D. W., Lasker, R. D., Bindman, A. B., and Lee, P. R. Containing costs while improving quality of care: the role of profiling and practice guidelines. *Annual Review of Public Health* 14:219–41, 1993.

12. *CPG Strategies: Putting Guidelines into Practice.* Chicago: American Hospital Association, 1992.

13. *Guidelines for Clinical Practice: From Development to Use.* Washington, DC: Institute of Medicine, 1992.

14. Kelly, J. T. The interface of clinical paths and practice parameters. In: P. Spath, editor. *Clinical Paths: Tools for Outcomes Management.* Chicago: American Hospital Publishing, 1994.

15. *Directory of Practice Parameters.* Chicago: American Medical Association, 1995.

16. *Directory of Practice Parameters.*

17. *Implementing Practice Parameters on the Local, State, and Regional Level.* Chicago: American Medical Association, 1993.

18. Aucott, J. N., Taylor, A. L., Wright, J. T., and others. Developing guidelines for local use: algorithms for cost-efficient outpatient management of cardiovascular disorders in a VA medical center. *Joint Commission Journal on Quality Improvement* 20(1):17–32, Jan. 1994.

19. Brown, J. B., Shye, D., and McFarland, B. The paradox of guideline implementation: how AHCPR's depression guideline was adapted at Kaiser Permanente Northwest Region. *Joint Commission Journal on Quality Improvement* 21:5–21, 1995.

20. Eagle, K. A., Mulley, A. G., Skates, S. J., and others. Length of stay in the intensive care unit: effects of practice guidelines and feedback. *JAMA* 264(8):992–97, Aug. 22–29, 1990.

21. Ellrodt, A. G., Conner, L., Riedinger, M. S., and Weingarten, S. Implementing practice guidelines through a utilization management strategy: the potential and the challenges. *Quality Review Bulletin* 18:456–60, 1992.

22. Ellrodt, A. G., Conner, L., Riedinger, M. S., and Wiengarten, S. Measuring and improving physician compliance with clinical practice guidelines: a controlled interventional trial. *Annals of Internal Medicine* 122:277–82, 1995.

23. Gottlieb, L. K., Margolis, C. Z., and Schoenbaum, S. C. Clinical practice guidelines at an HMO: development and implementation in a quality improvement model. *Quality Review Bulletin* 16(2):80–86, Feb. 1990.

24. Hu, T. W., Stotts, N. A., Fogarty, T. E., and Bergstrom, N. Cost analysis for guideline implementation in prevention and early treatment of pressure ulcers. *Decubitus* 6(2):42–46, 1993.

25. Myers, S. A., and Gleicher, N. A successful program to lower cesarean-section rates. *The New England Journal of Medicine* 319(23):1511–16, Dec. 8, 1988.

26. Watchel, T. J., and O'Sullivan, P. Practice guidelines to reduce testing in the hospital. *Journal of General Internal Medicine* 5:335–41, 1990.

27. Webb, L. Z., Kuykendall, D. H., Zeiger, R. S., and others. The impact of status asthmaticus practice guidelines on patient outcome and physician behavior. *Quality Review Bulletin* 18:471–76, 1992.

28. Weingarten, S., Agocs, L., Tankel, N., and others. Reducing lengths of stay for patients hospitalized with chest pain using medical practice guidelines and opinion leaders. *American Journal of Cardiology* 71(4):259–62, Feb. 1, 1993.

29. Weingarten, S., Ermann, B., Bolus, R., and others. Early "step-down" transfer of low-risk patients with chest pain. *Annals of Internal Medicine* 113(4):283–89, Aug. 15, 1990.

30. Zelenitsky, S. A., and Richard, A. Implementation of an aminoglycoside order review process in a central dispensary. *Canadian Journal of Hospital Pharmacy* 46(6):269–74, 1993.

31. Hendricson, W. D., Wood, P. R., Hidalgo, H. A., and others. Implementation of a physician education intervention: the Childhood Asthma Project. *Archives of Pediatrics and Adolescent Medicine* 148(6):595–601, June 1994.

32. Lomas, J., Enkin, M., Anderson, G. M., and others. Opinion leaders vs audit and feedback to implement practice guidelines. *JAMA* 265(17):2202–7, May 1, 1991.

33. Mittman, B. S., Tonesk, X., and Jacobson, P. D. Implementing clinical practice guidelines: social influence strategies and practitioner behavior change. *Quality Review Bulletin* 18:413–22, 1992.

34. Wise, C. G., and Billi, J. E. A model for practice guideline adaptation and implementation: empowerment of the physician. *Journal of Quality Improvement* 21:465–76, 1995.

35. Kelly. The interface of clinical paths and practice parameters.

36. Murrey, K. O., Gottlieb, L. K., and Schoenbaum, S. C. Implementing clinical guidelines: a quality management approach to reminder systems. *Quality Review Bulletin* 18:423–33, 1992.

37. Schriefer, J. The synergy of pathways and algorithms: two tools work better than one. *Journal of Quality Improvement* 20:485–99, 1994.

38. Shiffman, R. N. Towards effective implementation of a pediatric asthma guideline: integration of decision support and clinical workflow support. *Proceedings on the Annual Symposium on Computer Applications in Medical Care,* 1994, pp. 797–801.

39. Kellie, S. E., and Kelly, J. T. Medicare Peer Review Organization preprocedure review criteria: an analysis of criteria for three procedures. *JAMA* 265(10):1265–70, Mar. 13, 1991.

40. *Attributes to Guide the Development of Practice Parameters.* Chicago: American Medical Association, 1990.

41. *Guidelines for Clinical Practice: From Development to Use.* Washington, DC: Institute of Medicine, 1992.

42. VanAmringe, M., and Shannon, T. E. Awareness, assimilation, and adoption: the challenge of effective dissemination and the first AHCPR-sponsored guidelines. *Quality Review Bulletin* 18:397–404, 1992.

43. Hadorn, D. C., McCormick, K., and Diokno, A. An annotated algorithm approach to clinical guideline development. *JAMA* 267(24):3311–14, June 24, 1992.

44. Litzelman, D. K., Ditus, R. S., Miller, M. E., and Tierney, W. M. Requiring physicians to respond to computerized reminders improves their compliance with preventive care protocols. *Journal of General Internal Medicine* 8:311–17, 1993.

45. Hayward, R. S., Steinberg, E. P., Ford, D. E., and others. Preventive care guidelines: 1991. *Annals of Internal Medicine* 114(9):758–83, May 1, 1991.

46. Tunis, S. R., Hayward, R. S., Wilson, M. C., and others. Internists' attitudes about clinical practice guidelines. *Annals of Internal Medicine* 120(11):956–63, June 1, 1994.

47. Johnson, K. B., Hirshfeld, E. B., Ile, M. L., and others. *Legal Implications of Practice Parameters.* Chicago: American Medical Association, 1990.

48. Hirshfeld, E. B. Should practice parameters be the standard of care in malpractice litigation? *JAMA* 266:2886–91, 1991.

49. Garnick, D. W., Hendricks, A. M., and Brennan, T. A. Can practice guidelines reduce the number and costs of malpractrice claims. *JAMA* 266:2856–60, 1991.

50. Hyams, A. L., Brandenburg, J. A., and others. Practice guidelines and malpractice litigation: a two way street. *Annals of Internal Medicine* 122:450–55, 1995.

51. Kennedy, M. Ten strategies for making clinical guidelines and pathways work. *The Quality Letter for Healthcare Leaders,* Oct. 1995.

52. *Guidelines for Clinical Practice: From Development to Use.*

53. *Attributes to Guide the Development of Practice Parameters.*

54. *Directory of Practice Parameters.*

55. *CPG Strategies: Putting Guidelines into Practice.*

56. *Implementing Practice Parameters on the Local, State, and Regional Level.*

57. Brown, J. B., Shye, D. F., and McFarland, B. How the AHCPR's depression guidelines were adapted at Kaiser Permanente Northwest Region. *Journal of Quality Improvement* 21(1):5–21, 1995.

58. Herman, R. Harvard HMO improves pap smear screening. *QA Review* 1:2–3, 1989.

59. Peslin, S. Practice guidelines: an essential tool for managed care? *Managed Care Update* 9(2):6–12, 1995.

60. Hanchak, N. A. Using administrative data to evlauate the quality of care. *JCOM* 3:57–60, 1996.

61. Fifth report of the Joint National Committee on Detection, Evaluation, and Treatment of High Blood Pressure. *Archives of Internal Medicine* 153:154–83, 1993.

62. Bennett, P. H., Haffner, S., Kasiske, B. L., and others. Diabetic renal disease recommendations: screening and management of microalbuminuria in patients with diabetes mellitus. *American Journal of Kidney Diseases* 25:107–12, 1995.

Chapter 7

The Roles of Pharmaceutical Companies in Disease Management

Stan Bernard, MD, MBA

In the early 1990s, the pharmaceutical industry came under critical scrutiny—and even attack—from numerous sectors in the United States. Federal legislation and proposed government reforms targeted the industry and criticized it, particularly for the high prices of pharmaceutical products. This criticism came despite the fact that pharmaceutical companies, which were responsible for *discovering* over 90 percent of all drugs approved in the U.S. in the last decade alone, are required to spend on average over $350 million to develop and bring a single new drug to market.[1] Moreover, there was little appreciation that prescription drug therapy, particularly for chronic conditions, often eliminates the need for hospitalization and other costly interventions and is therefore tremendously cost-effective from the health care system perspective. The systemwide cost-effectiveness of pharmaceuticals represented the foundation for the industry's interpretation of the "disease management" concept. The pharmaceutical industry vigorously advocated the disease management approach to government reformers and managed care organizations. In fact, it was managed care which ultimately represented a far greater threat to pharmaceutical industry profits, policies, and prospects.

At the beginning of the 1990s, managed care controlled the distribution of the majority of pharmaceutical products in the United States. Sophisticated cost-cutting and drug utilization-control techniques implemented by pharmacy benefit management (PBM) companies and other managed care companies—including formulary lists, generic product substitutions, and discounted pricing contracts—were substantially reducing product sales and significantly eroding pharmaceutical profit margins. The industry tried to counter the managed care influence by offering "value-added services," such as free physician education programs and patient drug compliance programs, both to minimize managed care's focus on price and to obtain preferred status for their products on managed care formulary lists.

When those efforts largely failed, major pharmaceutical companies, led by industry vanguard Merck and Co., purchased the three largest PBM companies in an "if you can't beat them, buy them" strategic response. While there were many reasons for these acquisitions, industry observers recognized that these purchases represented an acknowledgment of the dramatic shift in the balance of power from pharmaceutical suppliers to large managed care buyers and signaled a new era for the industry.

Frustrated by such large purchasing power in the control of relatively few customers, the industry sought a strategic solution that would appeal to their customers' need to cut costs while maximizing the sales of pharmaceutical products. The proposed solution: disease management. The term *disease management* was originally coined in a Pfizer-sponsored report conducted by the Boston Consulting Group (BCG) and released in April 1993.[2] In the simplest terms, disease management is the application of business principles to medical practice. It involves managing and providing care to populations of patients who are at risk of or diagnosed with a specific disease through a comprehensive, integrated system that uses best practices, clinical practice improvement, information technology, and other resources and interventions.[3]

The BCG report called for a change in the way treatment for certain diseases is viewed. Traditionally, insurance companies processed and paid claims for specific services and products provided by hospital and physician providers, laboratories, pharmacies, and others. When managed care organizations (MCOs) came to the forefront in the latter part of the 1980s, they wanted to manage the health of patient populations at a minimum capitated cost. Financial claims data were the only information they possessed, because there was generally no electronic record of patient clinical data (that is, computerized patient records) at that time. They employed a strategy called *component management,* which emphasized price and utilization control by each category of provider or supplier—hospitals, physicians, pharmacies, and so forth. The idea was that by minimizing each of these budgets the MCO would reduce the overall health care cost for the employer or other payer (see figure 7-1).

• Reducing Pharmaceutical Use Can Increase the Utilization of Other Health Care Services

Several studies have demonstrated flaws in the component approach to pharmaceutical management: As the use of pharmaceuticals decreases, hospital and other medical costs often escalate far beyond the savings accrued to the pharmacy budget. For example, Drs. Stephen Soumerai and Jerry Avorn assessed the impact of 11 months of drug caps—a maximum of three reimbursed prescriptions per month—on Medicaid patients in New Hampshire.[4]

Although the use of pharmaceuticals was reduced by 35 percent, the number of elderly patients entering nursing homes increased by more than 50 percent. Moreover, overall Medicaid health care costs increased significantly. Similarly, Dr. Susan Horn and colleagues evaluated the impact of managed care pharmaceutical cost-containment strategies on the utilization of overall health care service utilization. In this longitudinal, prospective study in six U.S. health maintenance organizations (HMOs), the researchers examined a total of 12,997 patients having at least one of five diseases (arthritis, asthma, epigastric pain/ulcer, hypertension, and otitis media). The study found that for all conditions except otitis media, formulary limitations on drug availability were significantly related to higher rates of emergency room visits and hospital admissions.[5]

As a result, many in the pharmaceutical industry advocated adopting a disease management, systemwide approach to managing health care and its associated costs. They believed that if health plan administrators analyzed the impact of pharmaceuticals across the health care continuum by disease and not by budget code, they would document the cost-effectiveness of pharmaceutical products and actually increase, not minimize, their use. As demonstrated in figure 7-1, the interrelation of costs in the treatment of disease is the industry's key argument for advocating the disease management approach. Furthermore, by focusing on diseases as opposed to budgets, there can be an increased emphasis on the quality of care being given, which may not be apparent simply by looking at care costs.

Disease management strategies provide the groundwork for pharmaceutical companies and managed care plans to partner by aligning their incentives for mutual benefit. Disease management coordinates and integrates the elements of care, viewing the disease as a whole, where the success of one particular contribution can affect costs in other parts of the care continuum. Disease management gives a view across systems of what is being spent to manage patients with asthma, depression, and other conditions. In fact, although disease management is certainly not a new concept—there have been disease-specific carve-out management companies for years—it was the pharmaceutical industry that popularized the disease management movement in its earliest stages.

• Initial Managed Care Responses to the Disease Management Concept

As pharmaceutical manufacturers opened discussions with MCOs regarding participation in an integrated effort to manage disease, many MCOs were skeptical of their intentions. In many cases, these proposals were perceived simply as a new promotional tactic. Some MCOs maintained that they were already experts in managing patients with diseases and did not

Figure 7-1. The Two Approaches to Health Care Management

Component Management Approach (A)

Budget Focus

Budgets

Diseases	Hospital	Ambulatory Care	Physician Services	Laboratory/Diagnostic Services	Pharmacy
CAD	$$$$	$	$$$	$$$	$$
Diabetes	$$	$$	$	$$	$
Asthma	$$	$$	$	$	$
Cancer	$$$	$$	$$	$$	$$
Depression	$	$$$	$$	$	$$
AIDS	$$	$$	$$	$$	$$$
Total Costs	$	$	$	$	$

Disease Management Approach (B)
Systems Focus

Diseases	Budgets					Total Costs	Quality Measurements
	Hospital	Ambulatory Care	Physician Services	Laboratory/Diagnostic Services	Pharmacy		
CAD	$$$$	$	$$$	$$$	$$	$	↕
Diabetes	$$	$$	$$	$$	$	$	—
Asthma	$$	$$	$	$	$	$	→
Cancer	$$$	$$	$$	$$	$$	$	↕
Depression	$	$$$	$$	$	$$	$	↔
AIDS	$$	$$	$$	$$	$$$	$	←

need the industry's help. Other MCOs agreed that it was a logical approach that could have important repercussions, but most adopted a "wait-and-see" attitude toward the potential benefit of these proposals. A few MCOs challenged the industry to assist with patient management by accepting financial risk-sharing arrangements — not unlike physician capitation agreements — in exchange for preferred availability of their products to managed care patients.

For example, a managed care plan may request a pharmaceutical company that sells a cholesterol-lowering agent to provide "outcomes guarantees" based on the performance of its product in reducing cardiovascular events (for example, heart attacks) from elevated cholesterol. Therefore, the company would be at financial risk for a portion of the health care costs associated with any patients suffering a heart attack while taking its product; conversely, cost savings that accrued to the plan based on fewer heart attacks and reduced hospitalizations would be shared with the pharmaceutical partner.

However, if pharmaceutical companies are going to be held accountable for product performance in areas such as cardiovascular disease, they not only have to monitor patient response and compliance, but they also have to ensure that other cardiovascular risk factors are properly managed as well. What is their liability if cholesterol is effectively lowered by their product, but the patient has high blood pressure and diabetes, or smokes and maintains a high-fat diet and still has a heart attack? Suddenly the pharmaceutical company, which is best known for discovering and selling products, is partly responsible for managing patients' health. Although the company wants to be acknowledged as being responsible for achieving the best possible results, it must also enter into the business of helping MCOs to manage patients if it is going to be held accountable for product performance via risk-sharing agreements. This example highlights some of the potential challenges and different roles for pharmaceutical companies in the evolution of disease management programs.

• Classification of Disease Management Initiatives

One major reason that pharmaceutical companies' disease management initiatives have been met with skepticism by their managed care customers is that they each have very different ways of describing disease management. This author has designed the "Health/Disease Management Classification System," shown in figure 7-2, to clarify the confusion over disease management terminology. This system describes various levels of health/disease management initiatives by specific component areas of typical initiatives developed by health care organizations, including pharmaceutical companies.

Figure 7-2.   Classification System for Disease Management Initiatives

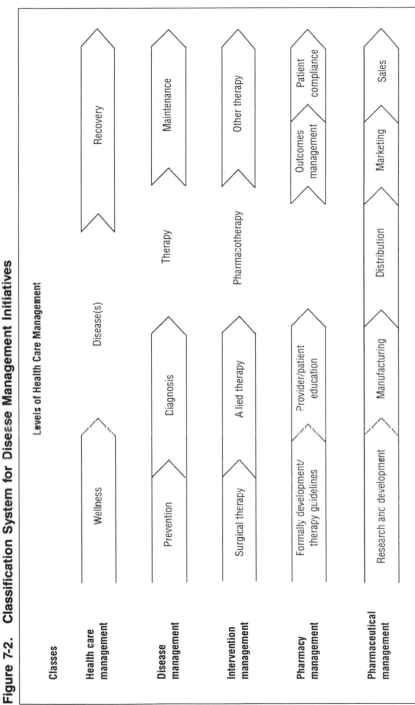

Health Care Management

This is the big picture of health care that is the ultimate goal of MCOs—a cradle-to-grave management not only of disease but disease prevention. Health management incorporates wellness, prevention of disease, disease management, and recovery phases for the patient population of a managed care plan. Although health maintenance is the stated objective of MCOs, widespread achievement of this objective for patient populations has been elusive. The vast majority of MCOs continue to focus on managing episodes of disease for individual patients for the projected time period that they will remain in that particular plan.

Only recently have HMOs, integrated delivery systems, and other care delivery organizations begun to implement comprehensive, population-based clinical programs targeting specific diseases. Lovelace Health Systems, the Mayo Clinic, and Kaiser have all been involved in disease management initiatives. Interestingly, the organizations responsible for managing health on a population basis are focusing first on preventing and managing diseases through disease management initiatives.

Disease Management

Disease management consists of the prevention of disease, the evaluation and diagnosis of patients with a particular disease, therapy, maintenance, and follow-up. It is a subclass of health care management. Historically, the primary organizations practicing disease management were the specialty carve-out companies that handled all clinical care for patients diagnosed with a particular disease or condition separately. These companies generally manage their own clinical providers and charge fees for their services.

Mental health and cancer specialty carve-out companies are the classic types of such organizations. More recently, Quantum Health Resources, Inc., has emerged as a leader in the management of specific disease states such as cystic fibrosis, hemophilia, and others. These organizations typically use a variety of tools, such as clinical practice guidelines, care process mapping, outcomes research, and information support systems, to optimize clinical operating efficiencies, minimize costs, and document favorable results for employers and other payers. When MCOs use their own providers and employ these same techniques internally to manage patient populations with specific diseases, it is termed a "carve-in" version of disease management, the usual characterization of disease management by MCOs (see chapter 4).

Intervention Management

Interventions are tools or techniques designed to support health or disease management initiatives or programs. They can take a variety of forms:

diagnostic interventions, therapeutic interventions, and maintenance interventions. Therapeutic interventions, such as provider education or patient compliance programs, are a pharmaceutical industry specialty. Intervention management, or, more specifically, pharmacotherapeutic management, is a subset of disease management, although most of the pharmaceutical industry uses the term interchangeably with disease management. This is a mistake and creates some of the confusion and skepticism on the part of MCOs when dealing with pharmaceutical companies.

Pharmacy Management

Pharmacy management is a subclass of therapeutic intervention management. Pharmacy-based interventions pertinent to disease management include formulary-based interventions, such as formulary management; drug utilization review; prescriber education; generic and therapeutic interchange; therapy-based interventions, such as therapy guidelines and compliance programs; and outcomes research, including database analyses and therapeutic decision-support tools.

Pharmaceutical Management

Traditionally, the pharmaceutical company's role in disease management has been as a supplier of medicines used to prevent, treat, or manage diseases. Most pharmaceutical companies have important and diverse disease management capabilities, particularly in the area of physician education and behavior modification, and are acquiring or developing broader capabilities. The industry has proven expertise in the development of medical educational tools and the use of sales forces to change physicians' behavior—a challenging task for MCOs. For example, if an MCO determines that its doctors are not diagnosing and treating cholesterol disorders early enough, a pharmaceutical industry partner can prepare the appropriate, customized educational materials, including educational seminars, brochures, and multimedia presentations, to train physicians on how to best treat these disease states.

Pharmaceutical sales forces have traditionally been a very powerful tool in changing physician behavior. MCOs can employ these representatives to make sure physicians follow the formulary or, more importantly, treatment guidelines. These representatives can also provide patient education and behavior modification programs and tools, especially compliance programs to improve drug utilization and maximize results.

Moreover, the drug industry has tremendous expertise in conducting rigorous, controlled clinical research. In a disease management partnership, MCOs can leverage this expertise for disease management tests, especially in the area of medical effectiveness. For example, it is valuable to MCOs to document the effectiveness of various interventions, including drugs in their "real-world" settings. In addition to clinical research, drug makers also have increasing capabilities in pharmacoeconomic or outcomes research, which MCOs can use not only to test the value of drugs but also to measure the cost benefits of a variety of different types of interventions. Obviously, pharmaceutical companies have extensive therapeutic area knowledge as well, having studied certain disease states in depth. Most important, the industry is well capitalized and has the financial resources to support disease management initiatives in areas that low-margin MCOs may not.

• The Evolution of the Pharmaceutical Industry in Disease Management

Pharmaceutical companies' disease management initiatives have evolved dramatically since the early 1990s, as shown in figure 7-3. The initial focus on industry-specific concerns has given way to more universal programs.

Pharmaceutical Management

To help address the needs of their MCO customers and to help differentiate their products, pharmaceutical companies began including value-added services with their managed care product offerings in the early 1990s. These services, which typically included packages of provider education, patient compliance, and administrative support programs, were the forerunners of the first pharmaceutical industry disease management programs. By the mid-1990s, most major companies had gone beyond traditional pharmaceutical management and added internal outcomes research or pharmacoeconomic departments to document the economic value of their products.

Pharmacy Management

The next major evolutionary step in the disease management continuum was the industry's acquisition of the three largest PBM companies: Merck's purchase of Medco, the SmithKline Beecham purchase of DPS, and Eli Lilly's acquisition of PCS. Several other strategic alliances between pharmaceutical and PBM companies followed these acquisitions. It was not necessarily the primary intent of these moves to augment the companies' disease management capabilities, but they had that effect.

The PBM companies supplement the disease management capabilities of the pharmaceutical companies by providing additional types of disease management interventions. For example, PBMs use different techniques including direct calls or visits by pharmacists, to change physician prescribing behavior. Such "academic detailing" could supplement the work of pharmaceutical sales representatives. However, the most valuable disease

Figure 7-3. Continuum of Disease Management Initiatives in the Pharmaceutical Industry

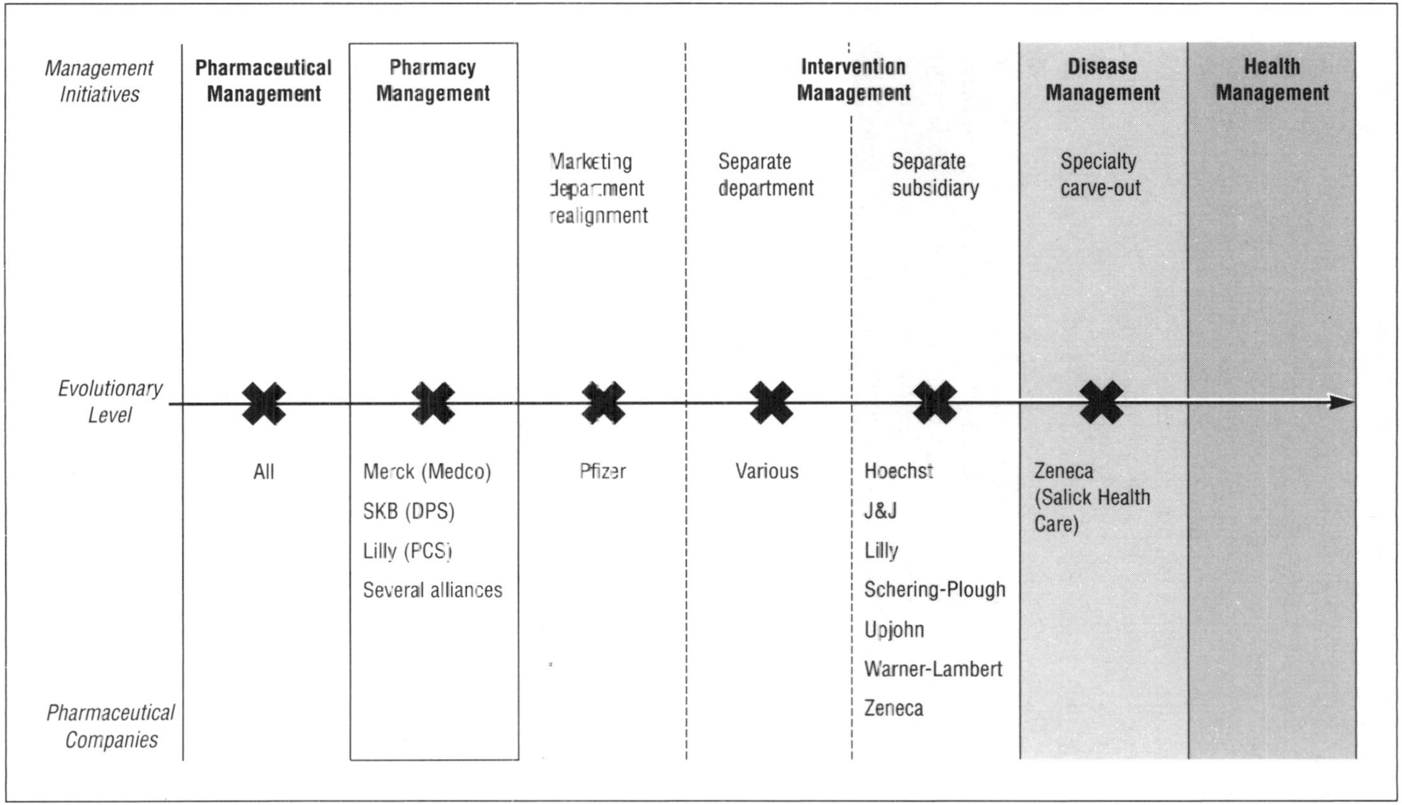

Management Initiatives	Pharmaceutical Management	Pharmacy Management	Intervention Management			Disease Management	Health Management
			Marketing department realignment	Separate department	Separate subsidiary	Specialty carve-out	
Evolutionary Level	✖	✖	✖	✖	✖	✖	→
Pharmaceutical Companies	All	Merck (Medco) SKB (DPS) Lilly (PCS) Several alliances	Pfizer	Various	Hoechst J&J Lilly Schering-Plough Upjohn Warner-Lambert Zeneca	Zeneca (Salick Health Care)	

management resource from PBMs is their extensive databases on the prescribing and use of pharmaceuticals, important information components for developing pharmacy-based disease management initiatives. These resources will become even more valuable as they become integrated with other health care databases. The integration and analysis of these disparate data sets will assist in the documentation of clinical, economic, and humanistic (for example, quality-of-life) outcomes.

Medco uses its extensive pharmacy database to identify and manage diabetic patients treated with insulin. It has partnered with Eli Lilly to introduce a "Diabetes Patient Support Program." Since the program's inception in 1992, Medco has enrolled over 195,000 patients from 415 plan sponsors.[6] The goals for the patients in the program include understanding and adopting self-management practices, improving glycemic control, reducing hospital admissions, and improving quality of life. Elements of the program are a drug utilization review program to enhance physician prescribing habits and avoid drug interactions, a newsletter to educate patients on self-management practices, toll-free telephone access to address specific patient information needs, patient self-assessment surveys, and physician survey cards.

Additional steps in the program include blood glucose self-monitoring, a hemoglobin A1C test program, a patient profile analysis to manage concomitant disorders, case management for high-cost/high-risk patients, and outcomes measures. A two-year outcomes analysis of 1,600 patients enrolled in the program demonstrated a reduction in total health care costs of $471 per patient per year. This decrease was the net result of a 13 percent decrease in hospitalizations, a 5 percent fall in outpatient visits, and a 1 percent dip in pharmaceutical costs, accompanied by increases of 2 percent in emergency room visits, 9 percent in physician visits, and 1 percent in other medical costs.[7]

Intervention Management

Pharmaceutical companies have formed a range of corporate structures to develop disease management intervention programs. Some companies, such as Pfizer, Inc., realigned their marketing departments into disease-specific groups. Many companies have formed separate disease management departments. And at least six companies have set up legally separate subsidiaries to develop intervention management programs to support the disease management initiatives of MCOs, government organizations, employers, and other health care organizations.[8]

Whatever the organizational structure, these initiatives share similar characteristics. First, the stated mission of such organizations is usually focused on improving health care quality while reducing its overall costs. Second, most of these organizations are composed of internally selected and externally recruited multidisciplinary professionals. Disciplines typically represented include medicine, pharmacy, nursing, case management, outcomes research/pharmacoeconomics, epidemiology, biostatistics, health informatics, business, marketing, managed care, finance, and others.

Generally the initiatives focus on developing a set of disease management "tools," or interventions, designed to support a managed care setting's overall disease management goals of standardized care, aligned incentives, efficient processes, and optimal outcomes. Pharmaceutical disease management organizations differ in three major ways: the level of corporate commitment, particularly regarding resources and funding; the extent to which the disease management interventions support product sales; and the quality of the disease management interventions being developed.

Greenstone Healthcare Solutions (GHS), a disease management subsidiary of The Upjohn Company, exemplifies the disease management strategy of a corporate spin-off entity. The overall mission of GHS is to develop innovative, technology-based tools and services to improve the quality of health care and enhance patient satisfaction.[9] Formed in 1995, GHS offers four categories of services: prospective health care, clinical practice optimization, therapy management, and data management.

Prospective health care includes programs to assess the health risks of members affiliated with an insurance or managed care plan and to encourage disease prevention and wellness. *Clinical practice optimization* assists medical directors with designing and implementing research-based clinical protocols. *Therapy management* helps to identify optimum treatment protocols and to enhance provider and patient compliance with such protocols. *Data management*, a cornerstone of all GHS services, provides tools and systems to integrate pharmacy and medical claims with patient demographics and clinical data.

GHS's primary target audiences are hospitals, MCOs, business coalitions, and insurance carriers. The company offers its products and services based on fee-for-service or risk-sharing contracts. It has been designed as a separate revenue-producing business with no direct Upjohn product ties.

Disease Management

To date, the vast majority of so-called disease management programs introduced by pharmaceutical companies would be better characterized as "intervention management" programs, primarily pharmacotherapeutic interventions. Prior to 1994, no pharmaceutical company owned or contracted with a group of providers to manage a population of patients at risk for or diagnosed with a particular disease — a major criterion for classifying disease management initiatives. However, that changed when Zeneca, Inc., a large British pharmaceutical and agricultural products company, purchased Salick Health Care Inc., an oncology disease management provider.[10] From a disease management perspective, Zeneca's acquisition was a more dramatic move than even Merck's purchase of Medco. Although Merck's action moved pharmaceutical manufacturers into part of the managed care industry, Zeneca's move represented the corporate transition from a pure supplier to a combination supplier-provider.

Unlike the pharmaceutical companies' purchases of PBMs that were initially intended to increase drug sales, Zeneca's purchase of Salick was designed to serve as a laboratory for understanding how best to differentiate its oncology drugs in a capitated managed care environment.[11] Fundamental to this quest was the leveraging of Salick's extensive database, which could facilitate outcomes research studies and oncology best practices research. Moreover, Salick's oncology carve-out service can serve as a valuable template for the development of disease management initiatives in other therapeutic areas.

Health Management

As of this writing, no pharmaceutical company has taken the next evolutionary step to become a health manager by developing or acquiring an HMO or other comprehensive health delivery organization. However, there have been several reports about plans for such actions. Pharmaceutical companies have established numerous strategic relationships for disease management activities with HMOs, most notably SmithKline Beecham's arrangement with United Healthcare. As part of its agreement to purchase the PBM division (DPS) from United Healthcare, SmithKline Beecham has access to United Healthcare's HMO database for six years.[12]

• Criteria for Assessing Pharmaceutical Industry Disease Management Programs

Given the preponderance of "disease management" programs and promotion put forth by the pharmaceutical industry, it is often difficult to evaluate the appropriateness and value of these initiatives. To facilitate the assessment of pharmaceutical industry–sponsored disease management programs, the author has created the "DM-10 Assessment Questionnaire." Listed in figure 7-4 are the 10 categories of questions that comprise the DM-10. A brief description of each question follows here.

1. *Where along the patient health care continuum is the disease management program designed to have its greatest impact?* This question helps to classify the disease management program and to determine the extent to which the pharmaceutical company has utilized disease mapping methodologies to identify the key clinical and economic "trigger points"

Figure 7-4. DM-10 Assessment Questionnaire™

1. Where along the patient health care continuum is the disease management program designed to have its greatest impact?
2. What disease states or conditions does the program target?
3. Who are the primary target audiences for the program, and what are they seeking?
4. What are the objectives for the disease management program, and how will it be measured?
5. What type of disease management service(s), product(s), or interventions(s) will be provided? Describe in detail the specific components of the program and how it will be customized to fit the needs of the target audience(s).
6. Who will design and implement the program and its components, and what is their track record?
7. Who will "own" the disease management program?
8. How will information be managed, and how will information technology be leveraged to achieve the program objectives?
9. What is the compensation structure to support the program?
10. What regulatory, legal, and legislative issues need to be considered, and how will they be addressed?

for a particular disease state. Does the disease management program demonstrate a health management orientation focusing on patient populations without a known disease, or a disease management orientation emphasizing patients with or at high risk for a specific disease? For example, Johnson & Johnson Health Care Systems has been developing health management programs that target specific patient populations, including senior citizens and women, and that initially emphasize identification, assessment, and stratification of risk followed by appropriate interventions.[13]

This approach is in contrast to most pharmaceutical initiatives, which concentrate on specific disease states and emphasize therapeutic interventions and measures. If companies take this latter approach, does the initiative focus on prevention, diagnosis, therapy, and/or maintenance of the particular disease state? More importantly, what are the key clinical and economic "trigger" or leverage points for the targeted disease condition, and how is the program structured to affect those trigger points for positive results? The latter question is especially relevant. Each disease has a different course that it generally follows. This course can be mapped to determine where interventions should be targeted to have the greatest clinical and economic benefit. The most sophisticated disease management programs are based on a thorough understanding of these "disease maps."

2. *Which disease states or conditions does the program target?* Pharmaceutical industry–sponsored programs generally target certain disease states that are characterized as high cost (for example, heart disease) or high

profile (for example, breast cancer) for their managed care and other customers; conditions that are inefficiently or ineffectively managed, resulting in increased resource utilization; those that primarily require pharmacotherapeutic treatment; and those that are usually chronic in nature. Most pharmaceutical company programs are based on the therapeutic areas in which the company has the most products and, therefore, expertise and resources.

For example, Parke-Davis, a division of Warner-Lambert, has been a leader in therapeutic management of epilepsy since its 1937 introduction of Dilantin (phenytoin), still the leading antiepileptic drug therapy. Parke-Davis has subsequently introduced several other antiepileptic medications. Leveraging its therapeutic expertise, resources, and partnerships (for example, Epilepsy Foundation of America) in this area, the company now offers the "Parke-Davis Seizure Management System" to help MCOs provide comprehensive, high-quality epilepsy care while reducing costs.[14] System components include a computerized risk-assessment analysis tool; customized treatment guidelines; guideline implementation support, such as sales representative support, mailings, and educational materials; patient education and compliance programs; and outcomes measurements.

Epilepsy is just one of the many therapeutic areas that pharmaceutical companies have targeted for intervention initiatives. The industry has either implemented or has in development several hundred other programs covering a wide range of conditions, including Alzheimer's disease; arthritis; cancers (such as breast cancer); cardiovascular diseases (that is, hypertension, hyperlipidemia, congestive heart failure, and angina); infectious diseases (ranging from AIDS to otitis media); migraine; osteoporosis; ulcers; and "women's health." To date, the most common disease states targeted by pharmaceutical companies are asthma, diabetes, and depression.[15]

3. *Who are the primary target audiences for the program, and what are they seeking?* The primary target audiences for pharmaceutical industry–sponsored disease management initiatives are MCOs, which currently influence or control the majority of the distribution and prescription of pharmaceutical products. By this definition, MCOs include HMOs, integrated delivery systems, insurance companies, hospital management companies, government agencies, PBM companies, and long-term care companies.

The key challenge for pharmaceutical companies is to be able to document the clinical and economic benefits of a disease management program within the one-year time frame that corresponds to the annual membership enrollment period of most MCOs. For example, if a disease management program can be shown to save money and improve or maintain the health of heart failure patients participating in a disease management program within a year, and if the benefits outweigh cost, it is likely the MCO will continue the program; if not, the program is likely to be eliminated.

Unfortunately, as long as employers continue to take a short-term perspective on containing health care costs, disease management programs will remain this way. A few sophisticated employers, such as John Deere, Digital, and Xerox, are looking past the one-year time frame, recognizing that although the MCOs are taking care of their employees one year at a time, the employer is responsible for its employees considerably longer, often throughout retirement. These companies and others are willing to give these programs longer than a single year to demonstrate their benefits economically. This perspective is particularly applicable to chronic conditions, such as osteoporosis and cardiovascular diseases, whose proper clinical management may result in economic benefits only over the long term.

Two other major stakeholders for disease management programs are providers and patients. Motivating physicians to participate and lead disease management initiatives often determines the ultimate success of such programs. Although financial incentives are helpful, pharmaceutical companies need to be able to demonstrate to physicians the clinical benefits inherent in their programs. Patients are the ultimate customers of disease management programs. Their program feedback to MCOs and employers can significantly influence the program's acceptance.

4. *What are the objectives for the disease management program, and how will it be measured?* Most observers would agree that disease management initiatives should have improving quality of care while reducing costs as their overall goal. But disease management programs need to have much more specific, *measurable* objectives. As shown in figure 7-5, disease management initiatives can be measured on numerous levels. Most people focus almost exclusively on outcomes measures, including clinical, economic, and humanistic (for example, quality-of-life measures). Although these are important, other variables also need to be considered.

To achieve positive outcomes repeatedly, processes need to be analyzed through best practices research and other tools to replicate beneficial results. Stakeholders in the program—including the managed care plan, providers, and patients—can be profiled by employing report cards, physician profiles, and patient surveys, respectively. Financial and technology audits can help determine the financial status and the information systems capabilities of disease management initiatives. Although the parameters listed in figure 7-5 are not exhaustive, they can assist in an overall assessment of the pharmaceutical company program and should be used where appropriate to determine whether the program has met its targeted objectives and how it competes with other such programs.

Figure 7-5. Measuring Disease Management Initiatives

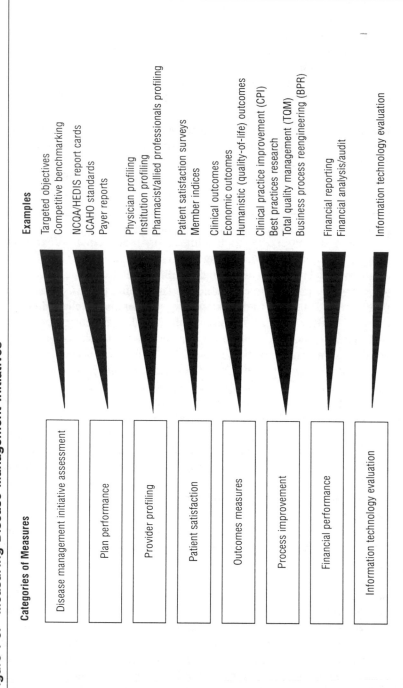

5. *What type of disease management service(s), product(s), or intervention(s) will be provided? Describe in detail the specific components of the program and how it will be customized to fit the needs of the target audience(s).* A typical pharmaceutical company offering represents interventions in a selected number of therapeutic areas, usually in those where the parent company has therapeutic expertise and products. The interventions can be classified into three major types of program components: design, implementation, and measurement/improvement.[16]

Program design components often center around clinical or therapeutic guidelines, usually based on established guidelines and developed in conjunction with managed care providers. *Implementation* tools, especially those developed to change physician behavior, are perhaps the industry's greatest strength. Such tools include provider education and compliance programs designed to increase practitioners' adherence to guidelines, formularies, and other health plan stipulations; and patient education and compliance programs to reinforce disease management initiatives among those who receive care. *Measurement and improvement* is the third category of disease management components. Most pharmaceutical disease management initiatives focus on clinical, economic, and humanistic outcomes research, an area in which the industry has increasing experience. More progressive companies provide more comprehensive measures as described previously. Whatever interventions are offered, they need to be tailored to fit the needs of the various stakeholders — the managed care organization, providers, patients, payers, and others.

6. *Who will design and implement the program and its components, and what is their track record?* Although pharmaceutical industry–sponsored disease management initiatives draw heavily on internal expertise and resources, there is a substantial need to augment these capabilities through third parties via strategic alliances, acquisitions, and outsourcing. Very few companies can develop, implement, and measure disease management initiatives on their own. This is particularly true for pharmaceutical companies, which do not provide direct patient care. Consequently, many pharmaceutical company disease management programs are an amalgamation of different organizations, components, and capabilities.

For example, GHS licensed 30 disease management programs developed by a unit of Lovelace Health Systems, a subsidiary of CIGNA Corp. and a leading developer of disease management programs, in an exclusive, 10-year arrangement. The agreement enables GHS to commercialize and implement disease management programs developed and validated by Lovelace.[17]

In assessing pharmaceutical company–sponsored disease management programs, it is important to know the capabilities and track record of the company and professionals leading the initiative, as well as their partners. What are their results? Who will be responsible for the various aspects of the program, and what is their accountability? Do they have past clients who would recommend them? Obviously, most pharmaceutical industry initiatives are in the early stages of implementation, but these are issues that need consideration.

7. *Who will "own" the disease management program?* Because disease management initiatives are often developed and implemented as a collaborative effort, it is important to establish which organization "owns" the rights to the program and the extent of those rights. Generally, the program can either be purchased by the MCO or the health care organization for which it was developed; owned by the pharmaceutical company that developed it; or owned jointly. For example, Group Health Cooperative of Puget Sound (GHCPS), a Washington State HMO, was assisted in its diabetes disease management program by two pharmaceutical companies, Eli Lilly and Boehringer Mannheim, which helped to develop patient education videos and outcomes studies. However, GHCPS owns the overall program, which incorporates many other disease management components as well.[18]

   For pharmaceutical companies that own and sell their own disease management programs, developing a disease management program entails a process not unlike the one used to develop and test a drug. The pharmaceutical company owns the program, but works with partners with different expertise to develop and test the product. For example, a pharmaceutical company may have an arrangement with an HMO to test clinical guidelines, work with a hospital system to prepare clinical care maps, obtain patient clinical data from an integrated delivery system, and license clinical decision-support tools from a software vendor. These different components are tested in a way similar to the manner in which drugs have to be tested for toxicology, pharmacology, clinical efficacy, and safety. Then the pharmaceutical company, acting as a general contractor, pulls the components together, packages the program, and commercializes it. More commonly, the pharmaceutical company acts as a partner or subcontractor and assists an MCO or other health care organization in the development of its internal disease management initiative.

8. *How will information be managed, and how will information technology be leveraged to achieve the program objectives?* Most experts recognize that the foundation of disease management programs is information management. Information management systems that underlie clinical, financial, and administrative data have the capability to drive virtually all aspects of disease management initiatives. However, information management is also the greatest challenge for disease managers. The current flow of electronic information, as detailed in figure 7-6, is based on the component management approach to health care, which is designed to provide a one-way flow of financial claims data from

Figure 7-6. Current Flow of Electronic Information

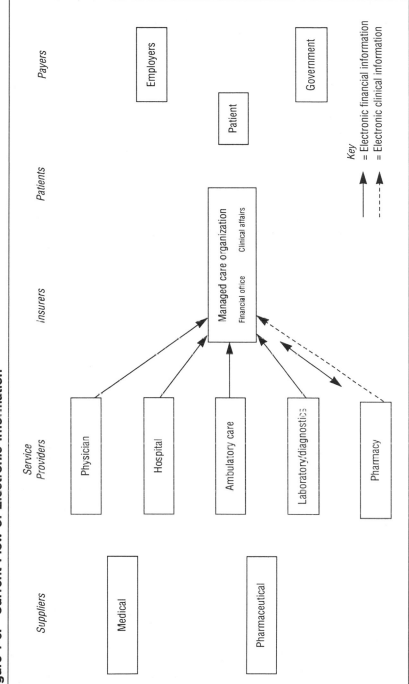

providers and suppliers to insurers (see chapter 1); the claims data from these different sources is rarely integrated.

The disease management approach really requires a flow of integrated clinical and financial data among the various health care stakeholders, including providers, payers, patients, suppliers, and insurers. Although many health care organizations are investing in computerized patient records, data warehouses, and other information technologies, there are only a small number with the kind of capabilities suggested in figure 7-7. Because of financial and other resource constraints, most MCOs will be phasing in integrated care systems over time.

The lack of integrated health care information is especially problematic for the pharmaceutical industry in two respects. First, the industry's whole premise behind disease management is based on having the integrated information to demonstrate the clinical and economic benefits of pharmaceutical products, the industry's most important type of disease management intervention. Using integrated health care data sets, pharmaceutical companies could potentially demonstrate that a cardiovascular agent actually reduces the number of myocardial infarctions, resulting in fewer emergency room visits, hospitalizations, cardiovascular surgeries, physician consults, and laboratory services. It also could be possible to integrate employer data to show benefits in higher employee productivity or reduced absenteeism.

Second, because the industry is not a direct health care provider, its access to patient data is restricted. Consequently, pharmaceutical companies often seek strategic partnerships with client or other health care delivery organizations to obtain such integrated health care data sets. Given the tremendous importance of information management in disease management programs, the industry has sought to expand its capabilities in collecting, integrating, analyzing, and communicating information with sophisticated information technology programs and systems. Increasingly, pharmaceutical companies are acquiring or aligning with health informatics companies to provide data and to enhance their informatics capabilities. For example, Eli Lilly has acquired the clinical networking firm Integrated Medical Systems, and Glaxo Wellcome has formed HealthPoint Inc. through a joint venture with Physician Computer Network in order to create clinical information products and services for disease management.[19]

In assessing initiatives, it is extremely important to determine the type of information that will be used; the source of the information; ownership of the raw and analyzed data; information flows and confidentiality of the data, especially patient records; the proposed benefits of the data analysis; and the duration and cost of the analysis. A general understanding of system architectures, database repositories, integration

Figure 7-7. Future Flow of Electronic Information

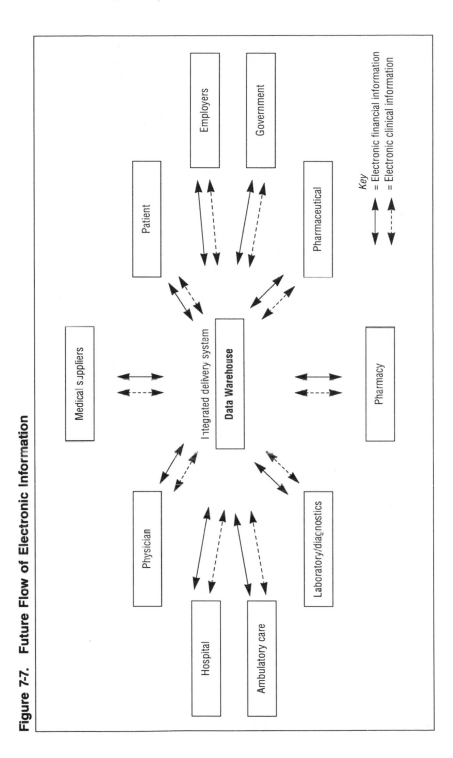

engines, analytical tools, user interfaces, and other information technologies as they relate to the disease management initiative is valuable as well.

9. *What is the compensation structure to support the program?* There is an extensive range of compensation options being considered as pharmaceutical companies implement disease management initiatives. Factors determining the type and extent of compensation include the category of disease management initiative; the nature and extent of services; characteristics of the disease state, including potential for carve-out, availability of clinical and financial data, and disease complexity; and experience and risk orientation of the disease management companies and their clients. The most important parameters in determining the compensation structure are the disease management category and type of services provided.

   For example, the most basic disease management programs offered by pharmaceutical companies (such as a package of provider education programs, patient education and compliance programs, and outcomes research studies) are being included as "value-added" options to enhance customer relationships or as part of a pharmaceutical contract incentive. Similarly, pharmacy-based programs offered by pharmaceutical company–owned PBMs are currently being provided free of charge as value-added components to differentiate their services. In the future, more elaborate pharmacy intervention programs may enable PBMs to charge a premium for such services.

   Dedicated disease management subsidiaries of pharmaceutical companies typically offer more advanced and comprehensive intervention management services and programs. Compensation options range from fee-for-service to risk-sharing arrangements, which may include performance-based incentives or participation in health care cost-savings agreements. For example, Parke-Davis has offered to risk share with MCOs through its seizure management program. Other types of "creative contracts" have been discussed as well. Pharmaceutical disease management carve-out companies, such as Zeneca's Salick Health Care, offer risk-sharing and/or capitation arrangements.

10. *Which regulatory, legal, and legislative issues need to be considered, and how will they be addressed?* In working with pharmaceutical companies on disease management initiatives, it is important to understand the role of regulatory issues in this highly regulated industry. The primary governmental agency overseeing the industry, the Food and Drug Administration (FDA), has not to date issued specific policies regarding disease management. The agency has adopted a "wait-and-see" approach regarding pharmaceutical initiatives into disease management. It has said, however, that it will continue to require companies to follow existing policies for product advertising and promotion.[20]

This latter point is pertinent for disease management programs. Pharmaceutical manufacturers are required to adhere to FDA-approved labeling, the product package insert that describes a drug's properties. However, this may be a challenging proposition for pharmaceutical companies involved in disease management.

For example, as part of a comprehensive disease management program, clinicians or managed care providers may develop or adopt clinical guidelines that encourage use of some pharmaceutical agents and that do not follow FDA labeling for those products. Some cancer products, for instance, may only be approved for one cancer, but are considered by the medical community to be the gold standard for other cancers as well. As partners or vendors in such programs, pharmaceutical companies are in a difficult situation. Evaluators of pharmaceutical disease management programs need to be aware of such potential restrictions and the company's policies so as not to jeopardize patients or the disease management initiative. This may affect companies differently depending on the relationship of the disease management subsidiary to the parent company.

Both the FDA and the Federal Trade Commission (FTC) have been closely scrutinizing the relationships between pharmaceutical companies and managed care companies. The FTC has already taken actions to ensure competitive fairness regarding the industry's vertical integration into the PBM business. The FDA has also held hearings related to managed care marketing initiatives.

Legal and legislative issues also need to be considered in working with pharmaceutical companies. Some of the most pressing current concerns revolve around the ownership and confidentiality of patient records and the extent of restrictions over managed care companies.

It is important for providers, payers, pharmaceutical companies, and others to explore each of these issues before entering into partnered disease management initiatives.

• Pharmaceutical Industry Prospects in Disease Management

There are inherent challenges and opportunities for pharmaceutical companies participating in disease management initiatives. Two major challenges involve financial feasibility and customer credibility. Companies that seek to use disease management as a tool to promote individual products may increase sales in the short term but run the risk of alienating their managed care customers. Conversely, companies used to high-margin technical products are unlikely to be enamored with less profitable, service-oriented interventions. Ideally, companies need to align their incentives with those of their managed care customers to bring value to both parties. Other hurdles to be overcome include the lack of access to patients, providers, and information unrelated to drugs; the lack of certain other capabilities and resources, including clinical management expertise and information technologies; the need to document the value of disease management initiatives; and potential regulatory or legal restrictions.[21]

Nonetheless, there are opportunities for pharmaceutical companies to play important roles in disease management. The industry brings to disease management an in-depth knowledge about specific disease states, a rigorous clinical research approach, a burgeoning outcomes management expertise, and effective provider and patient behavior modification techniques. The industry also has the financial resources to obtain those capabilities it may lack, as evidenced by its purchase of PBMs, its hiring of clinical professionals, and its increasing investment in information technologies. Furthermore, companies are motivated to be perceived as part of the solution to a deepening health care crisis. At the very least, the pharmaceutical industry has already played a critical role: It has increased awareness of the need for a systematic, integrated approach to managing patients.

References

1. Pharmaceutical Research and Manufacturers Association. *Opportunities and Challenges for Pharmaceutical Innovation.* Washington, DC: Pharmaceutical Research and Manufacturers Association, 1996, p. 12.

2. The Boston Consulting Group, Inc. *The Contribution of Pharmaceutical Companies: What's at Stake for America.* Boston: The Boston Consulting Group, Sept. 1993, pp. 143–57.

3. Bernard, S. Disease management: a pharmaceutical industry perspective. *Pharmaceutical Executive* 16(2):48–60, Mar. 1995.

4. Soumerai, S., and Avorn, J. Effects of Medicaid drug payment limits on admission to hospitals and nursing homes. *The New England Journal of Medicine* 325:1072–77, Oct. 1991.

5. Horn, S. D., and others. Intended and unintended consequences of HMO cost-containment strategies: results from the managed care outcomes project. *American Journal of Managed Care* 2:253–64, Mar. 1996

6. Gutman, J. Merck-Medco moves further into DM for diabetes, cardiovascular. *Disease Management News.* 1(17):2–3, July 25, 1996.

7. Gutman.

8. POV Incorporated. *Disease Management . . . And Its Impact on Business Strategy for the Pharmaceutical Industry.* Cedar Grove, NJ: POV, Inc., July 1995.

9. Greenstone Healthcare Solutions corporate brochure. Kalamazoo, MI: Greenstone Healthcare Solutions; (616) 323-4000.

10. Winslow, R. Zeneca sets purchase of 50 percent of Salick for $195 million; treatment data cited. *Wall Street Journal,* Dec. 23, 1995, p. B5.

11. Longman, R. Zeneca's PBM alternative. *In Vivo* 13(5):3–8, May 1995.

12. *SmithKline Beecham Annual Report and Accounts.* Philadelphia: SmithKline Beecham, Inc., 1994, p. 10.

13. Cassak, D. J & J Health Care Systems: beyond the supply chain. *In Vivo* 14(2):33–44, Feb. 1996.

14. Weiss, R. C. *Epilepsy: Improving Care, Lowering Costs.* Newark, NJ: Parke-Davis Healthcare Systems, 1996; (201) 540-2000.

15. POV Incorporated, p. 143.

16. Bernard.

17. Gutman, J., editor. Greenstone licenses 30 Lovelace DM programs. *Disease Management News* 1(9):1, Feb. 25, 1996.

18. Bernard.

19. Gutman, J. Drug giants look to link with informatics firms for DM purposes. *Disease Management News* 1(18):1, 5, July 10, 1996.

20. Pendergrast, M. Regulatory trends at the FDA—the long view. Presentation at the Pharmaceutical Executive Conference, Princeton, NJ, Oct. 16, 1995.

21. POV Incorporated, pp. 569–74.

Chapter 8

Disease Management in Managed Care Organizations

Joseph E. Biskupiak, PhD, MBA, Peter Chodoff, MD, MPH,
and David B. Nash, MD, MBA

It is believed that disease management may aid managed care organizations (MCOs) in their mission of providing high-quality, cost-effective health care, and it is this relationship that is examined in this chapter. The text first investigates the motivations behind the development of disease management by MCOs. Next, the current status of disease management in MCOs is considered, and a description of the elements necessary to engage in disease management is established. Examples of actual disease management programs at MCOs are described as well as potential partnership models. These examples illustrate how far disease management has advanced and how much further it still needs to go. After finishing this chapter, the reader should have a greater appreciation for the challenges involved in successful disease management in the managed care setting.

• A Natural Evolution

The development of disease management systems is a natural evolution for MCOs. MCOs are developing disease management programs as an extension of earlier efforts to fulfill their mission of providing high-quality, cost-effective health care. Even though pharmaceutical manufacturers may been early leaders in the development of disease management initiatives, the concept of improving the quality of health care delivered to patients along disease-specific lines did not necessarily originate with these manufacturers.

The authors would like to thank Mark Zitter of The Zitter Group for providing copies of the two proprietary reports entitled "The 1994 Disease Management Report on Diabetes" and "The 1994 Disease Management Report on Asthma" and for allowing us to report on the findings contained within. Without those two reports, it would have been difficult if not impossible to write a chapter on disease management at MCOs.

MCOs have struggled for a long time with the reputation of delivering substandard medicine (that is, low-quality health care) and being more focused on managing costs than care. Disease management programs hold the promise of helping MCOs deliver higher-quality health care at a lower cost than traditional fee-for-service insurance, which was the raison d'être for MCO formation.[1]

Forces Driving MCO Interest in Disease Management

As discussed in chapter 9, MCOs have participated in several forms of "first-generation" disease management via utilization review (UR), utilization management (UM), and, later, proactive forms of case management. Utilization review and its more prospective "cousin" utilization management, attempt to determine which services are medically necessary and appropriate under certain diagnoses and where those necessary services should be delivered. Unfortunately, these early efforts, which frequently focused on economic outcomes versus clinical outcomes, were not always as proactive as they could have been, and lacked the integration and sophistication of the newer forms of disease management. Eventually, the focus of MCOs, at least those that want to be survivors in the evolving health care marketplace, will have to be on quality improvement with a more appropriate balance between economic and clinical outcomes. Another important difference between UR/UM and today's versions of disease management is the focus on prevention and wellness initiatives. The original promise of the health maintenance organization (HMO) concept was that these organizations would reduce costs by focusing on early intervention and preventive care. These original basic principles of HMOs (now more broadly known as MCOs) are very similar to those of disease management.

Quality improvement requires that MCOs critically examine what happens to patients as they move through the system (that is, health outcomes and patient satisfaction achieved). It also examines how they can improve that progression to achieve optimal outcomes.

Although MCOs and disease management programs are ideally suited to one another, there are a number of forces (both internal and external) fueling MCOs' high level of interest in disease management. Internally, the goal of delivering high-quality, cost-effective health care is driving MCOs to develop and implement disease management programs. In some respects, disease management is being considered as the next "silver bullet" for many MCOs. Externally, their customers (that is, employer groups) are demanding that MCOs demonstrate that they can deliver high-quality care. A number of the major internal and external forces driving the interest in the disease management "movement" among MCOs are discussed in the following subsections.

Reduced Margins/Profits/Premiums

Although MCOs have performed exceptionally well financially during the past several years, competition has forced a rapid decline in premium increases. Last year, for the first time, MCO premium increases were lower than the increase in the general inflation rate.

However, unless MCOs can find ways to further reduce cost/utilization, the relatively flat premiums of recent years will be a thing of the past. Because UR, UM, and other MCO cost-containment efforts have been relatively successful, the law of diminishing returns dictates that MCOs find other means to reduce costs. Disease management is viewed as the next major cost-containment strategy by many MCOs.

Growth of Capitation

The expansion of capitation as a form of reimbursement for providers also has created a high level of motivation for providers to find new ways to both maintain and improve clinical outcomes while reducing costs. Increasingly, MCOs are being paid on a capitated—per member per month (PMPM) premium—basis by employers. Any cost savings achieved through a disease management program accrues to the MCO, or to its providers if the MCO decides to pass on the risk.

If disease management succeeds, all parties win. Patients are healthier, employees miss less time at work, and the MCO can pocket the savings resulting from not having to care for increasingly sicker members. Perhaps even more important, capitation opens the door to more creative forms of patient care than fee-for-service (FFS) reimbursement systems that may hinder the application of a variety of cost-effective interventions just because they do not fit into the existing reimbursement structure. There are many examples of how the old component system of health care delivery actually hindered the optimization of clinical, as well as economic, outcomes. Chronic illnesses, such as diabetes and asthma, are perhaps the best examples of this syndrome. The lack of reimbursement for patient education helped contribute to unnecessary exacerbations of these diseases and the resulting higher utilization of expense medical services.

Consolidation/Integration

The rate of consolidation in the managed care industry has accelerated, resulting in increased integration. Because disease management, in today's form, requires a high level of integration, the consolidation and integration of MCOs and other health care organizations has facilitated and will continue to help facilitate the growth of disease management initiatives.

Technology/Sophisticated Information Systems

The combination of improved profitability and consolidation has led to a significant investment by MCOs in more sophisticated information systems (ISs). It is important to realize that only MCOs with integrated information systems will be able to successfully execute the type of sophisticated disease management programs needed to achieve significant economic *and* clinical outcomes. These highly integrated information systems need to have several capabilities, including:

- Completely integrated medical and pharmacy claims databases
- Access to patient treatments and outcomes
- Tracking of patients and influencing care across various treatment settings
- Identification and notification of high-risk enrollees for preventive care

MCOs will also need to be electronically linked to physicians' offices, where much of the care delivery takes place. Although a completely electronic medical record would be a useful feature of an integrated IS, it is not an absolute requirement. A patient's diagnosis, treatment, and outcomes are the relevant data for disease management, and they do not need to be captured electronically.

HEDIS/Report Card Systems

As the interest of large employers in containing health care costs has grown, so has the demand for accreditation systems that allow both employers and employees to more easily compare different health plans. Increasingly, employers believe they can and should hold health plans accountable for their health care performance by demanding that MCOs obtain the accreditation imprimatur of the National Committee for Quality Assurance (NCQA) or other accreditation agencies. The NCQA is a private, nonprofit organization that seeks to assess and report on the quality of health care delivered by MCOs. It is governed by a board of directors that includes employers; consumer, labor, and MCO representatives; quality experts; state and federal regulators; and representatives from organized medicine. The accreditation process, which rates an MCO's level of compliance with NCQA standards, covers the following areas: quality management and improvement, utilization management, credentialing, members' rights and responsibilities, preventive health services, and medical records.[2]

It is important to recognize that this accreditation process measures an MCO's compliance with administrative matters regarding its operation. It is not a rating of the quality of care the MCO delivers. In order to answer the questions, "How do I understand what 'value' my health care dollar is purchasing?" and "How do I hold a health plan 'accountable' for its performance?" NCQA developed the Health Plan Employer Data and Information Set (HEDIS). A set of performance measures that attempts to answer the preceding questions, HEDIS covers five areas of performance, including quality of care, access and patient satisfaction, membership and utilization, finance, and descriptive information on health plan management. It has had the unintentional effect of being a major factor in encouraging MCOs to develop disease management programs in diabetes and asthma, as well as other diseases. Two performance measures in the area of quality of care regarding acute and chronic disease are the "asthma inpatient admission rate for pediatrics" and "diabetic retinal exam." MCOs, knowing that the quality of care they deliver will be assessed by these two performance measures, have implemented or are planning to implement disease management programs in asthma and diabetes to positively effect better outcomes in these areas.

Physician Readiness

Much of the fear, agony, and talk that accompanied the government's anticipated and infamous "health care reform" helped evolve the mind-set of many health care providers. Physicians who not too long ago were adamant concerning their position against the use of clinical practice guidelines (CPGs) are now much more open to their use. This changed mind-set has also been reflected in the growing involvement of physicians as entrepreneurs in new forms of health care delivery systems and physician-oriented MCOs. The days of the small "p" in physician–hospital organization (pHOs) may be over in that we are beginning to see more small "h" versions of the PhO.

Early Outcomes Data

The availability of some outcomes data from a number of the true first generation of disease management programs has helped encourage other MCOs to initiate similar initiatives. Although largely anecdotal, these early results have added that "little push" needed by some MCOs to gear up their efforts.

Recognition of Chronic Illness

MCOs have historically focused much of their cost-containment efforts on acute, episodic illness via UR/UM programs, volume price discounts from providers, and so forth. These same organizations have now reached the stage where they have to start addressing chronic illnesses. They are now beginning to develop the disease management systems needed to reduce the treatment costs associated with patients with certain chronic illnesses. MCOs, in an effort to further reduce utilization/costs, are developing disease management programs for those chronic diseases that have the following characteristics:

- High incidence in the target population
- Frequent utilization of specialty physician visits and emergency room visits
- Repeated inpatient hospital admissions
- Inappropriate drug utilization
- Improved clinical and quality-of-life outcomes possible through patient education and self-monitoring

Again, asthma and diabetes have been prime targets for the disease management efforts of many MCOs because both diseases possess many of the aforementioned characteristics. The case for improved management of asthma is very compelling given the direct costs of asthma care in the United States. In 1990, the direct costs of asthma were $3.6 billion, of which emergency room/hospital/outpatient accounted for 56 percent, drug use 30 percent, and physician fees 14 percent. Patients with severe asthma account for only 4 percent (0.5 million patients) of all asthmatics (15 million patients), but are responsible for more than 50 percent of the medical resources used in asthma treatment. It has been estimated that approximately half of these patients require such resources as the result of treatment failures. Many believe that disease management programs in asthma can result in significant cost savings.[3] Any MCO that reduces its asthma inpatient admission rate will probably save money and help its HEDIS rating.

Similarly, diabetes meets many of the previously mentioned criteria. The Diabetes Control and Complications Trial (DCCT), a 10-year controlled, randomized clinical trial launched in 1983 by the National Institute of Diabetes and Digestive and Kidney Diseases, assessed the safety and determined the benefits of intensive blood sugar control.[4] The DCCT showed that intensive treatment that keeps blood glucose levels as close to normal as possible slows the onset and progression of long-term diabetes complications, including eye (retinopathy), kidney (nephropathy), and nerve (neuropathy) disease. It should be noted that diabetes is the most common cause of blindness in adults in the United States. In addition, diabetes is the most common cause of end-stage renal disease in this country, with an estimated treatment cost to the federal government of $7.26 billion per year. Again, it is believed that disease management programs in diabetes can result in significant savings to health plans.

Simply put, asthma, diabetes, and other chronic diseases have finally "gotten on to the radar screen" of MCOs. They also have identified the concept of disease management as a way to reduce the cost of chronic diseases while maintaining, and perhaps increasing, patient quality of life.

• Considerations in the Implementation of Disease Management

Most MCOs are now developing and implementing their own disease management programs, focusing on CPGs for clinicians (see chapter 6) and on a variety of disease management interventions (see chapter 2). As these programs are designed, developed, and implemented, MCOs must address a number of factors that may potentially impede their success. These factors are discussed in the following subsections.

Short-Term versus Long-Term Focus

One of the major challenges facing MCOs is that of temporal focus, long term versus short term.[5] There are various time constraints in an MCO's environment. Most disease management programs require a long-term focus, but MCOs have membership disenrollment rates of 16.5 percent per year.[6] MCOs might argue that engaging in disease management programs is fruitless because of the length of time required for a payoff to be realized, when, in the short term, 16.5 percent of their current members will not be members in the near future.

This argument is flawed because it fails to recognize that MCOs will gain new members in the future that may have belonged to other organizations. Eventually, when the majority of the population receives its care in a managed care environment, MCOs will more readily recognize the value of disease management programs, even when the payoff is far in the future. Additionally, there are disease management programs with short-term goals that strive to avoid emergency room visits or inpatient hospital admissions. In the short term, it is probably more expensive to engage in disease management, because the organization will do more and spend more on patients; however, the long-term focus is to keep a population as healthy as possible and prevent chronically ill patients from progressing to more severe stages of their disease. The hope is that in the long run, this strategy will reduce costs by improving the health status of the MCO's enrollees.

Another confounding factor is that the competition in the marketplace seems to result in a continuing downward spiral in premium prices. Again, the MCO's focus is on the short term — namely, is a large employer group going to renew its contract for the coming year or go with a competitor offering a lower premium? In mature managed care markets (that is, markets where there is little difference in PMPM premiums), engaging in disease management programs may prove beneficial because these markets base competition not on price, but rather on the delivery of high-quality care (and the ability to demonstrate it). The price factor is interesting because of its dual and potentially conflicting role in disease management. On one hand, the current flat rate of premium price increases has motivated many MCOs to "take on" disease management programs for chronic illness, and the long-term payout on these programs may force MCOs to revise their thinking on disease management as a whole. In the meantime, it is obvious that MCOs are focusing on diseases that also hold the promise of short-term cost reductions. This temporal issue will play an important role in whether MCOs move on to address more complex diseases and whether they will actually make the leap from disease management into health management. These future transitions are discussed in chapter 12. It is, however, clear that in the long run the success of disease management and, eventually, population-based health management will hinge on what value society places on health care.

Carve-Ins versus Carve-Outs

Although MCOs have welcomed the assistance of pharmaceutical manufacturers or pharmacy benefit managers in their disease management initiatives, many do not want to totally carve out their disease management program to these organizations (pass on the disease cost/risk to providers) due to concerns regarding loss of control of their patients' treatment and loss of the opportunity to capture the reduced costs. One notable exception, aside from mental health and ophthalmology, which are traditional carve-outs, is Salick Health Care, founded in 1983 by nephrologist Dr. Bernard Salick. This organization has been successful in negotiating disease management carve-out contracts with managed care to provide cancer treatment.[7] The impetus to carve out various diseases versus merely contracting for various segments of a disease management program (a carve-in) depends on a variety of factors that include:

- The ability of the MCO to access and manage the data needed to implement a carve-out contract
- Potential conflict with existing contractual arrangements, for example, global capitation contracts with large integrated delivery systems, PHOs, and so forth
- The desire to maintain risk, along with the potential for profit from improved management of the risk

Clearly the jury is out on carve-outs. However, given the continued trend toward MCO consolidation and the increased ability/interest of MCOs in developing their own disease management programs, it is likely that most initiatives from non-MCOs will be in the form of carve-ins. (Carve-outs and carve-ins are discussed in more detail in chapter 4.) The issue of carve-ins/carve-outs is intertwined with the issue of "make versus buy." Many MCOs are recognizing that some of the components of disease management systems can and should be purchased for enhanced quality and/or cost-effectiveness. Disease management components purchased from external organizations also offer the added benefit of being regularly enhanced. This make-versus-buy decision is not dissimilar to those made concerning capital equipment, wherein the purchaser does not want to absorb the risk of rapidly changing technology. In several chapters in this book, the concept of sharing the risk of developing disease management programs with strategic partners is highly recommended. Chapter 11 addresses the potential of strategic business alliances in more detail.

Acceptance/Use of Clinical Practice Guidelines

Many of the disease management programs currently being developed and implemented by MCOs rely on providers' use of CPGs. Most of these efforts are focused on high-cost chronic diseases, such as diabetes, asthma, and, to a much lesser extent, hypertension. MCOs are implementing CPGs to standardize the management of targeted conditions (that is, reduce unexplained clinical variation) as an initial approach to disease management. Most of these CPGs also include patient education programs stressing the importance of lifestyle, patient self-management and testing, and drug compliance. Critics of disease management question whether MCOs will be successful in convincing physicians to adhere to these "best practices." Some of the early disease management programs that focused heavily on the use of CPGs by primary care physicians (PCPs) yielded disappointing results. It is worth repeating that considerable progress has been made in the quality and accessibility of CPGs. Although chapter 6 addresses the issues related to CPGs in some detail, there are additional issues to be discussed here.

Currently, 2,000 CPGs have been developed by various governmental agencies, academic medical centers, specialty societies, organized medicine, MCOs, and independent research centers. In addition, the American Medical Association (AMA) maintains a registry of approximately 2,000 practice parameters developed by 75 national physician specialty organizations.

Importantly, CPGs that are chosen to be incorporated into disease management activities need to possess certain attributes that will facilitate their use by clinicians. These attributes have been specified by the Institute of Medicine (IOM) and are presented in the following list:[8]

- *Validity:* Guidelines are valid if they lead to the health outcomes they project.
- *Strength of evidence:* A description of how the strength of evidence was weighed should accompany each statement in the guideline. These statements vary in the strength of their evidence and therefore in their acceptability. One must distinguish among care for which there is good scientific evidence, care for which there is good consensus but limited or no evidence, and care for which there is neither evidence nor consensus. It is interesting to note that in the Agency for Health Care Policy and Research's (AHCPR's) strength-of-evidence scheme, shown in figure 8-1, expert opinion is at the bottom of the list.[9]
- *Outcomes:* Guidelines should include an estimate of the expected health and cost outcomes, including patient preferences.
- *Reliability:* CPGs are reliable if (1) given the same circumstances, another group of experts produces essentially the same set of statements, and (2) the guidelines are interpreted consistently in the same set of clinical circumstances by different practitioners.

Figure 8-1. AHCPR Literature Quality-Rating System

>   I. Evidence from large, well-conducted randomized controlled trials (RCTs)
> II. Evidence from small, well-conducted RCTs
> III. Evidence from well-conducted cohort studies
> IV. Evidence from well-conducted case-control studies
> V. Evidence from uncontrolled or poorly controlled studies
> VI. Conflicting evidence, but tending to favor the recommendation
> VII. Expert opinion

- *Applicability:* The population(s) to which the guidelines apply should be explicitly defined.
- *Flexibility:* CPGs should identify areas of known controversy and discuss how patient preferences are to be identified and considered.
- *Clarity:* Guidelines must be concise, use unambiguous language, and be easy to follow.
- *Multidisciplinary process:* The guideline development process must include all members of the group providing services for the particular clinical circumstance.
- *Review:* CPGs must include statements defining the process by which they will be reviewed and kept up to date.

It is interesting to point out that although these attributes were developed for CPGs, many apply equally well to disease management programs.

MCOs that develop disease management programs using CPGs will need to be cognizant of the attributes that facilitate provider implementation. Similarly, developers of disease management programs will need to develop programs that possess many of these same attributes if they hope to have providers adopt and successfully implement their programs.

The Role of Case Management

Critics of disease management may consider it to be nothing more than glorified case management. Indeed, often the coordination of disease management programs is based on a case management approach. The role of case management in disease management programs is discussed in some detail in chapter 9. Although the role of the case manager has been well defined for many acute, episodic disease conditions, effectively dealing with the chronically ill in a prospective fashion is a relatively new challenge for case managers. The ability of MCOs to effectively utilize the case management function in disease management initiatives will hinge on the ability of case managers to adapt their roles and to acquire new skill sets, and on the sophistication of the information systems made available to case managers.

Case management essentially seeks to identify high-cost patients, both prospectively and retrospectively, and reduce the costs of their care. These patients are assigned a nurse case manager who functions as an educator to the patient and augments the care provided by the patient's physician. Prospectively, patients for surgical procedures are identified, and the case manager works closely with discharge planners to reduce the hospital length of stay. Case managers can coordinate the transition from the hospital setting to a lower-cost setting (such as long-term care facility, skilled nursing facility, rehabilitation hospital, home health care, and so forth).

Retrospectively, patients who have been admitted to the hospital frequently or visited the emergency room regularly are identified, and the nurse case manager develops a comprehensive ambulatory care program for them. The goal of this type of program is to reduce the use of hospital resources by the specific patient group. These programs typically have a patient education component that is provided by a visiting nurse in the patient's home or a hospital-sponsored education program in which the patient is enrolled. The patient also is educated regarding the value of self-monitoring his or her disease and the importance of drug compliance.

Because patients with chronic diseases are typically the more severely ill, the case manager is also responsible for ensuring that they have access to specialists and in-home medical equipment, when appropriate. The case manager can also act on the patient's behalf to design a treatment plan that goes beyond the health plan's covered benefits. Case management based on the retrospective identification of high resource use most closely resembles many of the features of current disease management programs. Case management of patients who have high resource utilization rates will probably result in improved management of the patients' health and reduce costs to the MCO. If a patient's use of the emergency room is reduced by having a case manager (that is, a nurse) call on him or her in the home to provide education on lifestyle choices, drug compliance, disease progression, and symptom recognition requiring medical assistance, these goals represent laudable outcomes for all disease management programs. Case management attempts to educate the patient and coordinate the care that is delivered across the continuum. Those MCOs that develop/expand their case management services will have a competitive advantage over organizations that do not recognize the importance and changing nature of case management in disease management.

Partnership Philosophy

As suggested earlier in this chapter as well as in chapters 2 and 11, the capabilities required to effectively develop and implement disease management systems are significant. Strategists say that organizations hoping to address major new initiatives within a rapidly changing environment should seriously consider spreading some of the development cost and risk to partners who have similar motivations and complementary capabilities. Many MCOs are, in fact, developing these partnership arrangements for disease management. Although the significance of adopting a partnership philosophy in the development of disease management programs seems reasonably straight-forward, it represents a major leap for some MCOs that have developed more of an "us-versus-them," vendor-oriented approach toward their provider networks. Again, given the potentially long-term nature of many chronic illness disease management programs, MCOs need to adopt a more allied approach to their provider relationships.

An often overlooked "partner" in discussions regarding disease management is the home health care agency (and to a lesser extent the home infusion provider). Most MCOs use home care agencies to provide care for patients that they are case managing. The agency acts as an important intermediary coordinating care and communication between the health plan, the patient, and the physician. It is important to remember that the need for disease management grew out of the lack of communication among these parties and is believed to be necessary because of the fragmented approach to health care in the United States.

Many home care companies have developed their own disease management programs and are offering them to MCOs on either a carve-in or a carve-out basis. Many of these organizations are offering "one-stop shopping" to MCOs by integrating a number of alternate-site delivery capabilities into one easy-to-access network that can be carved out and capitated by the MCO. One home care company, Protocall, based in Voorhees, NJ, offers a case management program in asthma. Once contracted by an MCO to case manage an asthma patient, Protocall sends an asthma nurse specialist to call on the patient and his or her family in the patient's home on a regular schedule. The nurse also contacts the patient's physician to inform him or her that Protocall has been assigned to case manage the patient for the health plan and to arrange for any standing orders for medications. The nurse is responsible for assessment and evaluation of the patient, patient and family education, nebulizer and peak flow meter use, and ongoing patient management and assessment. The patient is educated to recognize symptoms of his or her disease and to call on the Protocall nurse when the condition worsens. The Protocall nurse is empowered by the health plan and the patient's physician to coordinate and initiate the necessary medical care in whatever setting that care needs to be delivered. On the regularly scheduled visits to the patient's home, the nurse also collects a set of data (that is, outcomes measures) relating to the patient's asthma. Some of these measures include:

- Frequency of exacerbations
- Changes in severity or functional status

- Frequency of physician and emergency room visits
- Medication usage
- Work/school days missed

Protocall reports no knowledge of any of its customers currently using these data in any meaningful way. This case management program has all of the components of a disease management program. The only major part that is lacking is a transformation of the data into useful information that can be fed back to the health plan, patient's physician, and Protocall to modify the management of the patient. As this example illustrates, home care providers can and should be an important focal point of any disease management program, and any organization interested in disease management should consider the important role that home care can play. MCOs, as well as pharmaceutical manufacturers and pharmacy benefit management (PBM) companies, would be well advised to not only remember the important role that home care can play in disease management but to view their business arrangements with home care providers as a partnership versus a "vendor" relationship. Chapter 10 addresses the role of home care providers in the implementation of disease management initiatives.

• Managed Care's Current Attitude toward Disease Management

A recent Associated Press news article carried the following headline: "Disease Management/Next Trend?"[10] Many in health care believe that disease management is the latest fad, one that will eventually fade away. Others believe it represents a *paradigm shift* in health care from the traditional philosophy of only treating patients when they are ill to preventing disease and maintaining a patient's health.

Industry Survey

Surveys conducted by The Zitter Group, in San Francisco, offer some illuminating insights into the current status of disease management in MCOs. The results of these surveys have been summarized in two proprietary reports entitled *The 1994 Disease Management Report on Diabetes* and *The 1994 Disease Management Report on Asthma*. This section discusses the conclusions presented in these reports to highlight the current status of disease management across the managed care industry and then reviews specific examples of disease management at individual MCOs.

Over 50 percent of the 62 organizations surveyed by The Zitter Group, which included MCOs and PBMs, stated that they were either considering, developing, or implementing disease management programs. Interestingly, in the current political debate over reforming Medicare, an alternative plan released by Senate Democrats on October 2, 1995, included a provision that would allow Medicare to contract directly with chronic disease management programs. It is apparent that disease management will be present on the health care landscape in the short term. However, its long-term survival is dependent on its ability to make good on the promise of improving *both* clinical and economic outcomes.

Criteria Used for Selecting Disease States

In the Zitter surveys, a variety of criteria were identified that MCOs use most frequently to determine which diseases will be selected for the development of disease management programs. The most common responses included the following:

- Incidence of the disease
- Magnitude of treatment costs
- Amount of practice variation in treating the disease
- Employer requests
- HEDIS requirements
- The potential for documenting overall patient improvement

An additional criterion used to select diseases for disease management initiatives is the chronic nature of the disease. Importantly, chronic illnesses are seen as conditions where patients' management of their condition can significantly affect both cost and quality of life. Within this backdrop, diseases mentioned most frequently are asthma, diabetes, and hypertension. Asthma is the disease typically chosen first. In addition to the reasons stated earlier, there are several other common reasons that MCOs choose to develop an asthma disease management program, including the following:

- Asthma interventions typically yield outcomes in a relatively short period of time (recall the short-term focus of MCOs). This is due to the high incidence of emergency room visits and the high use of drugs. It is believed that many emergency room visits are unnecessary and that appropriate drug use would reduce the overall utilization of drugs. Additionally, literature has documented the ability of patient education programs to improve health status and quality of life.
- Asthma affects a large proportion of the population.
- Asthma is often cited by employers as an area of focus because of the large number of work- and school days lost as a result of the disease. Studies indicate that more than 10 million school days are "lost" to the disease annually, as well as more than 3 million workdays.

- HEDIS includes a measurement of "pediatric hospital readmissions for asthma." This single factor has created a frenzy of asthma "intervention" programs at MCOs.

Factors "Driving" Disease Management

In addition to the forces suggested earlier as enabling/motivating the development of disease management programs, the Zitter surveys discovered that MCOs are developing these programs primarily because of the influence of three factors: a process champion, accountability for clinical outcomes, and accountability for cost management. In the following discussion the latter two factors are grouped together.

Process Champions

The concept of a process champion was an interesting and somewhat unanticipated response to the question of influences. A *process champion* is an individual or group within an organization that has a strong desire to improve patient care related to a specific disease. The involvement of a process champion can go a long way in the development of a disease management program and most certainly helps sustain the disease management team discussed in chapter 2. In addition, identifying the process champions at an MCO is beneficial to pharmaceutical manufacturers and PBMs that would like to be part of the disease management process at an MCO.

It was also noted in the surveys that both clinicians and administrators within MCOs see the potential of disease management and are receptive to it. For clinicians, the prospect of standardizing the care of patients with chronic diseases — in other words, reducing the unexplained clinical variation in the management of these patients — was appealing. Administrators see the potential to document the quality of care provided and believe that it will lower treatment costs. MCOs also believe that employers will be attracted to disease management and make decisions about which health plans to offer their employees based on the existence of disease management programs. Clearly, MCOs and other health care organization view disease management as an opportunity to differentiate themselves from their competition.

Accountability for Clinical Outcomes and Cost Management

Interestingly, two of the three reasons cited for developing disease management programs are difficult to document, namely, outcomes and cost savings. The surveys found that almost all the participants were unable to fully evaluate the success of their disease management programs. The following quote from one of the individuals interviewed regarding a disease management program in asthma was typical of most MCOs: "We are still struggling with the program to see what kind of impact it has had." Almost all of the participants felt that the investment in disease management would pay off in the end, but there was a lack of documentation regarding improved outcomes and cost savings. Clinical outcomes measurements, although globally recognized as an integral part of disease management, were the most difficult to obtain. As indicated in chapter 3, the health care industry has been more geared to the measurement of economic outcomes than to the measurement of clinical outcomes.

Disease management requires a continuous quality improvement (CQI) approach. If an MCO cannot measure both the clinical and economic outcomes it hopes to achieve, as indicated by the Zitter survey, then are they really engaged in disease management? Probably not. As suggested earlier in this chapter, disease management as it exists currently at most MCOs is merely some form of practice guidelines for clinicians and a variety of demand management interventions that emphasize patient education, prevention, wellness, and so forth.

The two elements that were lacking in most disease management programs were *clinical health economics research* and *cost-of-treatment analysis*. It is not surprising that most MCOs cannot document any cost savings as a result of their disease management programs, when they do not even have the ability to establish what it currently costs them to treat patients with chronic diseases, and/or have not fully costed out the programs themselves. Indeed, the ability to simply identify members with chronic diseases is a major challenge for many health care plans.

U.S. Healthcare (USHC), a large for-profit individual practice association (IPA)–model HMO, based in Blue Bell, PA, has engaged in research to develop tools to provide a foundation for patient identification, classification, and risk-adjustment methodologies (U.S. Quality Algorithms Clinical Groups and USHC Membership Chronic Disease Database). Although USHC did not participate in The Zitter Group surveys, its research points out some of the difficulties in simply identifying members with chronic illness.

One of the problems the research uncovered was the difficulty that PCPs have in verifying a list of their diabetic patients without the assistance of a computerized medical record.[11] Although information from ICD-9 and CPT-4 codes from claims and encounter files, pharmacy data, utilization patterns of certain laboratory tests, and patient demographic data can all be used to identify potential members with chronic diseases, the presence of a chronic disease needs to be verified by review of the patient's medical record in his or her PCP's office. Without a computerized medical record, this can become a daunting task. One has to wonder whether the ability to review a patient's medical record favors the staff-model HMO over the other forms of HMOs in the absence of computerization. However, it is interesting to note that in a presentation of its asthma disease management program at a disease management conference, the Mayo Clinic, a staff-model operation, reported some difficulty in achieving desired results from its program.

Pharmaceutical manufacturers and PBMs that approach MCOs trying to market disease management programs with risk-sharing arrangements would be well advised to consider MCOs' lack of knowledge regarding treatment costs and their inability to identify all members with chronic conditions. Indeed, risk-sharing and capitation arrangements are very difficult to envision under these circumstances. If the pharmaceutical manufacturers and PBMs are truly interested in partnering with MCOs, perhaps they should consider working with the MCOs to identify members with chronic illnesses and their cost of treatment for the disease of interest. MCOs that are unable to determine their patient population and the cost of treatment for a particular disease should overcome their blanket suspicion of all manufacturers and PBMs and adopt a working relationship with one or two of these organizations that are truly interested in helping to achieve these goals.

One medical director in the Zitter surveys described health economics research as "looking at the total cost of all interventions and measuring the total impact on disease states." Many MCOs interviewed did not even discuss whether health economics research should be an integral part of their disease management program. Still fewer have put much effort into integrating this research into their disease management programs. Most were not planning to conduct any primary health economics research.

The Bottom Line—Integrated Information Systems

In spite of the current inability of most MCOs to document the effectiveness of their disease management programs, it was recognized by the participants in the Zitter study that MCOs that could effectively manage information within disease management would have a competitive advantage. Clearly, there is a lack of adequate information system capability at many MCOs; billing and reimbursement information systems that exist are simply not adequate to capture outcomes measures and analyze these data. Information systems designed to capture and analyze outcomes measures at MCOs were simply not needed until now. Although many MCOs would argue that the investment required for these information systems is prohibitive, this argument simply does not hold water.

If MCOs intend to survive these volatile times in health care, they simply must make the investment in information systems a high priority. Payers of health care (that is, employer groups) will be holding MCOs accountable for the outcomes they achieve. If MCOs do not collect and generate their own outcomes data, other third-party groups will collect and disseminate outcomes information concerning the MCOs (similar to the information published regarding mortality rates for individual hospitals and cardiac surgeons). Whether the MCOs agree with this information will be irrelevant: The marketplace will demand it, it will be supplied, and decisions regarding which MCOs to offer to employees will be made based on it.

If MCOs want information about the quality of care they deliver to be accurate, it would behoove them to begin collecting and disseminating that information themselves. It is interesting to note that the most successful MCOs in disease management (as well as in member satisfaction measures and HEDIS) are the ones that have invested most heavily in information systems. If MCOs are reluctant to make the investment in information systems that is necessary for proper disease management, they will simply have to collaborate with organizations that are willing to supply this capability. This is perhaps one of the greatest assets that firms marketing disease management programs can bring to an MCO. As discussed in chapter 11, many of the recent joint ventures in health care involve computer companies and MCOs. IBM has been especially aggressive in this area.

Because the ability to manage information within a disease management context is often viewed as a competitive advantage, many MCOs declined to provide specific information about their disease management systems in the Zitter survey. Disease management systems are viewed as proprietary, which is not advantageous to either the industry or, for that matter, to the health care of the population as a whole. If innovation in medicine is not freely shared among all providers, the public suffers. Certainly this has been the view of medicine toward new surgical procedures. Once a new procedure is developed, it is widely disseminated for all to use. The shifting of the burden for health care reform onto industry has created a highly competitive marketplace where "success" in health care is viewed as a highly proprietary asset.

Although competition has demonstrated its benefits in other industries, the jury is out concerning its long-term impact on health care. One could argue that the field of disease management would advance more quickly if all parties involved would share their successes and failures. It may also be argued that the investment in disease management requires parties to recover their investment by considering their system proprietary. Certainly for those organizations that are engaged in disease management but not directly involved in patient care (that is, pharmaceutical manufacturers and PBMs), this may be true. However, for health care providers, whose mission is to provide high-quality care to their members, this should not be the case. The delivery of high-quality care and the ability to document it should be a profitable endeavor. Further, this proprietary view assumes that any MCO can take a competitor's disease management program and successfully implement it, meaning that one disease management program fits all. This seems unlikely. A disease management program needs to be specifically developed to fit the particular needs of the MCO (its corporate culture, its care processes, and so forth) and its patient population.

As discussed in chapter 2, the implementation of disease management systems is very complicated. It is also interesting to note that to date the MCOs that have been most successful at developing and implementing disease management programs for their patients have made the details of these programs available. Perhaps it is only coincidence that MCOs that are still struggling to develop and implement disease management programs are the same ones that view their efforts as proprietary.

Pharmaceutical Integration

At most MCOs in the Zitter survey, formularies were *not* coordinated to disease management efforts. Well-designed disease management programs require that outcomes based on drug utilization be monitored on a regular basis. Although chapter 7 details the role of pharmaceutical companies and PBMs in disease management initiatives, it is worth noting a few additional observations here.

Most of the MCOs surveyed have adopted national practice guidelines and distributed them to their physicians. The practice guidelines contain only recommendations for the class of drugs to be used. Interestingly, pharmacy directors surveyed for the 1995 edition of the *Ciba Geneva Pharmacy Benefit Report* forecast that their pharmacy costs will continue to increase.[12] One would expect the use of closed formularies to rise as a cost-containment measure. It therefore seems likely that disease management programs in the future will contain recommendations for specific pharmaceuticals. Pharmacoeconomic studies that demonstrate the clinical and economic benefits of one drug versus another should be used to make formulary decisions. These same studies, as well as outcomes research studies that compare the effectiveness of alternative health care or medical interventions, need to be incorporated into the development of disease management programs. This will result in disease management programs that include specific recommendations regarding which medical interventions and pharmaceuticals should be used to provide patient care.

As can been seen from The Zitter Group's survey, disease management programs are currently in the earliest stages of development, and there is room for considerable improvement. A clear picture of the necessary characteristics that a disease management program should possess does emerge from the survey results. These characteristics are consistent with those discussed earlier in other chapters, especially chapter 2, including the following:

- An understanding of the course of the disease, including cost drivers
- Treatment based on the disease process rather than on the availability of reimbursement for a given therapy or component

- Patient education and compliance programs for chronic diseases
- Management of treatment that crosses care settings and provides full continuity of care
- Resource allocation to fund the most effective intervention regardless of treatment method or setting

Clearly, disease management represents an integrated approach to patient care for MCOs and is a natural evolution toward the original promise of the HMO. Disease management programs must, *at the very least,* address the following: information systems, utilization review, case management, formulary decisions, patient identification, PCPs' practice patterns, the role of specialty care physicians, patient education, practice guidelines, outcomes measurement, and benefit design. Most current disease management programs address only some of these items. The items that are most commonly overlooked are information systems; formulary decisions; and outcomes measurement, including evaluation of both the economic and clinical impact of the disease management program.

A program that possesses all of the listed items, however, is still not enough. *A well-designed disease management program must be based on the CQI approach.* As a CQI process, a disease management program should be a dynamic process involving:

1. Baseline measurement
2. Customized intervention
3. Outcomes measurement
4. Refined interventions

The *baseline measurement* would include the ability to identify the target population (that is, selected chronically ill patients); quantify the current costs of treatment for this group; and assess the clinical, economic, and patient quality-of-life outcomes the current treatments obtain.

The next step in the process would be the development of *customized patient-specific interventions* for the targeted group. One aspect of these interventions would be clinical protocols, based on nationally derived practice guidelines, that allow for local physician input. The interventions would have to be adjusted for patient severity, and need to be enforceable (that is, there needs to be some mechanism by which the MCO can get the physicians in its network to follow them). Another aspect of the interventions would be a patient education component. The intervention may utilize case managers and go beyond the covered benefits of the health plan. The intervention should have recommendations for preferred treatments and drugs.

The results (that is, outcomes) achieved by the interventions need to be quantified in *meaningful* outcomes. The focus needs to be on measures of importance to both the patient and the provider. Outcomes such as mortality; hospitalizations; preventable complications; and patient functional, psychological, and health status should be measured. These outcomes need to be evaluated by the providers to determine whether the interventions can be refined to achieve improved outcomes. The implementation of *refined interventions* would require additional outcomes measurement to assess their success. This evaluation and refinement should be an ongoing process for a disease management program.

• Examples of MCO-Based Disease Management Systems

For the reader, the question remains, what is actually going on in disease management at specific MCOs, and what is the scope of existing partnership models? Several examples will be presented in the following subsections. These examples represent disease management at various stages of complexity. In its surveys, The Zitter Group looked at eight elements of disease management that they felt were necessary components of disease management programs:

1. Disease mapping
2. Cost of treatment
3. Health economics research
4. Formularies integration
5. Practice guidelines
6. Patient education
7. Utilization review/management
8. Outcomes measurement and management

None of the disease management programs currently reported in the literature have all the elements of disease management (as defined by The Zitter Group) in place, nor do they possess all of the attributes discussed earlier. In spite of these shortcomings, there are reports of successful disease management programs. The common features of these successful disease management programs are practice guidelines, patient and physician education, high-risk patient identification, case management, and outcomes measurement.

Case 1: Health Net's Diabetes Program

Recently, Health Net, a Woodland Hills, CA–based network-model HMO, announced that the preliminary results of an outcomes study on its diabetes disease management program were very promising.[13] The preliminary results include declines in hemoglobin A1C levels and cost savings from reductions in hospitalizations.

Health Net has approximately 400 diabetics enrolled in its disease management program. Components of the program include clinical guidelines, automated lab test scheduling, patient education focusing on self-management and preventive care, and monitoring by both physicians and diabetes nurse specialists. In addition to the clinical endpoints in the program, the study also examined patients' quality of life. Health Net has identified 31,000 diabetics in its health plan and plans to send them patient education information as well as notifying their PCPs about the importance of monitoring. Health Net is currently deciding whether to offer the full diabetes disease management program to these diabetics.

Health Net's disease management program has several of the components discussed earlier. The program has a way to identify diabetics and influence their treatment through the physician network, and it contains a patient and physician education piece. The ability to determine the costs of treatment for the diabetic population is not known. That the HMO can state a cost savings from the program may simply be the result of being able to document a lower diabetic inpatient admission rate. Nonetheless, being able to measure the success of the program is noteworthy. The program also makes use of clinical guidelines and has measured patient quality of life.

One has to wonder how the patients in the program were selected. Do they represent patients with the highest resource utilization category? If so, it probably is not prudent to offer the full program to all 31,000 diabetics but rather to those who are responsible for high resource utilization. For the remaining diabetics in the plan, it would probably be more effective to offer some form of patient education stressing the value of patient self-monitoring and drug compliance. A physician education piece for patients' PCPs that emphasizes the need to see these patients on a regular basis to monitor their disease (for example, retinal eye exam) should also be developed.

Case 2: U.S. Healthcare's Asthma Program

U.S. Healthcare has developed a comprehensive asthma care program that possesses many of the components of a successful disease management program, although the organization refers to it as a patient management program.[14] This program has several stated goals that can be summarized into three main categories: improving asthma care, increasing member satisfaction, and reducing asthma treatment costs. The organization measures the success of its program based on the impact of asthma on hospitalizations. By using ICD-9 codes, USHC was able to identify 1,400 admissions for asthma and related diagnoses within its pediatric population and another 1,000 admissions in its adult population, among a membership of approximately one million in 1989.

The program has an educational component for both the patient and the PCP. Patient education comprises three parts. Upon their diagnosis, all asthmatics (or their parents) are sent written materials that are designed to assist patients with self-care and aid parents with pediatric care. The other two components of patient education are the assignment of a case manager and outpatient- and inpatient-intensive asthma training programs at centers of excellence, like the program provided by the National Jewish Center for Immunology and Respiratory Medicine in Denver. These two components are reserved for severely ill asthmatics. U.S. Healthcare determines asthma severity levels based on utilization data (hospital, specialty, and emergency department utilization). Severity can also be based on medication requirements and physician inputs, among other factors. One part of case management is the use of nurses who visit patients in the home to educate them and to evaluate the home environment for allergens.

Physician education consists of practice guidelines being distributed to PCPs and sponsorship of asthma care conferences at hospitals. The practice guidelines that USHC distributes are the "Executive Summary: Guidelines for the Diagnosis and Management of Asthma" developed by the National Institutes of Health as a component of the National Asthma Education Program. Included with the guidelines are a question-and-answer sheet that USHC developed and uses to determine whether the PCPs have read and understood the guidelines. PCPs receive financial incentives to return the completed question-and-answer sheet; USHC gives them additional compensation in its primary compensation model, which determines the PCPs' capitation rate, as well as providing continuing medical education credits. Sending a guideline to physicians in a managed care network is not enough; ensuring that they actually read the guideline and understand it is more important. U.S. Healthcare's additional compensation achieves this goal. Ultimately, however, the desired goal of sending a guideline to PCPs within a network is that they actually comply with it.

Another way that PCPs within USHC can obtain increased compensation is by having their primary care offices certified by USHC as a "Designated Primary Asthma Care Center." The goal is to improve the care delivered to asthmatics in PCP offices. In order to become certified, an office needs to conform to either structural or process elements that have been associated with improved treatment outcomes and are recommended by the National Asthma Education Project. Some of the items necessary for certification include availability of a nebulizer and/or a meter-dose inhaler for office treatment, availability of a loaner nebulizer, use of patient education materials, use of peak flow meters and patient-recorded diaries, PCPs' completion of the USHC's question-and-answer sheet, and screening of psychological and stress-related components contributing to the asthmatic's severity level.

Case managers overseeing the care of asthmatics have the ability to develop specialized programs for their patients. They may hire home health agencies that provide visiting nurses and respiratory therapists to call on the patient. They can utilize medical equipment vendors to supply patients with peak flow meters and nebulizers, as well as instruct patients in their use. They work with the PCP to coordinate care and make specialty referrals, and make phone calls to patients to determine whether their needs are being satisfied. Case managers can also make referrals to the centers-of-excellence educational programs. As mentioned earlier, the case manager is the central contact in coordinating the patient's care among USHC, PCP, specialist, and the home health agency and is empowered by USHC to create programs for the patient that go beyond the insurer's benefit plan.

U.S. Healthcare has also been able to document the successes of its asthma care program. In the Pennsylvania area, it has identified over 300 pediatric asthmatics with severe asthma. By employing case managers for this population, hospital usage for this group has decreased by 65 percent when comparing the patient's hospital usage for the year after entering the program to the year prior to entering the program. The organization estimates that it has saved over $200,000 in hospital costs with an investment of $46,000 in patient education and home health care. U.S. Healthcare is striving to collect additional outcomes measures, including patient satisfaction surveys and time off from school and/or work, and is also planning to survey physicians in its network to determine the impact of the asthma program on them.

Case 3: Group Health's Vaccination Program

The disease management programs described for Health Net and USHC are relatively comprehensive programs that include the following components: practice guidelines, patient selection criteria, intervention protocols for education and treatment, and outcomes management. However, all disease management programs need not be this comprehensive. A program that targets patients 65 years of age or older for an influenza vaccination may not sound like a sophisticated disease management program, but in reality it contains the same components as the other two and should be considered as such.

Group Health, Inc., is a staff-model HMO in the Minneapolis–St. Paul area with 300,000 members that developed just this type of program.[15] It consisted of walk-in influenza vaccine clinics, a patient education piece that was mailed to members age 65 or older, and a standing order for nurses to offer and administer influenza vaccine to this patient population. This seemingly simple disease management program was associated with a reduction in hospitalizations for influenza, pneumonia, all acute and chronic respiratory conditions, and congestive heart failure among vaccine recipients over the three flu seasons (1990 to 1993) the program's effectiveness was studied. Direct savings per year, after subtracting the costs of the program at $4 per person vaccinated, averaged $117 per person vaccinated. The total cumulative direct savings was estimated to be approximately $5 million.

For MCOs that want to develop disease management programs that have a high probability of generating a positive economic outcome, the message is simple: Focus on developing and implementing simplistic disease management programs that will have a short-term payoff. The experience gained from these types of programs will be invaluable when the organization decides to develop more comprehensive programs like those described at Health Net and USHC.

• Summary

MCOs are increasingly engaging in disease management initiatives. Both physicians and administrators at MCOs realize the potential value of disease management programs: Physicians hope to reduce unexplained clinical variation, and administrators look at the potential for cost savings. To date, however, few studies or MCOs can document these perceived benefits. Perhaps, as MCOs become more proficient at documenting outcomes, the benefits of disease management programs will be routinely demonstrated.

MCOs have many of the elements for disease management in place; however, these elements have not been integrated into coherent disease management programs. Information systems seem to be at the core of the problem. Capabilities such as the identification of members with chronic illnesses, electronically linked medical and pharmacy claims, access to a patient's treatments and outcomes, and cost-of-treatment studies would be greatly enhanced by the availability of more sophisticated and integrated information systems.

Disease management as it currently exists at MCOs resembles high-cost case management. Most programs focus on patients who are the high utilizers of health care resources (that is, hospitalizations, emergency room visits). Because of this focus, chronic diseases such as asthma, diabetes, and hypertension are typically chosen first for disease management program development.

Outcomes measurement and management are important to the disease management process and are typically the most difficult pieces of disease management to accomplish. Additionally, most disease management programs have little to no evaluation of their impact. Most current programs lack a CQI approach to their development and refinement.

In spite of the aforementioned limitations of current disease management programs, it is believed that MCOs will continue to develop more comprehensive and sophisticated disease management programs and become more proficient in documenting their impact. More recent advances in the sophistication of disease management systems have involved the development of comprehensive telephonic demand management systems based on enhanced call center technology. These call center/demand management systems are probably best represented by United Healthcare's OPTIM-24™, a 24-hour, seven-day-per-week telephonic aid to patients/MCO members that includes a broad spectrum of health information as well as triaging services. Variations of these phone-in health information/support services include a number of disease-specific case management services that proactively help chronically ill patients better manage their disease.

In addition to the inclusion of these new demand management components to existing systems, the recognition by many MCOs of the value of aligning with strategic partners is expected to play a critical role in the future success of MCO-based disease management programs. The economies of scale and new capabilities introduced through these partnership arrangements will enable MCOs to offer more cost-effective disease management systems by spreading the cost of development and risk associated with this new paradigm of health care delivery. It is expected that second- and third-generation disease management programs will continue to represent an important part of managed care's armamentarium supporting their twofold mission of providing high-quality, cost-effective health care to their covered populations.

References

1. Disease management/next trend? The Associated Press, Sept. 19, 1995.

2. *Standards for the Accreditation of Managed Care Organizations, 1994 Edition.* Washington, DC: National Cancer Institute, 1994.

3. Special report: managing asthma care. *Medical Economics* 13(7):[Supplement D. Business and Health], 1995.

4. The Diabetes Control and Complications (DCCT) Research Group. Effect of intensive therapy on the development and progression of diabetic nephropathy in the Diabetes Control and Complications Trial. *Kidney International* 47(6):1703–20, June 1995.

5. Hathaway, M. J. Managing care by managing diseases. *Managed Healthcare,* Oct. 1994, pp. S27–S30.

6. Group Health Association of America. *HMO Industry Profile, 1994 Edition.* Washington, DC: GHAA, 1994.

7. Zeneca-Salick deal offers promising new route into disease management. *Managed Pharmaceutical Report* 1(11):1–2, Jan. 1995.

8. Field, M. J., and Lohr, K. N. *Guidelines for Clinical Practice—From Development to Use.* Washington, DC: National Academy Press, 1992.

9. Konstam, M. A., Dracup, K., and others. *Heart Failure: Evaluation and Care of Patients with Left-Ventricular Systolic Dysfunction,* June 1994. Agency for Health Care Policy and Research, publication no. 94-0612.

10. Disease management/next trend?

11. Hanchak, N. A., Murray, J. F., McDermott, P., Hirsch, A., and Schlackman, N. The Membership Chronic Disease Database as a tool for health plan quality improvement. *Managed Care Quarterly* (Winter 1995).

12. Moss, K., editor. Survey shows continued gain for closed formularies. *Drug Outcomes & Managed Care* 2(19):4, Sept. 27, 1995.

13. Gutman, J. H. Health Net calls results of diabetes study strong. *Disease Management News,* Sept. 1995, p. 4.

14. Fabius, R. J., editor. *A Physician Executive's Guide to Patient Management for the '90s and Beyond.* Tampa: American College of Physician Executives, 1995.

15. Nichol, K. L., Margolis, K. L., Wuorenma, J., and Von Sternberg, T. The efficacy and cost-effectiveness of vaccination against influenza among elderly persons living in the community. *The New England Journal of Medicine* 331(12):778–84, Sept. 22, 1994.

Chapter 9

The Role of Case Management in Disease Management

Marcia Diane Ward, RN, and Julia A. Rieve, RN

• Introduction

Case managers have often been on the cutting edge of change as the health care industry has struggled to reform itself. Today, as the managed care industry continues to expand, capitation increasingly replaces fee-for-service methods of reimbursement, and disease management "catches fire," case managers have the opportunity to play an even more important role in helping to change how health care is delivered. This role is suggested by perhaps the shortest definition of disease management, which is offered by Dr. Edward Zalta, president of CappCare of California. According to Dr. Zalta, *disease management* can be defined as "proactive case management."[1] This chapter addresses how case managers can respond to the new challenges of disease management and how their function will likely evolve as proactive case management expands.

From a medical case management perspective, disease management can also be defined as an information-intensive series of clinical processes and services across the continuum of health care that identifies the medically at-risk population and professionally manages patients in a manner that improves care, promotes wellness, and manages/reduces cost. The concept and philosophy of case management fit very nicely with the principles of disease management, which are remarkably familiar to case managers. Disease management, albeit in a less systematic and integrated manner, has been practiced for centuries by health care providers. As indicated in chapter 1, the current concept of disease management first emerged in 1991 as a strategic response by the pharmaceutical industry to marketplace forces and the evolution of health maintenance organizations (HMOs) into managed care organizations (MCOs) and other forms of more proactive integrated care that have the potential to help maintain quality in an increasingly price-sensitive environment.

Historically, case managers have always strived to manage illness through a collaborative approach aimed at the delivery of high-quality, cost-effective health care. However, this early form of disease management was implemented primarily in the type of episodic, component-based delivery system described in chapter 1. Advances in technology, along with other new enabling forces in the industry, now promise case managers the potential ability to design and implement a more sophisticated form of disease management. As these newer systems evolve, case managers will be able to optimize a broader range of specific disease management interventions for targeted populations via greater access to standardized, more highly integrated clinical and financial data about their patients and patient populations. The increased sophistication, availability, and acceptance of clinical practice guidelines also promise to enhance the ability of case managers to provide true patient-centered care and wellness management—the ultimate goal of the professional case manager and, as mentioned earlier, the original concept/promise of HMOs. Depending on how case managers respond to the demands of disease management, they have the potential to significantly expand on the tools currently available to them.

Today, professional case managers, at every level of the multidisciplinary health care team, are well positioned to expand on their role as administrators of enhanced disease management protocols and care delivery over a continuum of time and delivery sites. The philosophy of case management within disease management remains essentially patient centered and holds that individuals within a defined population shall receive clinically and financially optimized care through processes and services coordinated by case managers. In the move toward a new frontier of health care delivery and disease management, case managers, with their patient advocacy heritage, are well positioned to be the hub of a plethora of clinical and non-clinical interventions, which must be highly coordinated and integrated if disease management programs are to be successful. As the process of designing, developing, implementing, and measuring the success of disease management programs has been detailed in earlier chapters, the primary focus of this chapter is to explore how case managers can adapt/enhance the role that they play within their individual organizations to help maximize the effectiveness of disease management programs.

• A Historical Perspective

Case management, which has developed over time to its present form as an essential component of the disease management process, was originally grounded in the roots of nursing and social work with a legacy as far back as the 1850s.

This early social services orientation evolved into a more disease-focused orientation with the advent of workers' compensation in the 1940s and, later, managed care in the 1980s. It gained swift momentum in the 1990s when national health care reform initiatives started to emphasize high-quality, cost-effective, patient-centered care.[2] This perspective leads many case managers to believe that disease management is simply a new view of an old concept.[3] Figure 9-1 depicts how today's case management fits into and has evolved within the managed care environment.

The early focus of MCOs was on the function of *utilization review,* which began with the understanding that health care must be more closely managed to obtain cost-effective results. Utilization review staff evaluated medical records and abstracted information that was then assimilated and developed into standards and/or criteria for acceptance or denial of medical claims. This phase of managed care was highly prospective and can best be described as the *discovery phase.*

As the shortcomings of utilization review became increasingly recognized, *utilization management* evolved. Utilization management emphasized the use of clinical guidelines and criteria (based on trends identified in the era of utilization review) to assess a patient's documented disease status and to determine appropriate levels of care. When a patient's disease documentation did not match clinical guidelines/standards, the information was shared with a physician. Utilization management staff attempted to encourage either the physician or the patient to conform with the clinical guidelines. The process was, to some degree, more perspective than utilization review, and can be referred to as the *conformity phase.*

The third phase of the evolution is represented by today's case managers. *Case management* was developed with the concept of coordinating care so that continuous discovery and conformity took place, and it added a very important new feature—individualized patient-focused care. It includes trend information and criteria to ensure high-quality, cost-effective delivery of care. However, case management in its most recent form has been based on a very restrictive episodic or component-style orientation to the treatment and management of disease. This phase may be labeled the *patient-centered/ episodic care phase.*

Disease management allows case managers and all members of the health care team to focus on the discovery, conformity, and coordination of a continuum of care across large populations with the same or similar disease process. It can be seen as the *population-focused phase.*

As discussed in chapter 1 and elaborated on in chapter 12, disease management has the potential to eventually evolve into *wellness management,* or health management. In this final phase of the evolution of managed health care delivery, case managers will be in a position to blend all of the aforementioned elements with as yet undiscovered elements to reach the ultimate goal—that of preventing disease. Perhaps this phase will become known as the *disease prevention phase.*

Figure 9-1. Managed Care Timeline

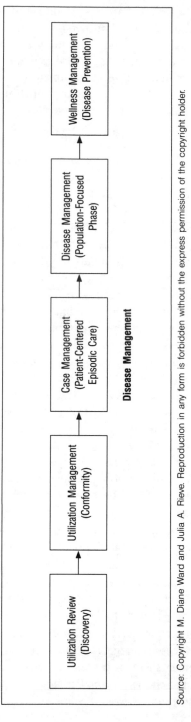

• A New Frontier

The concept of a "new frontier" holds a vision of a better place that is worth a great investment. The journey there will take time, courage, and commitment from organizations and health care professionals. The move into an era of truly integrated health care delivery is also a new frontier for case managers as advocates who are well positioned to serve the broader clinical, ethical, and societal needs of patients.

Health care reform has slowly and, at times, painfully moved this frontier in the direction of more integrated information systems capable of identifying and tracking the specific health care needs of targeted populations. The success of disease management will hinge to a large degree on both payers and providers having greater access to these more integrated clinical and financial databases. The opportunity to best pioneer this new frontier belongs to those organizations that have the expertise and resources needed to create these information systems. Case managers, as coordinators of care, should involve themselves in the design of such systems to ensure that they fully address the need to coordinate and track care delivery, outcomes, and so forth across a broad continuum of delivery locations.

The eventual availability of electronic global health records will eliminate time and distance limitations to patient record access and will facilitate a significant step forward in health care delivery as the year 2000 nears. Evolving information systems hopefully will include many new elements: longitudinal patient tracking and analysis capabilities, full data retention, continuum of care utilization data, accessible and up-to-date clinical pathways and protocols, and multidisciplinary documentation of care delivery.[4] Importantly, this greater access to clinical protocols and critical pathways will help enable the development of integrated databases for the purpose of outcomes analysis. These databases will also supply the information needed by case management specialists to more accurately evaluate disease management programs.[5] Again, it is important that case managers be part of the development teams that design these new systems.

As the industry evolves into the next phase of health care delivery, a new type of professional case manager must also emerge. Future case managers must be thoroughly knowledgeable about targeted diseases and specific treatment regimens. Case managers may well become recognized as disease management specialists if they take advantage of the opportunities available to them as the disease management movement continues to expand. As the responsibilities of this "new" case manager develop and change, it is conceivable that they may well incorporate or overlap with the functions of the specialized nurse practitioner and pharmacist.[6]

• Proactive Case Management

During the expected evolution of disease management, organizations will use the expertise of the nurse case manager. This proactive role is critical in the prevention and management of chronic diseases. Case managers are the essential link in the new health care delivery system. As comprehensive disease management programs become more common, case managers, who have historically been dedicated to specialized, culturally competent care coordination, have the opportunity to use their position as patient advocates to help shape the new frontier.[7] In fact, the pathway to the new frontier is already being traveled by many innovative case managers and their organizations.

Example: Risk Assessment and Case Selection

At Lovelace Health Systems, an integrated delivery system in Albuquerque, NM, case managers are taking an active role in designing and developing disease management programs. Karen Mannal describes why case managers in her organization fine-tuned health risk assessments for improved case selection from targeted populations: "We simply were not capturing definitive information capable of comprehensive member selection for proactive case management."

The case managers designed acuity scales that helped them determine case management goals and tailor individual care plans. "We have seen real progress in our case management program concerning its effect on our members' health status as we have worked together toward implementing disease management programs," says Mannal.

She also shared the success stories of two health plan members. An 80-year-old patient with a primary diagnosis of coronary artery disease and secondary diagnoses of chronic obstructive pulmonary disease and diabetes resulting in a below-the-knee amputation had frequent exacerbations of his illness resulting in numerous annual hospitalizations. On-site case management revealed his poor nutritional status, noncompliance with medication therapy, and living conditions that contributed to his lack of general wellbeing. According to Mannal, placement in a 24-hour-care facility produced improved health status, and this man actually thrived in the assisted-care environment. He has not required hospitalization in the past two years, and his quality of life has improved tremendously. His case manager is able to track his progress effectively through a case management software system.

The case management/disease management program at Lovelace Health Systems also intervened proactively for a 49-year-old plan member disabled with multiple sclerosis. Mannal describes her as fiercely independent and a writer for the disabled population. Living alone and preoccupied with her work, her general health status declined, and frequent calls to 911 resulted in costly interventions within the capitated health plan. Health risk assessments and acuity scales applied by her case manager indicated the need for intermediate custodial care with a later return home facilitated by a well-matched caregiver. As a result of these interventions, her frequent calls to

911 ceased, and the patient reported a high level of satisfaction with her current health status.

Example: Patient Education

When risk-assessment programs identify at-risk populations, new opportunities open up for organizations to use case managers to apply their skills toward promoting wellness and other disease intervention initiatives. As a result of the focus on disease management concepts by many MCOs, case managers in a variety of practice settings are now beginning to help design and implement educational, compliance-focused programs. The positive result of this type of proactive case management expertise within a comprehensive disease management system will ideally be enhanced cost management balanced with optimal clinical outcomes across populations.

Karen Keown, senior director of medical programs at United Health-Care Corporation in Minnetonka, MN, describes United HealthCare's approach to disease management as proactive case management intervention based on traditional nursing processes. "Nothing is new, just more focused on resource utilization and early intervention," she says.

United HealthCare consistently measures the impact of case management strategies on member behavior and perceived value. Its nurse case managers use a demand management approach to educate members about alternatives to high-dollar emergency room visits. When this educational process fails to direct members away from emergency room use, the health plan implements direct physician intervention. The commitment to outcomes analysis produces a well-balanced disease management system for cost-effective, measurable care. This example, as well as that of Lovelace Health Systems, illustrates the maturation of the case management nursing process in a new era of patient management.

Ideally, fully integrated disease management systems will eventually provide complete information about both individual patients and patient sub-populations. These new systems will enable case managers to access complete patient histories gathered and summarized from various sources within the integrated health system and, externally, from members of community health information networks. Libraries of up-to-date protocols and guidelines, from which care management plans can be carefully tailored, will also be increasingly available from these integrated, computerized information systems. Analysis and evaluation of patient health and/or disease progression against these protocols and guidelines will help generate the kind of health outcomes data that will significantly enhance both individual patient care planning and the refinement of population-based disease management initiatives. This level of proactive case management will be impossible without the empowerment of technology.

• The Process of Case Management within Disease Management Systems

Disease management was defined earlier in this chapter as focused, proactive case management. Although the clinical components of disease management include many of the basic processes of care management found in the historical episodic, component-oriented system of health care delivery, the level of integration of clinical and economic outcomes and the focus on early intervention are very different. Earlier chapters detailed the difference between component-style health care and disease management and outlined in some detail the process of designing, developing, and implementing disease management initiatives. The following discussion concerns the process of case management within a disease management environment and focuses on how case managers can help produce the best results from these programs for both the patient and their sponsoring organization.

Identification of At-Risk Members

After first determining which diseases to manage (see chapters 2 and 5), organizations must identify triggers and risk profiles for those targeted diseases. The ratio of population to membership must be assessed and risk profiles created. Although health risk appraisals are a standard in the wellness industry, those developed for purposes of disease management must be specifically designed to identify clinical triggers for given chronic diseases. Individuals at high risk or at acute episode are selected for disease management. The input of case managers in this phase of developing disease management programs is critical. As indicated in chapter 2, a team approach is needed to design and develop disease management programs. Case managers must ensure that they are members of these teams, if not the team facilitators.

Health Assessment and Evaluation of Identified Population

To develop appropriate customized patient care plans, case managers may need to further evaluate those members identified as at risk for chronic disease. For example, Independence Blue Cross in Philadelphia sends home health providers to do in-home clinical, psychosocial, and environmental assessments of selected plan members identified as at risk for asthma.[8]

Determination of Benefits

Determination of eligibility and benefits for at-risk populations is a key component of the case manager role in disease management. Payer source benefit structures tend to be relatively rigid in coverage in order to control costs, often creating circumstances in which either the care provided is more costly than alternatives or no service coverage is allowed. Case managers play an important leadership role in identifying opportunities to negotiate, create, and monitor exceptional benefits and service levels that enhance cost-effective, qualilty-care, team-driven disease management treatment plans. For example, BCBS of Michigan has implimented a coordinated care management program. The disease management program targets high-cost chronic disease management populations within its membership. Case managers are utilized to create, with other health care team members, extra-contractual treatment plans to provide prevention interventions, reduce future illness, decrease future costs, and improve member health status. Extra-contractual interventions may include smoking cessation, exercise and diet programs, cardiac rehabilitation, and individually designed self-management programs.

Development of Clinical Pathways and Disease Management Interventions

In recent years, many payers and providers have developed clinical pathways as well as new clinical and nonclinical interventions as components of their disease management programs. These disease management interventions, including clinical pathways, should be developed using academic research information as well as community-based "best practice" information. Again, case managers, as members of the disease management team, can and should have a leadership role in both the development and reassessment of these interventions.

Implementing the Disease Management Plan

Case managers must obtain all parties' agreement to participate in disease management programs. Those parties include the patient, payer, nonphysician providers, physicians, and case management team members. This "buy-in" element of disease management is often overlooked or underestimated by design teams. As suggested in chapter 2, the stakeholders of the disease management process must be made aware of the role they may individually play in the program and buy into their responsibilities. Case managers, because of their contact with many of the potential stakeholders (physicians, patients, allied health professionals, and so forth) are ideally suited to help identify strategies that will facilitate stakeholder buy-in.

Administration of Care Plan/Demand Management

Within the disease management environment, case managers are charged with the development of more *systematic* methods for educating members about their disease, explaining covered benefits, and promoting increased compliance with medication and treatment care plans. The care plans developed must address all necessary levels of care from ambulatory to acute and be integrated across the continuum. Flags and triggers, such as hospitalization, that signal the need for individual management must also be identified. A variety of member/patient contact methods may be built into the disease management program. These include member mailings, newsletters, telephone health information services, electronic medication management/ reporting tools, specialized case management services, and so forth. Collectively these tools are known as *demand management.* Demand management may be defined as "any organized effort or program designed to guide health care consumers into the most appropriate level of health care service by involving them directly in their own health care." Quite simply, the term was coined to cover a variety of interventions that may help reduce the "demand" for more expensive medical interventions. Again, case managers are ideally suited to help identify creative new demand management interventions and to oversee the implementation and/or administration of these new tools. Many payers and providers have already established sophisticated nurse call-in services to answer questions and advise members regarding health care.[9]

Compliance Monitoring and Management

The identification of specific actions for the population being managed requires compliance monitoring. Many chronic diseases require long-term compliance with therapy to prevent acute episodes. Evaluation of claims data and outcomes data analysis can provide compliance profiles. For example, at Kaiser Permanente in Atlanta, case managers telephone members at risk for hypertension to make sure they are taking their medication and keeping regular physician appointments for blood pressure monitoring.[10] For many case managers, the expanded emphasis on compliance may require the development of new skills in the areas of patient interviewing and/or problem identification.

Outcomes Measurement

Case managers must track both financial and clinical outcomes data for their targeted at-risk populations to determine the effectiveness of disease management treatment plans. These measurements should include financial, clinical, customer-satisfaction, and patient-compliance measures. As organizations begin the transition into disease management, they identify case management outcomes that can be compiled for both individuals and large patient populations.[11] Figure 9-2 illustrates how outcomes measurement is included in each stage along the continuum of care, including prevention, wellness, and disease management.

Figure 9-2. The Case Management Process

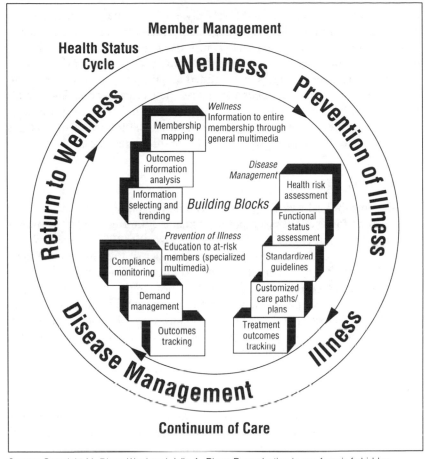

• Disease Management Tools

The expanded role of case managers in disease management is a natural progression. However, to implement the process outlined in the previous section and in chapter 2, case managers must develop tools that will help facilitate the effective management of large patient population groups. These tools of the trade can be divided into two major categories: patient-related tools and case management tools. In order to fully understand the relevance of these tools to the case manager's new role in disease management, the case manager's perspective of the process of disease management also needs to be examined.

Patient-Related Tools

Patient-related tools enable, and hopefully empower, the patient to participate as a partner in the disease management process with the case manager. This self-empowerment is especially important in cases involving chronic illness. Tools must be developed in such a way that patients, primary care providers, and case managers have immediate and ongoing access to them and to the outcomes data needed to assess their effectiveness. These tools also need to be user-friendly so that patients are encouraged to use them to effectively prevent and manage their disease. The following subsections describe some of the more widely used patient-related tools.

Report Cards

Report cards for health care organizations were established when the National Commission for Quality Assurance implemented the Health Plan Employer Data and Information Set (HEDIS; 2.0) in November 1993.[12] One way case managers can prove value and share the outcomes of their disease management efforts is to apply a similar evaluation model concerning the impact of the services they provide. Figure 9-3 demonstrates key elements to be included in a disease management–focused report card. By measuring similar indicators across organizations, case managers will be able to share their experiences with others in their profession and hopefully to improve the "science" of disease management.

Pathways

Clinical pathways are essentially traditional nursing care plans mapped to standardized protocols or clinical guidelines. Applying standardized, national

Figure 9-3.   Case Manager Report Card (Disease Management)

☑ Patient accessibility

☑ Patient satisfaction

☑ Resource utilization

☑ Disease outcomes

☑ Financial performance

☑ Prevention and wellness interventions

Source: Copyright M. Diane Ward and Julia A. Rieve. Reproduction in any form is forbidden without the express permission of the copyright holder.

guidelines to the development of clinical pathways creates an environment for more provider accountability because individual care plans now have guidelines against which they can be measured. The basic components of a disease management pathway are indicated in figure 9-4.

Demand Management

As suggested above, the collective use of risk appraisals, telephone health information services, and other prevention/wellness tools has become known as demand management. Many organizations have implemented nurse phone-in lines as a means of providing patient education and counseling. Nurses have traditionally been the first health care professional to talk to patients about their conditions. Case managers' ability to recognize early signs and symptoms of a disease process for prompt referrals to physicians, as well as their counseling skills, can positively affect patient outcomes.

Nurse telephone health information services and triaging have become additional tools in the disease management repertoire available to case managers. Fully informed consumers usually choose less risky and less costly options of health care delivery. The nurse case management counselor also helps patients determine potential self-care alternatives. The objective is to enable the consumer, in conjunction with the physician, to make a more informed decision concerning his or her health care.

Early statistics from major health plans reveal that members use nurse advisor lines for the following services:

- 63 percent to report symptoms
- 15 percent for general health information
- 4 percent for benefits information
- 3 percent for referrals[13]

Few members of the multidisciplinary health care team are more qualified than the experienced nurse case manager to move patients through the system with the least expense and the best outcome. Karen Berg, of Nurse On Call in Norcross, GA, describes her company's nurse advice software product as a "symptoms triage tool" for varied populations from primary care to pediatrics to geriatrics. Nurse On Call was designed exclusively by nurses and evaluated by specialty physicians for accuracy of content. Embedded decision-support logic prompts nurse reviewers with questions about urgency of symptoms and offers recommendations for treatment measures and care sites.

A conditioned disease inquiry and specific guidelines help ensure documentation of "an information-only call." These proprietary assessment tools help facilitate prevention of illness through the timely availability of coordinated patient education and general health information offerings.

Figure 9-4.   Case Management Generic Pathway: Basic Pathway to Identify, Disseminate, and Improve "Best Practices"

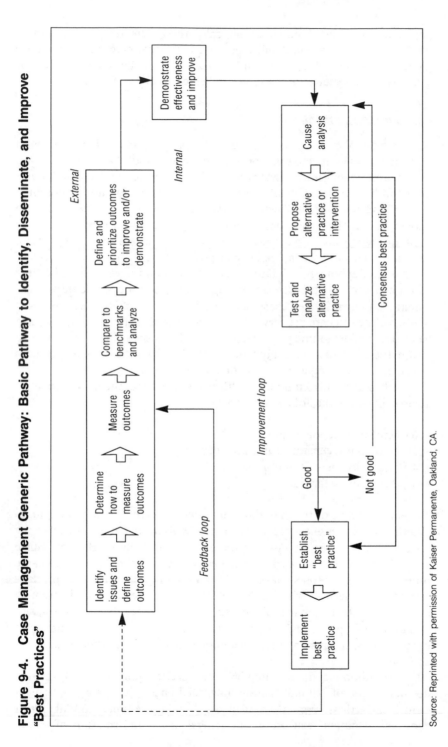

Source: Reprinted with permission of Kaiser Permanente, Oakland, CA.

Wellness and the prevention of disease "flare-ups" are also enhanced through patient compliance monitoring and timely follow-up from an acute episode of illness.

Education/Prevention/Wellness Programs

From the earliest days of professional nursing, prevention of illness and wellness education have been integral in this caregiver role. Today, financial value has finally been attached to the wellness ministry of nursing. Through the effective use of nurse case managers as patient educators, future patient populations can hopefully be spared much of the "dis-ease" of the past.

It is well recognized that a small number of diseases are responsible for the majority of medical costs for most health benefit plans. Programs that focus on prevention and early intervention for these costly conditions have the potential for vast savings because they go straight to the source of the largest claims.[14] It is also recognized that case management is a potentially effective means of balancing cost savings and access to a reasonable standard of quality health care.

The average lifetime medical cost in the United States is a staggering $225,000 per person, with a sizable chunk of that cost linked to health habits and lifestyle. Those who pay the bills, largely, employers and government, have a growing interest in keeping people healthy.[15] As employers seek to cut health care costs by encouraging workers to adopt healthful lifestyles, organizations can use case managers to monitor chronic diseases and to motivate improved employee lifestyles in the workplace through proactive education-oriented case management.

In 1984, following nine years of health care cost increases that averaged 19 percent annually, the city of Birmingham, AL, was searching for a way to control costs. With health expenses rising at twice the national average, it faced the prospect of medical benefits increasing from $7.6 million in 1984 to an estimated $31.3 million by 1992.[16] Working with the University of Alabama at Birmingham (UAB) and Wellness South, a Birmingham health care consulting firm, the city launched an aggressive wellness program for 4,200 employees. It also developed and implemented a self-insured, self-administered health plan that included a utilization review system, incentives to direct employees to hospitals with favorable outcomes and lower rates, and a health maintenance organization (HMO) option.[17]

The wellness program, operated since 1991 by the UAB School of Nursing, includes on-site medical screening and a health risk appraisal. Participation in the screening and appraisal was a prerequisite for entry into the health plan. After the screening, intervention programs were provided, when necessary, for weight loss, stress management, smoking cessation, blood pressure control, cholesterol reduction, fitness, and back care. The city offered incentives to encourage participation. In the last five years, the city's health care costs have been essentially flat.[18]

As the value of these types of health management programs continues to be documented, nurse case managers—through their natural role as educators, counselors, and wellness advocates—will be a valuable asset to promote wellness and prevention of illness.

Case Management Tools

Case management tools enable the case manager to assess, plan, coordinate, evaluate, and improve disease management-focused services. These tools must be developed by case managers and be fully integrated with other components of the disease management system in order for case managers to manage large patient populations effectively in real time. The following subsections discuss the five most common case management tools.

Health Risk Assessments

The potential effectiveness of health risk appraisals was implied in the preceding section and is expanded on in chapter 12. Health risk assessments are being individually tailored by organizations to meet specific screening criteria. Nurse case managers and medical directors are usually involved in the design process. Figure 9-5 lists the basic components covered by most health risk assessments. Case managers represent natural stakeholders/administrators of these assessment tools.

Computerized Patient Records

As stated earlier, technological advances will be an integral part of disease management's success. One of the most important areas for case managers is the patient record system. Computerization of this information makes a great difference to a program's efficiency and scope.

Figure 9-5. Components of Health Risk Assessment

- Cognition
- Emotional and psychological well-being
- Functional status
- Social work and support systems
- Economic status
- Environmental and safety issues
- Health behaviors and knowledge
- Medical history
- Medication regimen
- Disease process (short- and long-term goals)

Source: Copyright M. Diane Ward and Julia A. Rieve. Reproduction in any form is forbidden without the express permission of the copyright holder.

For example, case managers at Mount Vernon Hospital, a unit of Inova Health Systems in Alexandria, VA, access a computerized patient record system to obtain information about a patient's insurance coverage and benefit options prior to admission to the rehabilitation unit, explains Nancy S. Bennett, joint replacement case manager at Mount Vernon Hospital. All of this information is contained on one or two computer screens. This unique feature of the in-house customized software saves the case manager many steps in locating information from multiple points along the continuum, thus permitting faster and more accurate alternative care planning, and allowing case managers to save time.

Inova implemented the PHAMIS computerized patient record in March 1995. The system coordinates all patient information in a centralized, consistent manner so that all care providers have access to information as it is gathered. PHAMIS is designed to provide cost-accounting and quality-of-care clinical information for both individuals and aggregate populations across the care continuum.

The system's patient monitoring form contains patient demographics, including name, medical record number, diagnosis code, and physician. It also contains information used to track severity of illness and intensity of service that can be linked directly to cost–benefit and quality-of-care outcomes by individual patient or, again, for an aggregate patient population. For example, a patient recovering from total hip joint replacement develops a suboptimal postoperative hematocrit and hemoglobin that affects his or her ability to participate in physical therapy and slows positive progress along the continuum of care. Using the computerized system, the case manager can obtain "real-time" information regarding potential quality-of-care issues and make recommendations to avoid problems, to improve the patient's status, and to move the patient along the continuum in a timely manner. "From a disease management perspective, PHAMIS allows case managers to better manage multiple patients along the care continuum, allows me to develop time-saving alternative care options with my joint replacement patients. With PHAMIS, I can manage more patients in a virtually seamless manner," reports Bennett.

Case managers and other health care providers can now examine aggregate data to determine areas of best practice against which to benchmark similar disease management populations. According to Bennett,

> PHAMIS aggregate information allows the entire health care team to look at patient population data in order to develop methods to improve care. Case managers involved in disease management programs will find a computerized patient record system like PHAMIS invaluable. The system allows case managers to continuously obtain snapshots of clinical and economic outcomes for both individuals and aggregate populations, at any point along the continuum. Our joint replacement population

is the ultimate benefactor of PHAMIS. The system supports health care providers to successfully apply case management principles in a disease management model to continuously improve care.

Clinical Guidelines

Clinical practice guidelines were discussed in the previous section and in detail in chapter 6. Mount Vernon Hospital also uses a customer-focused system to develop its clinical guidelines, according to Ellen Stahl, a case manager who manages the hospital's head injury and stroke patient population. The model outlined in figure 9-6 was developed to formalize the various systems required to support patient outcomes analysis across a broad spectrum of disease populations. "Case managers skilled in a particular

Figure 9-6. Customer-Focused Systems Model

A. Five Customer-Focused Functions
   1. Provides the foundation for all case management programming
   2. Uses the concept of open communication in relationships, toward meeting mutual goals
   3. Promotes a "team practice" concept
   4. Defines those resources and personnel involved in the care process in terms of customer systems, which may be diagnostic or population specific as well as provider specific
   5. Defines ongoing and future opportunities for relationship growth and development, ensuring positive collaborative efforts that exceed program goals

B. Customer Systems
   1. *External customer system:* Those resources and personnel outside one's organization
   2. *Internal customer system:* Those resources and personnel inside one's organization
   3. *Nuclear customer system:* Those resources and personnel within one's immediate department or unit

C. Model Application
   1. Identify the parties in each customer system
   2. Assess and identify the strengths and weaknesses, in operational terms, within each system
   3. Prioritize the findings and relate to organizational goals
   4. Develop an action plan that addresses the necessary recommendations in all identified areas
   5. Develop an outcomes monitoring plan
   6. Develop outcomes monitoring tools

Effective collaboration + Diagnostic-specific resource knowledge + Clinical case management guidelines = Individualized and successful customer outcomes!

Source: Developed by and reproduced with the permission of Ellen Stahl, LCSW, ACSW, CCM, Mount Vernon Hospital, Inova Health Systems, Alexandria, VA (1996).

disease maximize patient care by improving coordination of care across the continuum and therefore continuously improve individual and aggregate patient outcomes," explains Stahl.

A case manager is able to use clinical guidelines through a collaborative approach across the care continuum. To use one-dimensional guidelines, case managers need to develop customer-focused tools that enhance the guidelines and bring them to life in actual day-to-day practice applications. The system used at Mount Vernon Hospital enables case managers to become effective system facilitators and information managers on behalf of both individual patients and patient populations. Communication is the active element of any guideline. The system serves as a template to achieve patient, physician, and case management goals.

"This system should be integrated with clinical guidelines because the guidelines alone cannot promote effective care management," notes Stahl. "The case manager role in disease management not only requires a clinical knowledge but also knowledge of how one utilizes a customer service process to obtain achievable outcomes in large population initiatives. Case management, as practiced within a disease management system, requires a specialized approach in obtaining collaborative response from across the entire continuum."

Selection Criteria

Indentifying and selecting patients for disease management is universal to all disease management programs. Risk identification is the cornerstone of every disease management program because this step is critical in discovering populations of patients that will benefit clinically and financially from having disease managed in a structured manner.

The case manager carries the pivotal role in the risk identification process by developing the selection criteria elements that trigger a patient referral for disease management. The four primary steps involved in determining risk include: (1) population-based major disease assessment by volume and cost, (2) individual patient risk screening through health status surveys, (3) risk acuity–level classification utilizing an acuity tool (figure 9-7), and (4) risk intervention opportunity utilizing clinical analysis and disease protocols and guidelines.

Examples of selection criteria may include patients who are placed on a new medication regimen related to a new diagnosis, such as a recently diagnosed diabetic whose medical treatment includes oral diabetic agents. Another example of selection criteria may include patients who encounter frequent interventions from an urgent care provider to alleviate chronic asthmatic episodes. A selection criterion specific to the worker compensation arena might be a patient who sustains repetitive work–related injuries resulting in nonproductive workdays.

Figure 9-7.   Acuity/Cost–Benefit Analysis Tool

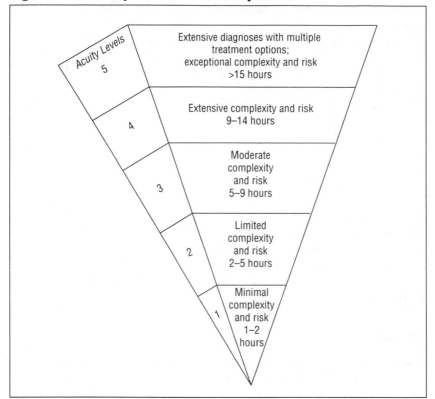

Outcomes Tracking

The term *outcomes* can be used in widely varying levels of abstraction, from very broad outcomes (such as health status or quality of life) to very specific outcomes (such as blood glucose or the ability to bathe oneself). Nursing-sensitive clinical outcomes are the focus of this section.[19] However, in considering the health outcomes steps discussed in chapter 3, nurse case managers should consider themselves major contributors, if not facilitators, for many of these outcomes tasks.

Nurse case managers are very familiar with outcomes documentation. They have always ensured that individual treatment plans were evaluated and that treatment outcomes were recorded. From nursing notes to case management reports, treatment outcomes were definitively stated. Variance from the plan and failure to comply were clearly documented. Nursing care plans were designed to capture such information. With disease management, population-specific outcomes data are made possible by the integration of information across the continuum and the capability for proprietary benchmarking that can be based on this information.

It may help to look at an example of the outcomes of noncompliance and the ultimate dollar cost to employers, health plans, and consumers. The following example involves a diabetic patient who failed to comply with medication therapy. The patient experienced diabetic complications and had to be hospitalized to regulate his insulin levels. Failure to comply with his medication resulted in hospitalization and staggering costs to the health plan and the employer. Unfortunately, the cost of such "high utilizers" ultimately trickles down to all health care consumers.

In a related situation, an estimated 50 percent of the approximately 1.8 billion prescription medications dispensed annually in this country are taken incorrectly, thereby negatively affecting therapeutic clinical outcomes. Between 2 percent and 20 percent of these prescriptions are never filled, and approximately 30 percent are not refilled. Significantly, medications with a propensity toward adverse side effects (antihypertensive agents) are most likely to evoke noncompliant behaviors. Noncompliance-related costs soar as nearly 10 percent of all hospital admissions and an estimated 23 percent of skilled nursing facility admissions are the direct result of prescription drug noncompliance.[20]

These illustrations make it clear that the consumer remains the greatest health care reform variable, and that the counseling role of the nurse case manager is vital to consumer compliance and improved clinical outcomes. Because case managers monitor and track variances from treatment plans and document outcomes information for analysis, they are well positioned to serve as patient educators and counselors. Although patient education is certainly no guarantee of behavioral change, early intervention and relationship building can create the opportunity for a personal and purposeful practice of wellness.

Ideally, the entire health care community should agree on a common language, understanding, and implementation of outcomes measurements so the possibility for misrepresentation and misinterpretation is minimized. Although no gold standard exists, the industry as a whole can benefit if individual organizations aggressively pursue the task of gathering raw data and transforming them into something useful and measurable, accepting the premise that imperfect data are better than no data at all.[21]

Organizations must also accept that not all desirable clinical outcomes will pass the short-term test of cost containment and that program comparisons must consider individual patient outcomes as well as cumulative aggregated data. In addition, organizations must understand that specific treatments yield given outcomes and that society will be faced with the choice of whether the outcome is good enough at the given cost. Outcomes studies illustrate only what might be accomplished with a specific treatment and

not whether it should be provided. Hopefully, the ethics of medical practice will survive in the era of automated health care delivery.[22]

Cost-Benefit Analysis

Cost-benefit analysis requires a unique approach to identifying and
documenting case management activities in a disease management arena.
In episode-based case management, cost–benefit analysis focuses on assign-
ing dollar value savings to individual-based intermittent interventions from
a single continuum of care perspective.

Disease management cost–benefit analysis is determined by population-
based case management, acuity levels, and the ability of the case manager
through individual interventions to prevent development of disease, reduce
disease severity, or prevent disease progression. The case manager is accountable for cost–benefit analysis and acuity management across the entire
continuum.

Figure 9-7 highlights a framework for applying cost–benefit analysis
to a disease management population. For example, a case manager managing a cardiovascular population would place a patient with cardiac transplant needs in the level five category as these patients generally have multiple
systems failure and require exceptional, lengthy hours of management. In
contrast, a patient with newly diagnosed hypercholesteremia would be placed
in the level one category because these patients generally have basic education needs that require minimal hours of management. (It should be noted
that the hours listed are examples only and not reflective of actual cases.)

• Evolution of Roles, Responsibilities, and Skill Sets

As suggested in the introduction to this chapter, the role of the case manager
in health care delivery has evolved and expanded considerably with the
growth of managed care. The shift from component-style delivery to comprehensive forms of disease management has created an opportunity for
case managers to make even greater contributions to the health care system
and to the patients for whom they have become advocates. It is expected
that these opportunities will expand even further as disease management
eventually evolves into health management. The ability of case managers
to fully capitalize on such opportunities will hinge to a large degree on
whether they *individually* and *collectively* recognize that new responsibilities and the potential need for new skill sets will accompany this expanded
role. The discussion in previous sections suggested a number of ways in which
case managers can use and capitalize on existing skill sets in different ways
to meet the challenges of new functions. For example, the familiarity that
case managers have with individual patient and caregiver needs can be a

major asset in the development of new population-focused demand management and treatment compliance tools.

In addition to the redirection of existing skills and experience, there may be a need for some case managers to add skill sets in order to maximize their effectiveness in the relatively new environment of disease management. For example, although case managers may be natural "collaborators" among other clinically oriented members of the health care delivery team, they may be less skilled at working with nonclinical members of the disease management development team. The facilitation of a team of individuals with frequently opposing philosophies and/or objectives may require the development of skills such as negotiating and focused listening. In another scenario, some case managers, who are more familiar with on-site nurse case manager functions, may have to adapt to the increasing use of patient intervention telephone systems and complicated computer information systems.

One of the potentially most critical areas of adaptation that may be required of many case managers relates to the huge gap that could exist between how care is coordinated in an individual patient-focused system versus a population-focused system. This gap may be exacerbated by the expected difficulty of balancing the clinical goals of disease with the economic goals of disease management. For this reason, it is highly recommended that case managers strive to be deeply involved in the initial setting of goals and objectives for disease management programs.

Of the role differences listed in figure 9-8, the shift to being a "developer of systems" versus a "user of systems" will also represent a significant challenge for many case managers. Establishment of goals and objectives for new disease management programs will restructure the traditional case manager role of individual patient advocacy and clinical optimization to a role in which a *balance* is sought between optimization of clinical and economic outcomes. Case managers will need to assess their individual skills relative to new tasks as disease management systems become more sophisticated. Although future case management responsibilities to the at-risk population may focus more on collective versus individual advocacy, the added emphasis on patient education and wellness counseling should enhance the contribution and effectiveness of case managers. Although case managers must expect, and perhaps accept, an evolution of their role and functions as the health care system changes, they also should actively provide thought leadership to help shape this new frontier. In reviewing figure 9-8, case managers must ask themselves, "How will this 'shift' affect what I do now or in the near future, and how can I best prepare for these changes?"

• Summary

Organizations that fail to recognize and incorporate the skills and clinical expertise of nurse case managers when developing and implementing disease

Figure 9-8. Evolution of the Role and Skills of the Case Manager to Disease Management Specialist

Prior to Disease Management	With Disease Management
Individual patient focus	Population focus
Clinically episodic intervention	Education, prevention, and wellness intervention
User of system	Developer of systems
Individual patient-based outcomes	Population-based outcomes
Prevention of hospitalization	Prevention of illness
Patient education for illness	Patient education for illness avoidance
Short-term, intensified case management relationship	Long-term, minimal to moderate case management relationship
Cost savings per patient	Cost savings per population
Case management activities primarily within payer domain	Case management activities across continuum of care and inclusive of entire multidisciplinary team

Source: Copyright M. Diane Ward and Julia A. Rieve. Reproduction in any form is forbidden without the express permission of the copyright holder.

management initiatives will also fail to reach the full potential of this exciting new phase in health care delivery. As disease management continues to evolve in response to the managed care environment, organizations have the opportunity to take a proactive role in the prevention and management of chronic disease through the judicious use of nurse case managers as participants, if not facilitators, of disease management development teams. The case manager is highly suited to coordinate and administer the necessary components of the disease management process. In fact, without case management, "true" disease management remains an elusive goal.

As disease management becomes the next generation of case management and the forerunner of specialty case management, case managers are becoming leaders in their organizations. Case managers are positioned to create, participate in, and sanction the unique and dynamic tools of their trade in the new realm of population-based disease management.

References

1. Zalta, E., Eichner, H. L., Henry, M. E., and others. New trends in disease management. *Managing Employee Health Benefits,* Winter 1994, p. 1.

2. Learning Tree University. Introduction to Case Management Seminar. LTU Extension, Chatsworth, CA, 1995.

3. Peterson, C. Disease state management. *Managed Healthcare,* May 1995, pp. 45–48.

4. Remmlinger, E., Ault, S., and Hannahan, L. Information technology implications of case management. *Journal of Healthcare Information Management and Management Systems Society* 9(1):21–28, May 1995.

5. Remmlinger, Ault, and Hannahan.

6. Zalta, E., Eichner, H., and Henry, M. Implications of disease management in the future of managed care. *Medical Interface,* pp. 8, 12, 66–77, 1994.

7. Ward, M. D., and Rieve, J. Disease management: case management's return to patient-centered care. *Journal of Care Management* 1(4):7–12, Dec. 1995.

8. Use disease management to reduce costs through prevention. Moving from episodic care to care across the continuum. *Case Management Advisor* 6(8):105–7, 1995.

9. Todd, W. E. New mindsets in asthma: interventions and disease management. *Journal of Care Management* 1(1):37–44, 52, 1995.

10. Use disease management to reduce costs through prevention.

11. Ward and Rieve, pp. 7–12.

12. Zablocki, E. Employer report cards. *HMO Magazine* 35(2):28, Mar.–Apr. 1994.

13. Preventive medicine: strategies for quality care and lower costs. *Business and Health* (sponsored by SmithKline Beecham) 13(3).Supplement A, 1995.

14. Preventive medicine: strategies for quality care and lower costs.

15. Preventive medicine: strategies for quality care and lower costs.

16. Preventive medicine: strategies for quality care and lower costs.

17. Preventive medicine: strategies for quality care and lower costs.

18. Preventive medicine: strategies for quality care and lower costs.

19. Zielstorff, R. D. Capturing and using clinical outcome data: implications for information systems design. *Journal of the American Medical Informatics Association* 2(3):191, 1995.

20. Smith, D. L. The effect of patient noncompliance on health care costs. *Medical Interface* 6(4):76–78, Apr. 1993.

21. Banja, J., and Johnston, M. V. Outcomes evaluation in TBI rehabilitation. Part III: Ethical perspectives and social policy. *Archives of Physical Medicine and Rehabilitation* 75:19–26, 1994.

22. Banja and Johnston.

Chapter 10 _____

Home Care and Disease Management

Sharyn S. Lee, RN, BSN, MS

As the evolution of disease management penetrates the health care system, effective home care represents a key element in the development, implementation, and ongoing success of this approach to health care maintenance. Although the growth of home care has already been fueled by existing cost-containment efforts, the paradigm shift that must occur for home care companies to further develop and excel will require a clear understanding and commitment to a new method of service delivery.

This chapter focuses on how the growth of disease management affects the home care industry, which opportunities and challenges may be involved, and what home care's role is and will be within the continuum of care.

• Industry Overview

Before one can understand how home care fits in with disease management and the continuum of care, it is necessary to look at the services that comprise home care, how the industry has grown and why, and current perceptions of home care.

Home Care Services and Delivery

Home care is a very personal kind of health care. In all other delivery models, the patient is required to travel to a location where care is rendered. Whether this is a physician's office, an acute care hospital, an ambulatory clinic, or some other type of facility, the patient is cared for in an unknown environment. In return for access to care, patients typically give up independence and control. For example, patients admitted to an acute care setting are asked to don hospital gowns, leave all valuables at home, and so forth, eliminating or minimizing their personal identity. Their individuality is diluted, and they often express feelings of powerlessness.

When home care services are used, however, providers literally take the required technology into the patient's home and modify the treatment plan to accommodate and integrate the care within these surroundings. Practitioners must consider themselves "guests" in the home, and all services are provided in the privacy of this environment. Instead of the patient adapting to the environment (as in all other care settings), home care providers adapt their services to be as compatible as possible with the setting and the patient's/family's unique cultural, physical, emotional, social, and financial needs.

Today, home care is vast and varied, ranging from unlicensed personnel providing personal services to highly skilled practitioners with advanced degrees and expertise administering clinical interventions that were at one time available only in an acute care setting. Home care represents both services and products, including infusion therapy and home medical equipment.

The structure of home care services generally includes at least two of the services shown in figure 10-1. Many agencies overlap these services and, with integration of services being driven by the managed care and health maintenance market, "merger mania" has resulted in the consolidation of many companies and services within the industry. Although the figure lists the many services that make up home care, integration has resulted in three main product lines — home health, home infusion, and home medical equipment — largely provided through one company, or at least coordinated by a lead agency in the "network concept." Often overlooked are home care agencies that provide hospice care, which has earned a place as a key service that is provided in terminal patient situations, no matter what disease or condition is involved. Hospice provides palliative medical care and supportive social, emotional, and spiritual services to the terminally ill and their families.

In general, the service offerings of skilled nursing and personal care (offered by at least 90 percent of surveyed agencies) lead the list of the 10 most commonly offered home care services. Physical therapy, occupational therapy, speech therapy, and home infusion (each offered by at least 75 percent of agencies) also have large patient populations. Similar findings resulted in another 1995 survey by Fazzi Associates for the National Association for Home Care, which asked managed care organizations (MCOs) which home care services they requested most frequently.[1] Responses indicated that nursing, infusion therapy, and physical therapy were the three most frequently used services.

The History and Evolution of Home Care

First established in the 1880s, the number of U.S. home care agencies* had grown to approximately 1,100 by 1963 and topped 15,000 in 1994. The

---

*The term *home care agencies* here refers collectively to home health agencies, home care aide organizations, and hospices.

Figure 10-1.   **Categories of Home Care Services**

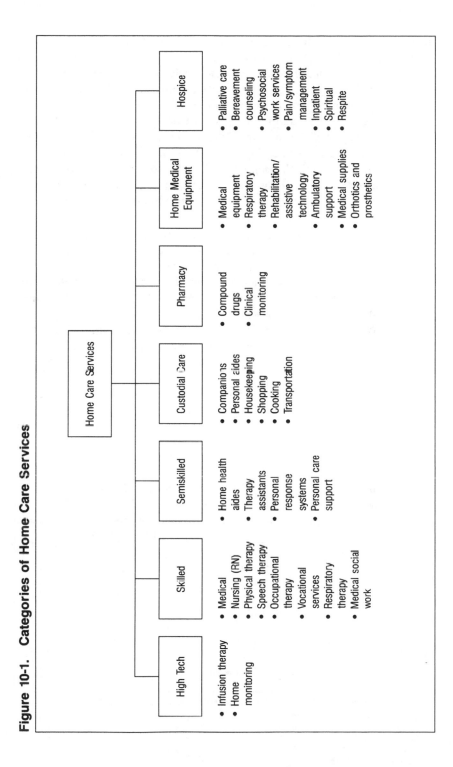

National Association for Home Care identified a total of 15,027 home care agencies in the United States as of March 1994. This number includes 7,521 Medicare-certified home health agencies; 1,459 Medicare-certified hospice agencies; and 6,047 home health agencies, home care aide organizations, and hospices that do not participate in Medicare.[2]

As suggested by these numbers, the Medicare enactment of 1965 significantly accelerated the industry's growth by reimbursing for home care services, including skilled nursing of a curative or restorative nature; some therapies such as physical, occupational, and speech; services to disabled young Americans (since 1973); and hospice care (since 1983). The numbers of Medicare-certified agencies doubled between 1967 and 1980, rising to 5,983 by 1985. Prior to 1987, the predominant type of agency was the public health agency, which represented more than 75 percent of Medicare-certified providers. However, after a 1987 lawsuit was brought against the Health Care Financing Administration (HCFA) for unreliable payment policies, the number of hospital-based and propriety agencies grew faster than any other type of Medicare-certified agency, currently accounting for more than two-thirds of the 7,521 such agencies providing care.[3]

Regardless of the payer, home care is growing at an annual rate of 10 percent to 15 percent and currently represents a $30 billion industry, although it comprised only 3 percent of total U.S. health care expenditures in 1994, as shown in table 10-1.[4] The number of U.S. home care agencies increased by 16 percent overall in 1994. The greatest growth occurred in the South Central region of the country, and only three states (California, Tennessee, and Nebraska) experienced a decrease in their number of agencies.

Table 10-1. National Health Care Expenditures (1994)

	Percentage of Service Expenditures
Hospital care	42
Physicians' services	21
Nursing home care	9
Drugs and other medical nondurables	9
Other professional services	6
Dentists' services	5
Home care	3
Other personal health care	2
Vision products and other medical durables	2

Source: Office of National Health Statistics. *Basic Statistics About Home Care,* 1994.
Note: Percentages do not total to 100 because of rounding.

Reasons for Growth and Its Effects

As already stated, the U.S. home care industry has seen rapid growth, especially in the last decade. This growth, and the predominance of skilled nursing and personal support services, can be traced to the paradigm shift taking place in the health care industry as a whole.

First, technological advances have encouraged the development and increasing complexity of available services. Many product manufacturers have used technology to make equipment portable and streamlined enough to be adaptable for home use.

Second, reduced lengths of stay in acute care and other settings have increased the referrals to home care agencies. As patients are discharged with more needs, the complexity of those needs has fueled the growth of agency diversity and integration of services. Not only are patients' treatment plans more complex, their needs require both product and service. A single treatment plan may include a combination of skilled nursing; one or more therapies; home medical equipment and high-technology adjuncts, such as home infusion therapy; and telemedicine capabilities.

No end is in sight for this shift toward home care services; in fact, it is expected to grow over the next 20 to 50 years. Important demographic and public policy trends suggest that dependence on family caregivers will continue to increase substantially, as elderly patients are discharged home from acute care facilities with increasingly complicated conditions and with case management plans requiring detailed supervision and monitoring.[5]

Although the influx of patients has been a boon to the home care industry, it also presents several challenges. The growth in sheer number of visits, severity of illnesses treated, and diversity of skills needed by practitioners has increased the need for both attracting and training qualified caregivers. The introduction of extended services, including new disease management tasks, adds significantly to this management task. High technology and disease state management require licensed clinical professionals to provide for patients with higher acuity care needs and to participate in the multidisciplinary teams delivering comprehensive care across the continuum.

Juxtaposed with this situation is the desire of managed care companies to reduce the number of providers necessary to coordinate and provide home services. As mentioned earlier, this desire has resulted in industry consolidation and service integration across distinct product lines, placing a premium on the need for sophisticated management and information systems to coordinate the care being delivered by various providers.

As care delivery in alternate settings continues to evolve, home care options must be made known to health care partners who will play a pivotal role in directing the provision of disease management services. Both the public and many health care professionals still think of home care in terms of the public health nurse or visiting nurse services. Surveys suggest that MCOs and referral sources have only a limited understanding of the capabilities, depth, range, and breadth of services provided by home care agencies.[6]

Although many reports highlight the challenges of family caregivers, families often struggle with difficult care situations because they have no or limited knowledge of home care resources and their accessibility. Because hospital lengths of stay are continually decreasing for all illnesses and conditions, discharge planners and social workers do not have the time they once did to assist families in identifying home care resources and discussing options for care and the financial aspects of purchasing home care services.

All of these challenges require a revision in the way patients have been managed historically. Disease management programs can help improve the efficiency and quality of home care delivery, creating a more seamless care experience for patients and helping agencies to improve both efficiency and quality of care delivery.

• Home Care and Disease Management: A Clinical Pathway Model

The successful development and implementation of home care disease management clinical pathways requires a multidisciplinary team approach that considers the variety of ways a patient can be admitted to home care. Because home care is typically at the end of the process in the spectrum of care, the home care agency and MCO have a unique and creative opportunity to derive clinical pathways responsive to a number of entry mechanisms.

For example, when developing a clinical pathway in the acute care setting, the constellation of clinicians impacting care and the mechanism by which the patient enters the system is straightforward. The hospital pathway is applied in a controlled environment, where diagnostic, physical, and laboratory data are key components in pathway progression. In the home care setting, the patient's admission may follow a hospital discharge, or result from direct referral from a physician, case manager, subacute facility, or specialty practice group. As a result, the terminology and severity indices at the initial home care evaluation visit must incorporate both an appreciation for the disease and referral processes and the referral's impact on the initiation of care.

The following model may be used in structuring a clinical pathway process. The process may be incorporated by the home care agency for its own use in managing patients; used in conjunction with MCOs or physicians; or be modified easily for incorporation in a continuous care pathway, such as a hospital-home pathway. The model addresses development, implementation, and evaluation.

Developing Clinical Pathways

Figure 10-2 outlines the elements that must be considered in developing a clinical pathway. The model is suggested as an integral tool for disease management, as it captures and addresses the components of care, such as nutrition, medications, and so forth, and incorporates them into a sequence of home care visits.

Step 1: Deciding on a Clinical Pathway

Looking at the development model in figure 10-2, first, a home care agency must identify the population for which a disease management clinical pathway is appropriate and why such an initiative should be undertaken. Frequently, evaluation of ICD-9 codes or diagnosis-related groups (DRGs)

Figure 10-2. Clinical Pathways Development Plan

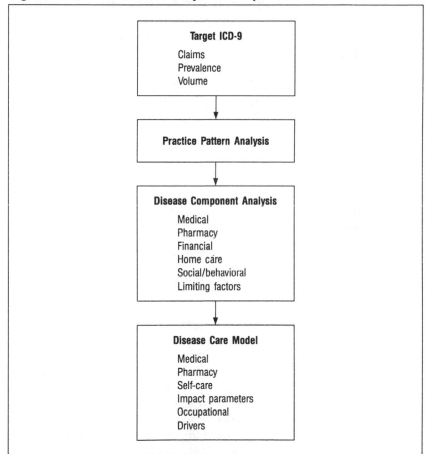

provide much information about the incidence of a disease or condition within a specific group, population, or database. A clinical pathway may be desirable to address health care claims costs within a specific population, such as diabetes, medical cardiac diagnoses, or orthopedic procedures; or a payer, physician, or hospital may request the home care agency to participate in disease management planning and home care implementation. Specific corporations that are noted as centers of excellence or disease-specific companies may also look to the home care providers to complement a disease management program and develop clinical pathways for the home care component in order to provide a fully integrated disease management program along the continuum.

Home care agencies that want to develop disease management programs must investigate both the internal and external environments, and should ask the following questions:

- What is our motivation for developing disease management programs within our organization?
- Who will spearhead this effort, and how much time will be necessary to initiate it?
- What is our financial and human resource capacity for this initiative?
- What are our limitations in time and financial commitment?
- Which aspect of our strategic plan, business growth, and development will be satisfied with this approach?
- How will we market this approach, and to whom will we sell?
- What market research should we conduct (both internally and externally) to ensure that we effectively develop this product line to our existing business?
- What is the competition doing?
- How will we differentiate our program?
- Will a disease management program solve current problems for ourselves, physicians, payers, and employers?
- Should we consider alliances?

Step 2: Reviewing Pertinent Data

If the answers to these and similar questions, including the central question of whether appropriate clinical and economic outcomes are being achieved, reinforce and sustain the organization's interest in developing disease management programs, the next step is to review the practice patterns in the home care intermittent visit record reports. As there are few practice guidelines in home care for specific diseases, a home care agency developing clinical pathways for a disease will likely conduct retrospective chart audits to formulate the visit-specific interventions of the pathway. Interviewing staff who provide home care, in addition to analyzing physician orders and parameters, will facilitate the development of the pathway components to be included in the plan. If the agency is developing programs in conjunction with another organization, such as a payer or hospital, interviewing patients who have received services for the disease is extremely helpful.

In establishing a hospital–home care program for cardiovascular disease, the author spent time in the hospital outpatient clinic, meeting with patients who had received home care services in the past. Because patient involvement is key in disease management programs, patient feedback regarding previous home care experiences was invaluable in structuring a meaningful pathway approach. Patients described their experiences, and offered valuable suggestions for the program's structure. Their insights included aspects of nutrition, activity, medication management, emergency information, and communications, with both positive and negative examples.

This retrospective review should also provide the basis for the development of the core team, which should include as many disciplines as appropriate for the disease. At the least, access to consultants and specialists who will assist in documenting the process of care and interventions will be very helpful. As home care information systems increase in sophistication, ease of access to and retrieval of data will streamline the development process. Currently, many home care agencies' data-retrieval systems are manual or semiautomated, increasing the labor intensity of chart reviews and disease pattern intervention analysis.

The key purpose of analyzing all these data is to ensure that the pathway will include components consistent with reasonable practice guidelines and include emerging data and standards for care.

Step 3: Identifying Components of Care and Limiting Factors

Once the data from step 2 are organized, a disease component analysis is performed, and the components to be included in the model are selected. As many aspects of the patient/family situation as possible should be incorporated into the framework of the model. The impact of medically oriented interventions; pharmacy, social, and behavioral considerations; requirements for equipment; safety issues; and community resources available should be evaluated for their appropriateness to the home care pathway.

Factors that may limit or reduce the effectiveness of the proposed program are addressed during this phase. The agency must look at the realities of the proposed program and address the following questions:

- Are we able to provide all or most of the care components we have identified?
- Will it be necessary (and costly) to purchase or subcontract to provide complete care?
- Is the patient population in our service area large enough for the program?

- Will referral sources support the program by adding this as a recommended or required service for their members or patients?
- Has the competition already captured the available market?
- Will we be paid for the program? If so, how and by whom?
- Do we have the necessary and appropriate resources to continue to develop this approach?

The agency needs to consider limiting factors carefully and decide at this point whether to continue work on the program's development or redefine its objective.

Step 4: Refining the Pathway

If the decision is made to continue with the program, the next phase of development involves incorporating a multidisciplinary approach, components of care, and intervention guidelines into the pathway. The pathway should state a plan for the number of visits (intermittent home care is measured by visits, usually defined as two hours or less), guidelines for interventions to be accomplished on each visit, and the types of clinicians or therapists expected to be included in the visit structure.

In addition to including specific medical orders and nursing interventions that relate to the disease process, patient self-management and learning opportunities are a differentiating component of home care clinical pathways. Whether the patient has been newly diagnosed or the pathway complements the patient's knowledge base for a chronic, recurring condition, the home care agency has a great opportunity and obligation to incorporate age-appropriate education. The patient's and family's ability to learn and assimilate information is greatest in the home, where the health care professional can incorporate the multisocial, environmental, and financial impacts of education into the plan of care. Appropriate educational materials may include some excellent literature already in the public domain. The American Diabetes Association, the American Lung Association, and other groups publish materials in many languages. These publications, as well as those from pharmaceutical companies, home medical equipment companies, patient education materials within the industry, and materials provided by payers, should be incorporated in the plan for interventions as appropriate.

The disease model also should allow for stratification of the interventions based on the patient's severity of illness. A complex asthmatic requires a higher-level intensity of home care services and more visits than a moderately complex patient with the same diagnosis. The potential impact of other diseases must be incorporated into the model and addressed within the framework of the pathway. Many patients have multiple conditions, such as diabetes with renal disease, or complications/conditions that exacerbate the severity of the presenting diagnosis. A mechanism that distinguishes the care required when comorbidities exist will enhance the value of the process and provide clear data by which outcomes and variances can be measured.

The home care agency's development of a disease management clinical pathway involves not only the clinical aspects of the disease state, but an evaluation of both the characteristics of the home care management process and the agency's ability to incorporate a disease management program into its existing organization. In structuring the model, the agency assumes the responsibility of thinking creatively and the opportunity to manage its business in a less self-contained, more integrated manner.

Implementing Clinical Pathways

Once the pathway is created, it is made available to appropriate patients, preferably in a pilot program. Many simultaneous activities will be required in order to ensure a successful pilot test. Figure 10-3 depicts the implementation

Figure 10-3.   Clinical Pathways Implementation Plan

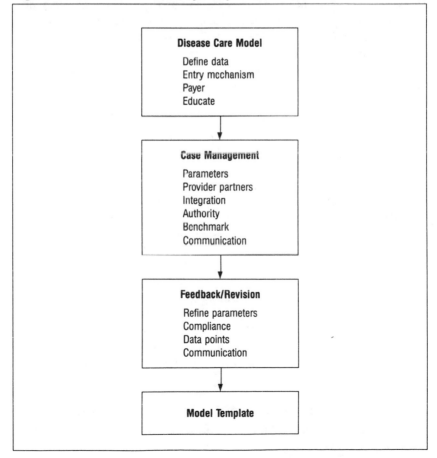

plan scheme, which includes the disease care model, case management, feedback/revision, and a model template.

Step 1: Building the Disease Care Model

Once the model or plan of treatment has been developed, the data that will be collected for monitoring purposes and entry mechanisms (admission criteria) need to be formulated and communicated both internally and to desired referral sources. This process involves identifying the data to be collected and the methods by which outcomes are to be determined, variances recorded, and communication relayed, as well as building these elements into the program implementation procedures.

At this point, a focus group or management development team is key to securing payer and practitioner buy-in, which will result in use of the pathway for appropriate patients. Payers, supportive medical directors, and primary care physicians should be solicited to participate in the continued review and development of the process, helping the home care agency personalize it for their patients. In addition to referral sources, internal personnel, select clinicians, provider partners, and patients should be invited to participate in the process.

The development team's clinician group and the implementation team of agency clinicians expected to provide the nursing care within the pilot must be involved in clearly identifying what data are to be collected. Whereas certain data, such as vital signs, will be collected as a matter of course, based on the agency's policies and procedures, the following questions should be considered when framing the data-collection mechanisms for the clinical pathway pilot program:

- What is the goal of the pilot program?
- What is important to monitor to determine its success or measure the differences in care as compared to other nursing activities conducted with patients not in this program?
- How will variances be measured and reported?
- In the model, is the number of nursing visits assumed?
- If so, how will cost data be examined?
- What demographic data collection will be included?
- Are data relative to admissions criteria for the program important? (Criteria must be determined and thoroughly understood within the home care agency and referral sources in order to capture diagnosis(es) data in the trial.)

The process of education within the organization and among the clinician participants is critical during this time. Specific clinicians qualified to implement the program with patients should be identified, and care of the patients in the pilot limited to these clinicians.

Step 2: Integrating Case Management

Case management parameters need to be defined and integrated into the program. The collaboration of both agency (internal) case managers and payer (external) case managers will enhance the definition of responsibilities and communication throughout the pilot phase.

Establishing clearly defined roles for the home care case manager in implementing a disease management program is paramount to its success in both the initial pilot phase and the ongoing management approach. The home care case manager must be clearly identified as the project leader and given commensurate authority. His or her decision-making and coordination roles must be understood within the agency and among payer and provider partners. The case manager must be empowered to admit patients to the pilot program, monitor the patients' progress, and participate in the patients' ongoing progress. As a decision maker, the case manager should be expected to play a key role in data management, problem solving, and communication with the constellation of clinicians, physicians, and other partners in ensuring compliance with the program.

Step 3: Monitoring Feedback and Revisions

The case manager, also considered the project manager, should be responsible for quickly managing changing indicators in the pilot, and initiating revisions or clarifying changes as the pilot progresses. This feedback and revision step is critical. For instance, in a cardiac medical home care program, the necessity for electrocardiograms (EKGs) to be done on each visit may be proven to be excessive from a cost–benefit standpoint. However, the capability for home EKGs to be done must be available within the visit structure of the program. The case manager must also be able to monitor compliance within the agency, in conjunction with provider partners, and by the patients in the program. Compliance issues range from those of completing nursing documentation notes to visits occurring on time and per protocol for the program.

By viewing the pilot phase as a "work in progress," communication, enthusiasm for suggestions, and intermittent changes that affect the outcomes will be met with optimism and a high degree of personal investment from the participants.

Evaluating Clinical Pathways

The clinical pathway evaluation plan is illustrated in figure 10-4. The steps to complete the program — evaluating effectiveness, identifying continuous quality improvement (CQI) needs, and evaluating outcomes — are summarized.

Figure 10-4.   Clinical Pathways Evaluation Plan

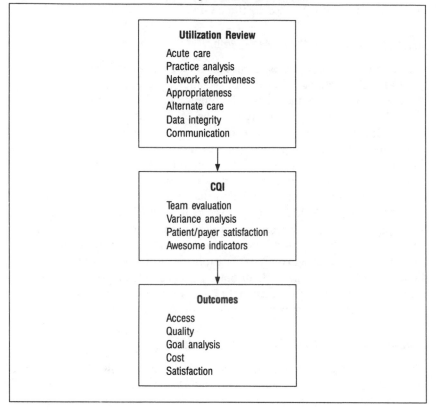

Step 1: Evaluating Effectiveness

This step involves a utilization review, whose components reflect the following areas:

- *Acute care:* It is necessary to determine whether the disease management program reduced the number of admissions to acute/subacute care and whether it impacted emergency or urgent care admissions. The review also should examine whether patient referrals from acute care facilities were appropriate to the clinical pathway plan. In addition, in measuring the acuity levels of patients admitted from acute care facilities, were the admissions criteria appropriate for patient inclusion into the home care disease management program? If not, changes must be planned to ensure that patients are properly identified.
- *Practice analysis:* This refers to both the visit activities and components of the pathway. Review of the visit–visit goals (that is, the goals to be achieved in each meeting or appointment with the patient) and the achievement

of each intervention within the visit structure will assist in modifications to the model. If, for example, the patient and caregiver were expected to "return demonstrate" the proper use of a nebulizer and compressor for the asthmatic patient on visit 2, and review of patient outcomes from the pilot program indicated that 60 percent were unable to meet that expectation, the model must be modified. In this case, additional training materials, more time preparing the patient on visit 1, or changing the expectation of the outcome to visit 3 is necessary.

- *Network effectiveness:* Much of the success of disease management depends on the effective interaction and integrity of all clinicians and professionals participating in patient care. This will often require that a network of providers be incorporated into the clinical pathway model. During the utilization review process, it is necessary to evaluate the effectiveness of provider partners as it relates to the achievement of outcomes.
- *Appropriateness:* Review of appropriateness measures a number of aspects, including whether the components of the model were appropriate, achievable, and measurable; whether patients were selected appropriately; whether there were enough patients in the pilot phase to make predictable, reasonable decisions regarding the integrity of the model as a viable tool; and whether changes to admissions criteria are necessary to ensure that future patients are chosen appropriately. This review also encompasses appropriate utilization of resources, other providers, and the overall structure of the program.

Step 2: Ensuring Continuous Quality Improvement

CQI is essential in all health care initiatives, particularly those relating to disease management. Home care agencies must include ongoing quality initiatives in their programs, and, given the outcomes-oriented structure of disease management initiatives, CQI is almost built into the model automatically.

Specific quality review relates to both team and data evaluation. At the conclusion of a pilot program, a formal team evaluation is in order. The aspects to be included in the team review are exhaustive, and include everything from communication to protocol-specific analysis. If the home care agency developed the disease program in conjunction with another organization or group, its evaluation of the program, member satisfaction, and future investment to continue this and other programs should be included in CQI activities.

Patient satisfaction with all aspects of the program is imperative in evaluating its overall success. The mechanism to evaluate patient satisfaction may be as simple as telephonic or written evaluation tools, or as complex as focus groups. A focus group review will provide both experiential and anecdotal data, as patients in disease management programs frequently have numerous experiences in a variety of health care settings because of their disease.

Step 3: Measuring Outcomes

Finally, the measurement of all outcomes will complete the evaluation stage in the pilot program. Simply stated, outcomes measurement asks: "Did we do what we said we would do, in the time frame we said it would be completed, and at a cost that was greater or lesser than we stated it would be in terms of revenue, quality, and satisfaction?"

Clinical outcomes and goals achieved are derived as a function of the expectations stated in the pathway. Deviations in clinical outcomes may be determined objectively, and variances described in terms of the patient, the system, or the process. A patient variance, for example, may include a patient's inability to achieve a goal within the expected time frame as a result of noncompliance with the plan. A system variance may result from equipment malfunction, whereas a process variance may indicate an inherent problem with the plan itself, as in the earlier example of return demonstrations for asthmatics.

The objective measurement of *quality outcomes* is dynamic, precise, and still seemingly elusive in many ways. Quality is patient and setting specific, defined in individual terms, and, in terms of the aggregate, present in all health care environments. Clinical pathways provide a definition of quality, and a program's quality may be expressed as a component of practice guidelines or by referencing length of stay, number of visits, satisfaction, or variance analysis.

Communication outcomes and the communication process will be measured and qualified/quantified (directly and indirectly) based on outcomes of the program as a whole. In disease management programs, clinicians perceive their roles as an integral part of the process. By definition, disease management incorporates the continuum of care, thus elevating the role of each clinician in terms of the overall achievement. This effect enhances the clinician's personal and professional self-esteem, increasing the investment each is willing to make in the program.

Financial outcomes are measured in terms of actual costs, cost savings, and cost–benefit analysis within the program. With appropriate data management, valid financial outcomes are an expected result of the disease management initiative. Too often, however, comparative data (from care rendered outside a specific program) is unavailable, rendering cost-savings comparisons weak or questionable.

Currently, measuring financial outcomes is, at best, limited to the evaluation of a program's short-term impact. The adoption of disease management in home care is too recent to evaluate the long-term impact of resulting programs. Regardless, there is an urgent need to attempt to measure even the short-term value and cost savings of a focused disease program within the home care setting. Such measurements can include several types of data.

Payers who seek home care assistance in implementing disease management programs frequently capture financial data based on claims paid by patient and by DRG. In attempting to measure costs, a preprogram and postprogram analysis will yield cost comparisons and assist in projecting cost trends as the result of the disease program.

The initiation of disease management programs yields reductions in hospital lengths of stay, particularly when the implementation of the program is an adjunct of the hospital's pathway and is designed to fit in with the hospital's program. The days-saved value is calculated on preprogram length of stay compared to length of stay for the same diagnoses following the program's introduction.

The cost savings for eliminating unplanned hospitalizations and emergency room visits are formidable and should be captured in the financial analysis. Typically, the frequency of emergency room use or emergent hospitalizations is well known by both payers and patients!

Comparison of preprogram to postprogram costs (over a specified time period) will also demonstrate the impact of the disease program. In one situation for a large mid-Atlantic payer, cost-savings analysis for 100 congestive heart failure (CHF) patients in the six months following initiation of a CHF disease management program demonstrated savings of nearly $200,000 resulting from reduction in emergency room visits. An 18-month data review proved that the program saved the payer an additional $125,000 in emergency room and hospital costs.

Clinical pathways are an effective and required tool to ensure that the disease will be appropriately managed, that all of the care components have been considered, and that the role of the multidisciplinary team has been included at appropriate intervals to ensure quality without excessive utilization. Clinical pathways developed for and by home care agencies have the unique property of standing alone, or being assimilated into the continuum of care wherever the patient enters the system.

• Meeting Payer Needs

For home care professionals, working effectively with all types of payer groups is a marketing and business strategy that consumes a majority of time and strategic investment. They work diligently to understand MCOs, their needs, and the role home care may play in the future for plan members.

As noted at the beginning of this chapter, however, it is important to impress on MCOs the true value of home care services and the cost-effectiveness of care rendered in the least costly setting—the home! Although the recognition problem is in part due to the cost of home care services in the total scheme of things—home care accounts for about 3 percent to 5 percent of a payer's expenses—there are a number of strategies that agencies may employ in working with MCOs interested in the value of disease management for their members.

Thinking Like a Managed Care Organization

In order to effectively work with MCOs, home care agencies must work to discover their needs and problems. Whether the home care agency is a national, regional, or local organization, trying to imagine the position of the MCO is imperative to both access and opportunity. Managed care initiatives are changing rapidly, but two objectives remain consistent:

- Increasing market share
- Demonstrating quality, satisfaction, and innovations that support the ability to increase market share

Home care agencies that are able to demonstrate their ability to assist the payer to achieve these goals will be rewarded by increased business and partnerships that position them for the future.

Providing Solutions to the Dilemmas of the MCO

The 80/20 rule (80 percent of the [costs, problems, or expenses] are borne by 20 percent of the [members, diagnoses, physician providers, home care providers, hospital affiliations]) applies almost universally in business and health care, including MCOs. Home care agencies seeking to provide solutions to an MCO's problems should ask that MCO the following questions:

- What is the most frequently occurring problem in managing the home care needs of your plan members?
- What 10 DRGs have the highest costs within your organization?
- What communication methods do you use with your best home care agency?
- What are the two things you like most about your preferred home care provider?
- What are the two most frustrating aspects of dealing with home care providers?
- What kinds of communication structures work best for your organization?
- What are your expectations in this regard?
- What outcomes data are you currently receiving from your home care agencies?
- What would you like to see provided? At what intervals? How should it be displayed?
- What is the most important value this agency can provide to assist you during the next 90 days?
- What can this agency do to earn a preferred relationship with you?
- What disease management initiatives are currently under way and planned for the future?

- What employer groups or clients are you targeting in your marketing efforts?
- How might we work together to capture them as new clients?

Offering to Develop a Disease Management Pilot Program

The concept of a pilot program is generally a time- and expense-limited opportunity for the home care agency to demonstrate its ability to deliver value and implement a program that is meaningful and beneficial to the MCO and its members. Pilot programs are generally perceived as nonthreatening to payers, and only require them to endorse a proposal with limited exposure to their organizations.

• Reimbursement Trends in Home Care

The mantra of reimbursement in managed care for home care services is typically "authorized number of visits." Unlike the Medicare model of reimbursement, savvy MCOs sanction home care services by authorized visit structure and typically include everything that is to occur under the "per diem" concept of services. With this approach, the home care agency must provide all services for one daily price. The costs are calculated for all of the care delivered and equipment and products used for a particular patient.

This approach is new to most home care agencies. Care provided in a disease management model clearly outlines the components of care that will be included, the number of visits in the model, and variables that will reduce or increase the cost to the payer. This organized approach includes factoring in costs for products, dressing supplies, and equipment and should allow the home care agency a margin of safety in pricing its disease management program for payers. A range of visits or an absolute number is specified by the home care agency and prepares it for "bundle billings" reimbursement. In this structure, one bill is submitted for the total program and is reimbursed at a single fee. Home care agencies that have carefully itemized their costs of care, supplies, and equipment and have managed them effectively will benefit from this simplified one-invoice billing approach.

Many managed care payers, when surveyed for this chapter, indicated that payment by authorized visits was their approach to home care reimbursement. They also indicated that "sole source providers," organizations that can do it all, are attractive partners in a disease management approach.

Ninety percent of payers surveyed indicated that disease management programs are a focus of their approach to care in 1996. Thirty-five percent indicated that at least one program (typically, asthma care) was already in the pilot program stage or fully implemented in 1995.

Fewer than 30 percent perceive home care companies as leaders in the development and implementation of disease management programs. However, they were receptive to considering home care agencies as key partners in program development. MCOs' understanding of the value of home care is limited to the provision of nursing, infusion therapy, and physical therapy, as indicated earlier.

• Summary

Disease management programs in home care represent unique opportunities for new business development, new management strategies, improved care delivery, and excellence in managing chronic diseases in the most appropriate and least costly setting. The constellation of services that may be managed, coordinated, monitored, and delivered within the home will continue to expand, enhancing the ability of home care organizations to impact care across the continuum.

References

1. Fazzi Associates. What managed care companies want and expect from home care. White paper presented at National Association for Home Care, Washington, DC, 1995.

2. National Association for Home Care. *Basic Statistics about Home Care.* Washington, DC: NAHC, 1994, p. 1.

3. NAHC.

4. NAHC.

5. Council on Scientific Affairs. Physicians and family caregivers. *JAMA* 269(10):63, Mar. 10, 1993.

6. Lee, S. S. Unpublished case management survey report, Nov. 1995.

Chapter 11

Strategic Alliances

Warren E. Todd, MBA

The preceding chapters paint a picture of disease management as an evolutionary form of health care delivery that is highly complex in nature and that has inherent requirements typically beyond the capabilities and resources of any single organization. As there are many who question whether health care providers are capable of consistently delivering high-quality care within their own single dimension of expertise and experience, the idea of these same providers taking on the coordination of multidisciplinary and multi-organizational care necessary in any true *system* of disease management raises great concern and doubt. The sheer complexity of developing, implementing, and managing comprehensive disease management systems is compounded by the high level of risk associated with the development of any new service in a rapidly changing marketplace.

Actuarial experts, the "risk managers" of our industry, would clearly advise any organization that the sharing of risks in this environment is a must. Disease management cries out for the identification of risk partners and almost demands the creation of business alliances. As will be suggested later, many health care organizations have already discovered the need for strategic business alliances and are working to identify potential partners. The rapid pace at which organizations are "partnering" (advice against the use of this word for legal reasons is given later in this chapter) will invariably

---

In the search to find material for this chapter, it became evident that a book by Robert Porter Lynch represented the definitive source for guiding the uninitiated through their first alliance experience. The frequent reference to and use of material from Mr. Lynch's *Business Alliances Guide* is a testament to the quality of this work. It is recommended to anyone who is involved in creating, managing, or working with business alliances. Having spent three years working on alliances in the area of disease management, and many years prior to that in other areas of health care, this author still finds it extremely useful to revisit Mr. Lynch's guide on a regular basis. A tour of this book would also benefit more experienced deal makers and alliance managers. A second recommended reference is *Working Together* by Seth Allcorn (Chicago: Probus, 1995). This book nicely complements Lynch's work, addressing the dynamics of human behavior as it relates to the formation of alliances and integrated delivery systems.

create additional problems for disease management developers if these alliances and partnerships are entered into without the necessary knowledge and expertise needed to ensure both the selection of the right partners and the management know-how to enable the alliance to survive.

This chapter addresses both the opportunities for strategic alliances and the obstacles that organizations face when they choose to use such alliances to enhance their competitive position in the marketplace. Ideally, the reader will complete this chapter with a better appreciation of the complexities of forming and managing strategic business alliances and will have gleaned sufficient knowledge to significantly improve the probability of developing successful alliance relationships.

• Factors Driving the Growth of Strategic Business Alliances

From the 1950s through the 1980s, the early American colonial experience with strategic business alliances was exported and taken to a unique level of sophistication by the Japanese. The Japanese have both formal (*keiretsu*) and informal (*shudan*) forms of business alliances. In the Japanese culture, control—an important component of many traditional U.S. management cultures—has taken the form of coordination, not subservience, with close personal relationships developed between top executives being critically important in the functioning of Japanese alliances.[1]

This early history of American and Japanese experience with business alliances is now being revived by many modern corporations. A good example of American alliance ingenuity was recently demonstrated by United Airlines and McDonald's: United is offering McDonald's Kids Meals™ on its North American flights.[2] Corning of Corning, NY, has 22 alliance ventures in 12 countries with earnings contributions from equity alliances accounting for 35 percent of the company's net income in 1992.[3] The rapid growth of alliances was highlighted in a 1991 survey by Dataquest and Arthur Young of over 700 CEOs of start-up and fast-growing companies. According to this survey, nearly 90 percent of the companies surveyed had begun forming alliances, up from 81 percent in 1990 and 73 percent in 1989. In contrast, a 1988 study by Booz-Allen & Hamilton showed that at that time only 17 percent of American business executives saw alliances as effective, compared to 74 percent of their Japanese counterparts.[4]

The increasing movement toward alliances is decidedly a trend of the 1990s. During the 1970s, U.S. companies were focused on diversification strategies. This trend gave way to "merger/acquisition mania" fueled by investment bankers in the 1980s.[5] Interestingly, the majority of these acquisitions ended in disaster as a result of culture shock. The failures of the 1980s have created an environment in which many companies now view strategic business alliances as a "safer" alternative. Some experts view the growth of strategic alliances as a preacquisition strategy for many organizations. Nevertheless, a study by Venture Economics in 1991 tracked the formation of over 5,000 alliances and estimated that at least twice that number went unreported.[6]

The climate favoring the formation of strategic business alliances is especially evident in the health care industry. Of the three fundamental vehicles for business growth — internal expansion, acquisition, and alliances — the formation of strategic alliances is more appropriate in an environment characterized by rapid change and uncertainty, especially after a decade of less-than-stellar performance from mergers and acquisitions. Simply put, if a new cooperative venture structure is going to fail, alliances are inherently less risky than full-blown mergers or acquisitions. The major forces favoring the continued growth of alliances in this country include:[7]

- The accelerated pace of technological change
- The availability of a broader range of technological capabilities
- Industry and economic maturation
- Shorter product life cycles
- Larger capital requirements
- Higher-risk ventures
- Entry by new firms
- The need for multiple proficiencies that no single firm can possess
- Deregulation and open trade agreements

Perhaps one of the most basic and powerful forces driving change in the U.S. health care delivery system lies in one of Naisbitt's megatrends, that is, the global economic boom of the 1990s.[8] With the economic forces of the world surging across national borders, the danger that rising health care costs may prevent us from maximizing our position in this new global market is both real and frightening. Companies burdened with rising health care costs will simply not be competitive in the world market. Disease management represents one potential solution to these costs.

Faced with the need to be more competitive in a larger marketplace, it is interesting that the formation of alliances as a vehicle for increased competitiveness and corporate effectiveness is, in some respects, a return to the past, when earlier international business dealings were achieved largely through the formation of cartels. The new alliances, or cartels, may be called by a different name — *consortiums* — but they still represent a type of alliance for maximizing the resources and capabilities of organizations with complementary strengths and weaknesses.[9] Burrus, in his *Technotrends,* addresses the need to revisit how we manage as well as the need for major shifts in our corporate culture, should we hope to succeed in the new global economy and in the development and implementation of new means of managing health care (that is, disease management) (see table 11-1).[10]

Table 11-1.   Changing Value-Chain Assumptions

Old Model (Each organization aims to maximize its own profit.)	New Model (Each organization aims to maximize total value-chain success.)
1. Strategies/plans are developed independently.	1. Business/operational planning is coordinated.
2. Information sharing, and joint problem solving is limited.	2. Information is widely shared, and problems are solved jointly.
3. Accounting, measurement, and reward systems are separate and unsynchronized.	3. Accounting, measurement, and reward systems are consistent.
4. Salesforce pushes products on salespeople's terms.	4. Selling is a consultative process.
5. Resources are inefficiently utilized.	5. Resources are shared.

Source: Ashkenas, R., Ulrich, D., Jick, T., and Kerr, S. *The Boundaryless Organization.* San Francisco: Jossey-Bass, 1995, p. 200.

The issue of management readiness is addressed later in this chapter. Meanwhile, the need for rapid adaptation to change is further suggested by the following maxims:[11]

- If it works, it's obsolete.
- Past success is your worst enemy.
- Learn to fail fast.

Although the factors fueling today's expansion of business alliances may be unique, it is comforting to know that the history of this country provides numerous examples of successful alliances. As early as 1776, at the signing of the Declaration of Independence, Benjamin Franklin inadvertently promoted the concept of alliances, commonly referred to as *unions* in those days, when he stated "We must hang together, or assuredly we shall all hang separately."[12] Later, a highly complex network of strategic alliances was created by Thomas Edison to develop the infrastructure needed to bring electricity to America. As recounted by Lynch, Edison faced a triple threat in that he had to deal with a new company entering new markets with new technology.[13]

More recently, Paul Lawrence of the Harvard Business School expressed his belief in the future of business alliances via his prediction, "In the decades to come, managers will either be part of an alliance or competing with one."[14] Peter Drucker seemed equally disposed to the promise of business partnerships when he predicted that cooperative partnerships will become the dominant form of business in the future.[15]

• Alliances Defined

Rigsbee describes two basic types of alliances. The first, *cotton candy partnering,* looks good and tastes good, but is mostly fluff and dissolves into nothing after a short period of time. The second, *integrity partnering,* involves organizations with integrity, that is, organizations that continually seek superior approaches to make their business or company even more powerful.[16] This implies careful selection of partners—the most difficult part of building strategic alliances.

There are other definitions offered for an alliance as well. Kaluzny and colleagues, in *Partners for the Dance,* offer the following definition: "Alliances seek to achieve sharply focused, swiftly attained goals, relying on the complementary strengths of the partners involved."[17] One must be careful of language. Frequently, *partnering,* or the formation of strategic business alliances, is confused with *partnerships.* Whereas a partnership is contractual, alliance or partnering activities might simply mean working together to build a product.[18] Roger B. Tompkins defines partnering or a strategic business alliance as "a relationship which occurs when two or more people (or companies) voluntarily commit to help each other as part of achieving what each wants to achieve independently."[19] A strategic business alliance involves a situation wherein one company is taking advantage of another company's strengths and vice versa. Ideally, alliances arise out of mutual need and a willingness among and between organizations to share risks and costs, to share knowledge and capabilities, and to take advantage of interdependencies to reach common objectives.[20] Alliances must ideally satisfy three basic criteria:

- They must be long-term relationships.
- They must be built on close operational ties.
- They must have true vested interest in each ally's future.

The basic aim of alliances is to gain competitive advantage, leverage critical capabilities, increase the flow of innovation, and improve flexibility in responding to market and technological changes.[21]

There are several different types of alliances, including:[22]

- *Strategic alliances:* These are typically informal business relationships that include operational linkages and mutual vested interests. Although long term in nature, separate management is left intact.
- *Equity alliances:* These are more advanced in that one company generally takes a minority interest in another.
- *Franchise alliances:* These are systems of multiple alliances in which partners are linked together through interlocking license agreements.

- *Joint ventures:* These are formal business relationships uniting two or more companies, resulting in the formation of a new, separate business entity. The new company is staffed by separate management.

Unfortunately, the form of strategic alliance, or the "structure of the deal," is frequently the reason many alliances fail, in that deal makers tend to rush into deciding what "structure" will be used for an alliance before resolving whether there is both a strategic and an operational fit between the organizations. The failure to use adequate methods and processes to conceptualize the organizational form of a strategic alliance frequently leads to its eventual failure. This is covered in more detail later in the chapter.

Spectrum of Alliance Types

Lynch has developed a simple method of viewing different forms of alliances on a spectrum, as illustrated in figure 11-1.[23] One of the significant benefits of this spectrum is the categorizing of alliance types into three very different types of corporations: external, extended, and internal. As Lynch so astutely points out, the extended corporation is highly complex in that it requires a style of management in which most organizations have no experience. In the internal and external categories, traditional management techniques are still valid.

Value Chain

In addition to Lynch's visualization of the different types/categories of alliances, the "value-added" concept of organizational cooperation is very important. Ramarez offered a definition of the "value chain" in the *Harvard Business Review:*

> Increasingly the strategic focus of successful companies is not the company or even the industry but the value creating system itself, within which different economic actors — suppliers, business partners, allies, customers — work together to coproduce value.[24]

The value-chain concept reflects the core driving force behind strategic business alliances. Very simply, it represents the mind-set and process by which organizations are linked together to create products and services that have more value in combination than separately. Ashkenas and colleagues, in *Boundaryless Organizations,* stress the need for companies to loosen external boundaries, that is, the forces that divide organizations from their customers, suppliers, and other stakeholders.[25] Table 11-2 details the differences between the "old model," in which companies aim to maximize their own profits, and the "new model," in which companies aim to maximize total value-chain success.[26]

Figure 11-1. The Strategic Spectrum

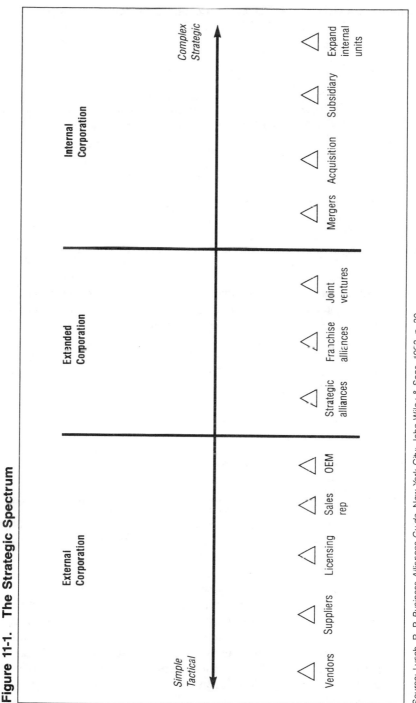

Table 11-2. Needed Shifts in Corporate Culture

From	To
Management	
Management	Leadership
Control	Commitment
Decision by command	Decision by consensus
Negative reinforcement	Positive reinforcement
Culture	
Cost/growth/control	Quality/innovation/service
Corporate groups	Partnerships/alliances
Periodic improvement	Continuous improvement
React to change	Initiate change

Source: Burrus, D., and Gittines, R. *Technotrends.* New York City: Harper Business, 1993, p. 315.

The value-chain concept, essentially the foundation of strategic alliances, implies that the alliance partners understand the needs of their customers. Simply put, one cannot go about enhancing "value" without understanding what values are important to one's customers. The alliance strategies created by alliance partners cannot be established without a thorough understanding of their customers. Treacy and Wiersema suggest that true market leaders are distinguished by their ability to "tune into the values of their customers and to create an environment and management system wherein each employee works to create value for the customer."[27]

Lateral and Integrative Alliances

Another helpful way to categorize alliances in the health care arena is offered by Kaluzny and colleagues. They suggest that alliances may be categorized into two general types. The first is *lateral,* where similar types of organizations with similar needs or dependencies come together to achieve benefits, such as economies of scale, enhanced access to scarce resources, and increased collective power. These types of strategic alliances have formed among hospitals based on common religious preferences, clinical focus, or geographic distribution. The second type of health care alliance is described as *integrative,* in which organizations come together for purposes largely related to market and strategic position and to securing competitive advantage.[28] This category has also been described as a "stakeholders' alliance." Many of the alliances formed for the purpose of developing and implementing disease management initiatives can best be categorized as integrative alliances.

• The Basics of Strategic Alliances

Although this chapter provides many specific tools needed to form and maintain successful strategic alliances, Rigsbee addresses a core concept that is so simple and basic that it is frequently overlooked: "Partnering begins in the mind of an individual. . . . Partnering is both an activity and a *mind-set*."[29] Unfortunately, the corporate mind-set of many of today's managers is geared more to seeing their environment as a world of competitors, not alliance partners. It is suggested that a successful business alliance must begin with individuals who "want to partner." Now this sounds pretty straightforward and seems hardly worth further discussion. However, many organizations that enter into alliances and partnerships do so because it seems like the right thing to do, but deep down they do not really believe in it. Many managers and deal makers do not realize that underneath the outward expressions of partnering they would actually prefer to "go it alone" as in the past. Few managers are reflective enough of their own motivations and business styles to realize that they may not make good long-term partners. This chemistry of strategic alliances and partnering is critical and is addressed in detail later in this chapter.

Although the motivations behind alliances may be as numerous as the alliances themselves, the core impetus is frequently one of the following:

- To achieve a strategic goal
- To reduce risks while increasing rewards
- To leverage expertise or resources

Although the increasing number of alliances being formed in this country may be partly a reflection of dissatisfaction with mergers and acquisitions, there are many important advantages to business alliances, including the following:

- Alliances are typically easier to create.
- Alliances are invariably easier to operate.
- Alliances are usually less risky and require less up-front capital.
- Alliances are relatively easy to establish.

The disadvantages are also quite straightforward. The two most important deal with changes in management style. Alliances require very different management skills and control methods than those for mergers and acquisitions. Given the intangible nature of these obstacles, it is very easy for companies to underestimate how difficult it is to develop and manage alliances.

Importantly, none of the potential long-term benefits of strategic alliances can be achieved without the development of a new form of leadership within organizations, along with the ability to build a team-oriented

culture within an organization. As suggested by Moody, "leadership in partnering goes beyond signing up to work together on and/or 'head up' a specific
project."[30] Teamwork is essential to the success of business alliances. Most
teams initially fail because purpose, objectives, and structure are not clearly
defined and because unrealistic expectations of empowerment are created.[31]
Success in disease management alliances will necessitate the alignment of
the values, cultures, expectations, and systems of the respective partners.
A careful engineering of leadership mechanisms and team-building principles will be critical in such undertakings. As indicated in chapter 2, most
organizations are not truly prepared to take on these changes. In addition,
the success of alliances, partnerships, integrated delivery systems, and other
forms of value chains and extended organizations will eventually hinge on
interpersonal relationships.[32] The reasons for most alliance failures reflect
this lack of attention to the management/interpersonal aspects of alliances:

• Entering alliances for short-term financial reasons
• A lack of trust among partners
• Uneven commitment and imbalance of power
• Failure to inform or involve middle management in the alliance
• No clear understanding of goals and expectations
• A lack of mutually accepted performance measures

Basic Rules

In *Growth Partnering,* Hanan suggests four basic rules for successful
partnering:[33]

• Set mutually agreeable objectives
• Create mutually participative strategies
• Make mutually validated measurements
• Prepare a partnered profit plan

The addition of two more "rules" could be suggested. The fifth would
be to assess leadership culture/skills and team management expertise. Actually, the very first step that any organization should take in considering the
development of disease management alliances is to conduct an audit of its
corporate culture, leadership style/skills, and management systems. This
inherently forces the organization to look inward and to be truly honest and
reflective concerning its core management competencies. Barker, in *Future
Edge,* suggests a number of paradigm shifts that will go into creating the
new culture necessary for the management of strategic business alliances.[34]
Barker sees the need for management to be less reactive and more anticipa-
tory, with more emphasis on opportunity identification and problem
avoidance than on problem solving. He further suggests that the "future

is where our greatest leverage is," and offers an interesting question: "Why is it that intelligent people with good motives do such a poor job at anticipating the future?"[35] Of course, the book goes on to explain why this is frequently true.

The proposed sixth rule is derived from the thinking of Treacy and Wiersema in *Discipline of Market Leaders*. This rule is external in that it suggests "creating the cult of the customer" and is an extension of the value-chain concept addressed earlier.[36] The importance of the value-chain concept was perhaps understated before and is deserving of further emphasis in this section. One powerful endorsement of the value chain is Michael Porter's *Competitive Advantage*. For organizations that are seriously considering the formation of strategic alliances as a core strategy for their future growth, Porter's book is recommended. Although every organization is essentially a collection (or chain) of activities that are performed to design, produce, market, deliver, and support its product or service, the extension of this chain to include complementary business partners is potentially very powerful, albeit complicated.[37]

• Forming Successful Alliances

The development of a successful alliance requires both careful selection of alliance partners and equally careful analysis of whether the alliance members satisfy three basic "fit" criteria—strategic fit, operational fit, and chemistry fit. Without a good match in these three areas, the alliance is likely doomed to failure. Lynch also outlines eight essentials for successful partnering that are discussed in the following subsections.[38]

Complementary Critical Driving Forces

Every successful alliance is maintained based on the strength of the *driving forces* that brought the organizations together in the first place. These forces may be strategic, resource oriented, technology based, market driven, risk based, or financial. In addition, many alliances are created because of the threat of lost market share, competitive intrusion, or even a potential hostile takeover (see figure 11-2). For example, alliances between a well-known national center-of-excellence health care provider and several home care organizations were driven by several basic forces that included:

- The leveraging of a worldwide reputation (strategy)
- The need for stronger marketing and sales capabilities (resource)
- The need to access local/regional markets (market)

Ideally, a more favorable alliance environment exists if these driving forces are driven more by opportunity than by problems. It is also important to

Figure 11-2. Driving Forces Keeping an Alliance Together

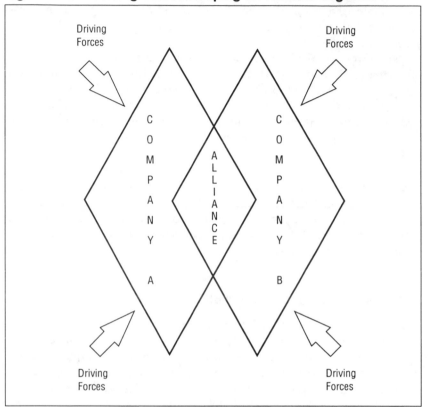

Source: R. P. Lynch. *Business Alliances Guide.* New York City: John Wiley & Sons, 1993, p. 69.

realize that the forces that brought two companies together in the first place will most likely change over time. Companies that anticipate what their driving forces will be in the future will have the best chance for success. The more numerous or the stronger the driving forces for all organizations involved in an alliance, the better.

Complementary Strengths or Strategy Synergy

Potential partners should have strengths that complement each other's weaknesses. It is the strategic synergy that will/should provide the alliance with *the leverage effect of one plus one equals three.* As important as synergy is, potential alliance partners should be wary of the unrealistic "halo effect" that can be created when alliance partners become too enamored of the strategic synergy of a potential alliance and skip over operational realities that may negate the basic validity of the alliance. It is critical that potential alliance partners objectively assess their respective strengths and weaknesses. In addition, the alliance must create a clear, well-defined strategy of its own.[39]

Great Chemistry

It is people—not contracts and strategy statements—that enable alliances to be created and to prosper. Unfortunately, the lack of "great chemistry" is too frequently the reason for alliance failures. Tom Benson, vice-president of Mitsubishi, notes that "people pretty much operate based on their values, and the key to partnering is to somehow align the values."[40] The secret to determining whether great chemistry exists between two organizations is to ensure that both top and middle management have sufficient opportunity to observe the value system of their potential alliance partner(s). Lynch wisely suggests that alliance negotiations take place in a variety of business and social environments in order that managers can be observed in different settings.[41] His example of managers having great chemistry on the golf course but not in the boardroom or in stressful situations is very well taken. It is guaranteed that at some time over the course of an alliance, stress will be introduced into the relationship. It is best to find out how a partner reacts to stress up front. Rigsbee has a good analogy on this basic chemistry issue: "Partnering, like a marriage, will not change people."[42] He goes on to suggest that the alliance stakeholders from each company be given a chance to adapt to the alliance.[43] Too much change too quickly can be fatal to success. The importance of sorting out the values and chemistry issues cannot be overstated. As Lynch points out, "Companies with mediocre values do not make good partners.[44]

Win/Win Attitude

A quote from John F. Kennedy nicely sums up the importance and difficulty of developing a win/win business relationship: "We cannot negotiate with those who say: what is mine is mine, and what's yours is negotiable."[45] The negotiation process should be considered more of a design process than a bargaining process if a win/win mind-set is to be achieved.[46] A double win requires that managers continuously seek flexible solutions that maximize gain and value for both partners.[47]

In attempting to achieve this critical win/win situation, it is essential that alliance negotiators recognize and deal with the basic differences between the organizations. Lynch suggests that the gaps between the organizations be identified and dealt with. Figure 11-3 suggests a number of different dimensions that should be assessed for potential alliance partners.

Spending too much time on the technical details of the agreement versus the broad issues is not advisable during the negotiation process. Legal counsel is frequently brought into negotiations too early in the process. Lawyers too

Figure 11-3. Assessment Dimensions for Potential Alliance Partners

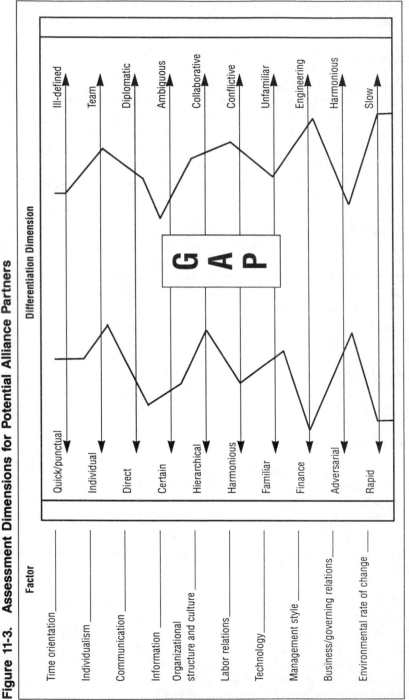

Source: Lynch, R. P. *Business Alliances Guide.* New York City: John Wiley & Sons, 1993, p. 116.

often have an "acquisition mentality" that tends to force too much attention on detail and "exit strategies." After all, a lawyer's primary job is to protect the client from unreasonable risk. As noted by Lynch, "alliances never fail because of the quality of the legal agreement."[48]

Operational Integration

All too frequently, the "deal makers" involved in finalizing the alliance agreement fail to involve middle management. One of the reasons for the success of Japanese firms in alliance building is their involvement of middle managers in the negotiation process. This may seem like an expensive and time-consuming step, but it is cost-effective in the long term. All too frequently, middle managers cringe when they hear of a "new deal that the boss just negotiated." In addition to the knowledge that middle managers bring to the table concerning whether the alliance will actually "work," their involvement in negotiations helps ensure buy-in throughout the organization.

Growth Opportunity

Any successful alliance should, by its very nature, create an opportunity for placing the participating companies in a leadership or growth position. This point may seem intuitive but it is frequently overlooked by many companies. If the probability of achieving excellent rewards is only marginally higher with the alliance, it may not be worth the effort.

Sharp Focus

If alliance partners cannot clearly delineate expected results, milestones, methods of management, and resource commitment, the alliance should expect to encounter difficulty. The first steps toward attempting to achieve this clarity is to have the alliance team develop a *statement of principles* that includes the following:

- The basic spirit of the alliance
- The purpose, goal, strategic mission, and values
- The scope of the alliance
- Key objectives, responsibilities, and operational milestones
- Methods of decision making, communication, and management
- Technology inputs and resource requirements
- Financial philosophy
- Project-specific subjects
- Anticipated structure of the alliance
- Means of transformation

Commitment and Support

Alliances require both top management and middle management commit-ment to these principles in order to ensure success. In addition, the creation of an alliance champion and alliance management team will help increase the probability of success. The alliance management team must be skilled at managing conflict and have a built-in plan for transformation for the alliance over time.

One view of strategic alliances, offered by Kaluzny and colleagues, is valuable in its suggestion that alliances be viewed in terms of a life cycle. Steps along the way may be listed as:[49]

1. *Emergence:* The type of people involved in this phase must have strong strategic planning/marketing experience, as the selection of potential part-ners can be a complicated process.
2. *Transition:* Once partners are identified and the partner development process is begun, negotiating activities will eventually shift to collabora-tion, that is, when the organizations start to use "we" versus "you/me." This is a delicate transition to make, and many alliances are lost because the negotiators do not know when to stop negotiating. In this phase it is important to beware of the negative influence that lawyers can have on "process."
3. *Maturity:* In business, certain types of people are great at developing new concepts and initiating new businesses. These same people can be equally bad at managing a business on a day-to-day basis. The alliance team should have people at the maturity phase who are operationally oriented and have the mind-set to manage the details of the alliance.
4. *Critical crossroads:* The driving forces of any alliance will change over time. The alliance team must be prepared to recognize critical crossroads within the relationship in order to avoid disaster. Renegotiation of the alliance relationship is typically necessary at these crossroads. Ideally, as indicated earlier, it is helpful if the changes in the driving forces can be identified up front.

This life-cycle viewpoint is useful in that it creates the need to develop different management solutions to the various stages of the life cycle and forces the organization to recognize the critical differences between the differ-ent stages. Ideally, alliance partners should preplan strategies for each stage.

• Alliance Pitfalls

A number of reasons for the failure of alliances were offered earlier in the chapter. It is also worth noting that the "seeds of alliance failures" are frequently sown early in the negotiation process. Many of these can be avoided. Lynch suggests that organizations be aware of "six deadly sins:"[50]

- Allowing deal makers to violate key rules during the negotiation and deal structuring phase
- Focusing on details versus core issues
- Using a "six-gun" style to negotiate the deal
- Failing to gain *both* top and middle management support
- Completing the deal without an operational plan
- Failing to maintain a win/win environment

Implied throughout this chapter, but probably worth a specific mention, is the importance of avoiding certain partners. Three warning signs of bad partner choices are companies that really do not want to partner, companies that need others to survive, and companies in which there is an overabundance of big egos. It is also worth noting that not all alliances are made in heaven. Lynch lists several "alliance traps," which are highlighted in figure 11-4.[51] Finally, like anything in life, change will be inevitable and alliances will be in a better position to ensure ongoing success if a few problem-solving rules, such as the following, are established:[52]

- Deal with problems quickly.
- Work through problems together and do not blame the other party.
- Make a commitment to action; do not procrastinate.
- Communicate, communicate, communicate.
- Keep your partner whole, that is, demonstrate that you care about your partner's winning.

Figure 11-4. Alliance Traps

> 1. "The Fake"—Competitive companies pretend interest in an alliance to get information.
>
> 2. "The Steal"—Company takes technology and information after an alliance breaks up.
>
> 3. "The Squeeze"—Financial constraints force one alliance partner to turn over data and technology to the other.
>
> 4. "The Float"—Alliance partner gets cold feet and leaves joint venture in limbo.
>
> 5. "The Bleed"—Partner takes processes and applies them to a joint venture with another competitor.

Source: Lynch, R. P. *Business Alliances Guide.* New York City: John Wiley & Sons, 1993.

• Alliances and Disease Management

As indicated earlier, the complexities of developing and managing disease
management programs will almost demand the formation of strategic alliances among complementary organizations. Although disease management
is still a relatively new concept, there have already been numerous strategic
alliances formed in the health care industry. This trend is supported by table
11-3, which lists a number of success factors needed for disease management
development and implementation and goes on to rank five pharmacy benefit
management (PBM) companies on their ability to meet these success criteria.

One only has to look at the "weak" areas to envision that some of these
companies may benefit from the development of a strategic alliance. For
example, concerning the disease portfolio success factor, companies B and
C were rated weak in this area. Should these two organizations rush out
and acquire these capabilities or develop them internally—or should they
acquire them via a strategic business alliance? A real-life example of this
scenario is offered by the recent strategic alliance between Greenstone Healthcare Solutions (a division of Upjohn/Pharmacia) and Lovelace Health Systems.[53] In this alliance, Greenstone, a disease management organization that
focuses heavily on providing data management capabilities (among other
things), formed an alliance with Lovelace Health Systems, a well-known and
respected physician-oriented, integrated health care delivery system in Albuquerque, NM. Under the arrangement, Lovelace will develop the disease portfolio indicated in table 11-3. Actually, Lovelace will be developing up to 30
disease-specific disease management programs over a three-year period.
Lovelace Health Systems benefits from the infusion of funds needed to

Table 11-3. Disease Management PBM Success Factors and Ranking

Success Factors	PBM Companies				
	A	B	C	D	E
1. Disease portfolio	Strong	Weak	Weak	Medium	N/A
2. Clinical rationale	Strong	Strong	————————————→		
3. Integrated database	Weak	Strong	Weak	Strong	Weak
4. Analytical capability	Medium	Medium	Weak	Strong	Weak
5. Information systems	Medium	Medium	Strong	Medium	Medium
6. Implementation ability	Strong	Medium	————————————→		
Overall rank	1	2	3	4	5

Source: Health Industries Research Company, Palo Alto, CA, Sept. 1994.

redirect the necessary resources to develop and test these new disease management protocols, as well as from the "acquisition" of needed data management and analytical capabilities from Greenstone. Greenstone benefits from the alliance by gaining access to high-quality clinical practice guidelines. This is an excellent example of how the right kind of alliance can help further the growth of disease management. Without it, neither organization would have been able to generate the kind of truly integrated disease management program needed to be successful.

Another example of the use of strategic business alliances in disease management involves the National Jewish Center for Immunology and Respiratory Medicine of Denver. National Jewish, a recognized center of excellence in the treatment of severe asthmatics from all 50 states and numerous foreign countries, had developed a strategic initiative to offer its clinical expertise and disease-state knowledge to managed care customers in the form of a disease management program. The marketing strategy involved the creation of alternative potential revenue streams via the development of a disease management program that could be offered in communities outside of Denver. In effect, National Jewish would be offering existing clients what they had been asking for, that is, help in preventing the need to refer patients to expensive treatment programs like the center-of-excellence one provided in Denver. To implement this strategy, National Jewish needed to repackage some of its educational programs and create new ones. In addition, it had to develop a number of strategic alliances that would help provide some of the "basics" needed for a comprehensive program. Through the development of seven strategic (and, in some cases, not-so-strategic) alliances, National Jewish was able to acquire the following resources/capabilities that were missing within its own organization:

- Capital funding for program development
- Home care provider services
- Data analysis and management
- Community-based provider support for patients
- Comprehensive marketing and sales support
- Alternative-site clinical expertise
- Additional differentiated program components

The number of strategic alliances being formed in health care and in the disease management arena are increasing exponentially. Some of the more interesting alliances that have been publicly announced include:[54]

- Continental Health Care Systems, a supplier of mobile commuting solutions for health care organizations, and Proxim, Inc., a supplier of wireless data communications products, have formed an alliance with the purpose of developing point-of-care patient data entry.

- Columbia/HCA Health Systems and NovaCare have joint-ventured in selected markets to combine their inpatient and outpatient rehabilitation services into a single jointly owned company.
- Glaxo Wellcome, one of the country's leading research-based pharmaceutical companies, has formed a partnership named Healthpoint G. P. with Physician Computer Network, Inc., one of the leading providers of health care information systems. The partnership's goal is to integrate Glaxo's health care and clinical information technology expertise and Physician Computer Network's information and distribution expertise to provide solutions for health care providers, payers, and suppliers.
- IBM and CappCare have formed an alliance to combine CappCare's growing expertise in clinical practice guidelines and physician information services with IBM's hardware and software delivery capabilities to provide greater access to a variety of clinical health care data.
- Caremark, Inc., formed one of the earliest disease management alliances with Pfizer and a consortium of three other pharmaceutical companies.
- Hoffman-LaRoche and Millenium Pharmaceuticals formed a collaborative venture to focus development efforts on drugs for obesity and diabetes.
- Value Health and Johnson & Johnson entered into a five-year research and development alliance to develop disease management products and services.
- Nova Nordak and Johnson & Johnson's LifeScan subsidiary entered into a worldwide diabetes disease management alliance that will offer a total diabetes management package, including physician support, patient education, and behavior modification.
- SmithKline Beecham and EDS entered into a joint-venture marketing agreement to reduce health care costs by eliminating waste and duplication through electronic transmission of data.
- Caremark International and Blue Cross of Idaho formed a new for-profit PBM that will provide a variety of services to prospective customers. This represented one of the first long-term partnerships between a payer and a PBM.
- Merck's Medco Containment Services subsidiary and American Home Product's Wyeth-Ayerst formed a joint-venture company to develop and market disease management programs.
- Caremark International and Technology Assessment Group formed an alliance to develop disease management programs in a number of chronic disease states.
- Medco and Cedar Sinai, S.A., entered into a long-term licensing agreement in which Medco will provide certain know-how that Cedar Sinai will use to establish a company in France.

Although many of these alliances relating to disease management and joint ventures clearly involved pharmaceutical manufacturers and PBMs, other organizations wishing to tap into the potential benefits of disease management have the opportunity via the formation of appropriate alliances. It is also expected that managed care organizations (MCOs) will increasingly recognize the value that can be created by forming strategic alliances with pharmaceutical companies and PBMs. Furthermore, based on the early work initiated by academic medical centers and premier physician groups such as Lovelace Health Systems, it is also likely that the industry will see alliances develop between academic medical centers, payers, and pharmaceutical companies.

• Conclusion

It is difficult to imagine the development of any organization's infrastructure for the purpose of alliance building without revisiting many of the basic concepts proposed by Hammer and Champy in *Reengineering the Corporation*. They suggested that organizations need to move beyond asking "How can we do what we do faster?" or "How can we do what we do better?" or even "How can we do what we do at a lower cost?" to the more basic question of "Why do we do what we do at all?"[55] Unfortunately, many health care organizations have not asked themselves this basic question. Too frequently, they are more interested in seeking out the latest potential solution to problems than in assessing their basic reasons for existence. As organizations approach the business of forming strategic alliances, this is an excellent time to step back and look at these strategic questions. Although the formation of strategic alliances for disease management may represent a more viable vehicle for business growth with less inherent risk than mergers or acquisitions, they are no less prone to failure. When the dust settles, it will be necessary for disease management developers and alliance managers to recreate an atmosphere that makes "their business" and "your business" into "our business."[56]

This author's strong belief in the need for creating strategic alliances for the purpose of developing and implementing disease management programs is hopefully conveyed throughout this chapter. Certainly, the recent cover story in *Nations Business* suggests that the potential benefits of strategic alliances goes well beyond the health care industry.[57] Although it may be too early to suggest any kind of a trend, it appears that many organizations that were early adopters of disease management are revisiting their "first-generation" programs and are looking to alliances of one type or another to help create second- and third-generation programs. Another hint of a trend appears to be a softening of MCOs toward the development of alliances with pharmaceutical companies. Should this trend continue, important resources and capabilities will become available to the industry. A third trend to watch is that involving the increasing role of business and business coalitions in direct contracting with health care providers.[58] Considerable alliance development is to be expected from this sector of the industry.

Two other segments of the industry also appear to be growing as alliance candidates. The first are the product manufacturers. The second are physicians. Both of these groups appear to be adapting/increasing their role in the industry and in disease management.

Finally, the continued consolidation of various segments of the industry, including the increased sophistication of integrated delivery systems, holds the promise of enhanced computer and data coordination. In the final analysis, it will be data/computer integration that will make or break disease management.

The challenge facing disease management developers is a significant one in that a host of new management issues must be addressed concurrently. Disease management, as a relatively new concept in health care, represents, by itself, a major challenge for providers, payers, and suppliers. Couple this with the need for strategic alliances and its added complexity, and one ends up with a very significant challenge for the industry. Ideally, the scope of the threats facing the industry, and the country, will be extensive enough to generate a more persistent effort behind the concepts of both disease management and eventually population-based health management.

References

1. Lynch, R. P. *Business Alliances Guide.* New York City: John Wiley & Sons, 1993, p. 15.

2. Rigsbee, E. R. *The Art of Partnering.* Dubuque, IA: Kendall/Hunt Publishing, 1994, p. 5.

3. Rigsbee, p. 6.

4. Lynch, p. 7.

5. Lynch, p. 16.

6. Lynch, p. 18.

7. Lynch, p. 40.

8. Naisbitt, J., and Aburdene, P. *Megatrends 2000.* New York City: Avon, 1990.

9. Burrus, D., and Gittines, R. *Technotrends.* New York City: Harper Business, 1993, p. 266.

10. Burrus and Gittines, p. 315.

11. Burrus and Gittines, p. 13.

12. Rigsbee, p. 3.

13. Lynch, p. 12.

14. Lynch, p. 1.

15. Lynch, p. 18.

16. Rigsbee, p. 6.

17. Kaluzny, S., Zuckerman, H. S., Ricketts, T. C., and Walton, G. B. *Partners for the Dance.* Ann Arbor, MI: Health Administration Press, 1995, p. 3.

18. Rigsbee, p. 7.

19. Rigsbee, p. 8.

20. Naisbitt and Aburdene.

21. Naisbitt and Aburdene, p. 4.

22. Lynch, p. 25.

23. Lynch, p. 30.

24. Ashkenas, R., Ulrich, D., Jick, T., and Kerr, S. *The Boundaryless Organization.* San Francisco: Jossey-Bass, 1995, p. 196.

25. Ashkenas and others, p. 192.

26. Ashkenas and others, p. 200.

27. Treacy, M., and Wiersema, F. *Discipline of Market Leaders.* Reading, MA: Addison-Wesley, 1995, p. 178.

28. Kaluzny and others, p. 8.

29. Rigsbee, p. 1.

30. Moody, P. E. *Breakthrough Partnering.* Essex Junction, VT: Oliver Wight Publications, 1993, p. 169.

31. Moody, p. 168.

32. Allcorn, S. *Working Together.* Chicago: Probus, 1995, p. 9.

33. Hanan, M. *Growth Partnering.* New York City: AMACOM, 1992, p. 67.

34. Barker, J. A. *Future Edge.* New York City: William Morrow and Company, 1992, p. 27.

35. Barker, p. 18.

36. Treacy and Wiersema, p. 178.

37. Porter, M. E. *Competitive Advantage.* New York City: The Free Press, 1985, p. 36.

38. Lynch, p. 6.

39. Lynch, p. 90.

40. Rigsbee, p. 20.

41. Lynch, p. 96.

42. Rigsbee, p. 23.

43. Rigsbee, p. 19.

44. Lynch, p. 112.

45. Lynch, p. 110.

46. Lynch, p. 110.

47. Lynch, p. 111.

48. Lynch, p. 127.

49. Kaluzny and others, p. 3.

50. Lynch, pp. 50–54.

51. Lynch, pp. 172–74.

52. Lynch, p. 302.

53. Genesis Group Associates, Inc. *The Genesis Report/MCx.* (special report) Vol. 2, No. 3, Feb. 1996, p. 31.

54. Genesis Group Associates, Inc.

55. Hammer, M., and Champy, J. *Reengineering the Corporation.* New York City: Harper Business, 1993, p. 4.

56. Hanan, p. ix.

57. Maynard, R. Striking the Right Match. *Nations Business,* May 1996, p. 26.

58. McManis, G. L., and Pavia, L. Partnering—the ultimate alliance. *Healthcare Forum Journal,* Sept./Oct. 1991, p. 20.

Chapter 12

Beyond Disease Management: Population-Based Health Management

Kent W. Peterson, MD, and Dennis P. Kane

The authors of the previous chapters have suggested that disease management represents a dramatic shift in the way that we deliver health care and that the success of this new "paradigm" is yet to be determined. Although we are hopeful that the success of disease management will ultimately be achieved via the sensibilities of strategic alliances, the rapid growth of technology, the consolidation of the health care delivery system, and the ultimate stakeholders' (that is, *us*, the real consumers of health care) increased recognition of the importance of lifestyle changes, logic does not always prevail. The biggest challenge will be for disease management to shift from a focus on individuals and products or events to populations and systems.

Despite almost universal references to "health care," "health insurance," "health benefits," and "reforming the health care system," the unfortunate truth is that all these terms are misnomers. The United States has a medical care system focused on diagnosis and treatment of those with disease (or at least "dis-ease"), not a health system that addresses the needs of the healthy.[1] However, powerful, effective technology now exists to prevent illness and maintain health.

The schism between health and medical care goes back to the ancient Greeks, who worshipped Aesculapius's two daughters — Panacea, the goddess of cure, and Hygeia, the goddess of health and well-being.[2] For almost two millennia, dual systems addressed these needs — barbers and surgeons carried out Panacea's mission, public health and hygiene advanced Hygeia's cause. Today, as unrelenting cost pressures force dramatic reform of our fragmented medical care system, comprehensive approaches to *population health management,* as well as the continued treatment of the sick, must be adopted if managed care, disease management, demand management, and integrated 24-hour health care are to be effective. In essence, we *must manage health risks as well as medical care costs.*

Disease management can and should evolve into population-based health management. As illustrated in figure 12-1, disease management is a part of

Figure 12-1.   Population-Based Health Management

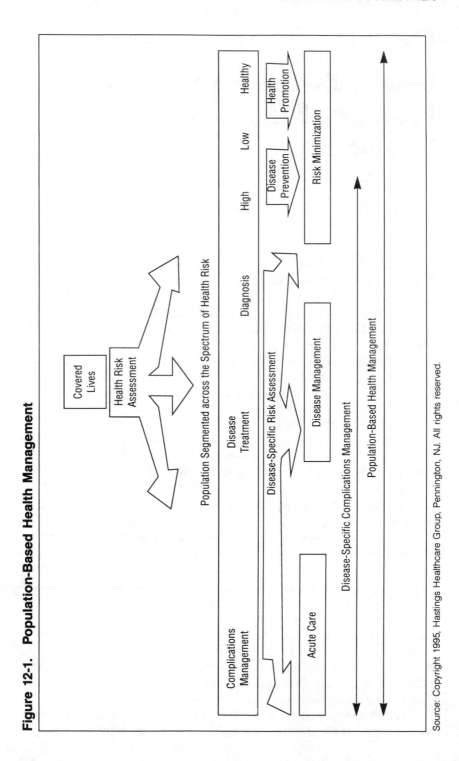

the overall health management process, which takes the concept of disease management to the next level. Whereas disease management is focused on diseases, complications, and specific interventions such pharmaceuticals, health management integrates all components for a physiologic system or the whole patient/population.

• Health Management: An Overview

Health management can be defined as the optimization of clinical, financial, and quality-of-life outcomes accomplished by management of the entire range of health risk for a population. As suggested by this definition, the objectives of health management include:

- Optimizing functional health and well-being
- Minimizing health risk factors
- Preventing specific diseases in at-risk populations
- Facilitating the early diagnosis of disease
- Maximizing clinical effectiveness and efficiencies
- Avoiding preventable disease-related complications
- Eliminating or minimizing ineffective or unnecessary care
- Measuring outcomes and providing continuous assessment and improvement

The keys to success with population-based health management are the systematic collection of health status, health risk, and severity data and the linkage of this information to clinical and economic outcomes data for the purpose of determining the predictors of health, disability, illness, disease, complications, and probability of eventual outcome. As with disease management, health management requires an integrated system of health care interventions to be successful.

This chapter reviews the underlying concepts and terminology of health management, emphasizing risk management as a fundamental approach. It then discusses tools of prospective health care, including:

- Economic risk analysis
- Screening and early disease detection
- Health risk assessment
- Behavioral approaches to risk reduction and health optimization
- Economic and other incentives
- Demand management and self-care
- Anti-aging and mind–body–spirit medicine
- Occupational medicine/corporate health

• Building the Foundation for Population-Based Health Management

Next, the discussion turns to how these tools can be applied in workplace settings through integrated health care that addresses marketplace demands and population needs. An illustrative 24-hour care model builds on occupational medicine–workers' compensation services.

Economic Risk Sharing

As discussed in chapter 1, the dramatic market-driven health care reform now taking place is primarily driven by rising medical care costs. The traditional medical model—which was unquestioned until only a couple of decades ago—was physician driven, focusing on diagnosis and treatment of the sick without regard to costs. The early managed care model, which has taken the traditional model's place, still focuses on the diagnosis and treatment of individual patients, but it employs practice protocols, medical guidelines, case management, and price discounts. The recent focus in this current era of disease management is still largely on the management of costly diseases, the subject of most of this book.

We are now on the brink of a new era, a *mature managed care model,* that broadens the focus from individual patients to total populations of covered lives. This model balances concern for the numerator (few people with costly illness) with the denominator (many people who are well and not using the system) in the health care equation. The people in the denominator are those whom managed care organizations (MCOs) want to attract and retain as members. Under a mature managed care model, the focus broadens from the *few* with diseases to the *many* with risks, from the relatively *few* patients to the *many* members, from the *few* utilizers to the *many* nonutilizers of medical care.

As discussed in chapter 2, approximately 20 percent of a population accounts for 80 percent of total medical care costs. Disease management aims at reducing the risk of disease progression by reengineering and coordinating the many elements of medical care—in short, supply-side intervention. In a mature managed care era, organizations must integrate the management of medical costs with the management of health risks. Among the healthy 80 percent of the population, many are already well on their way to becoming the costly 20 percent.

The natural history of disease can now be altered using tools designed to identify those at high risk and to deliver targeted risk-management interventions. Preventing disease means preventing medical care costs. The emerging world of capitation requires economic risk sharing. Revenue is fixed, but costs are variable. Fortunately, many low-cost prospective health care tools are available that represent a smart investment in containing immediate and future medical care costs. Eight of these tools are described in detail later in the chapter.

Basic Concepts and Terminology

From a continuous quality improvement (CQI) perspective, every medical diagnosis and every episode of medical care represents a failure — a failure of prevention. The stages of illness we pass through from healthy physiologic functioning to disabling disease are as follows:

1. Healthy physiologic functioning
2. Diminished physiologic functioning (within normal limits)
3. Minor variation from normal
   - Laboratory test values
   - Physical examination
4. Detectable or measurable abnormality
5. Perceived symptom or difficulty ("dis-ease")
6. Early diagnosed illness
7. Disabling disease

Every illness prevented (at the earliest stage possible) represents less expense for medical care within a total population.

Travis's Illness–Wellness Continuum, shown in figure 12-2 formalizes and extends the idea of "high-level wellness" first espoused by Halbert Dunn.[3,4] At the left-hand side (illness), the domain of medical care and disease management, the focus is on minimizing disability, alleviating symptoms, and detecting those few patients with signs of early illness. The furthest that the traditional medical model can reach is the middle of the continuum, where many people in a population have increased risk of disease.

The right-hand side of the continuum extends into the domain of high-level wellness — of peak performance, maximum reserve capacity, creativity, flexibility, and adaptability. This world, seldom addressed by medical professionals, strives for an optimal state of health consistent with the World Health Organization's definition of *health* as "a state of complete physical, mental and spiritual well being, not merely the absence of disease."[5] To achieve this, a wellness model appropriately shifts responsibility from the provider of medical care to the individual, who must be empowered to be responsible for his or her own health through awareness, education, and personal growth.

The tools of population-based health management include primary, secondary, and tertiary prevention.[6] *Primary prevention* means preventing disease before it has an opportunity to begin; examples are immunization, sanitation, nutrition, the ergonomic design of workplaces, and healthful, safe home or work environments. *Secondary prevention* detects diseases early before they can spread; examples include medical symptom history questionnaires

Figure 12-2.   Illness–Wellness Continuum

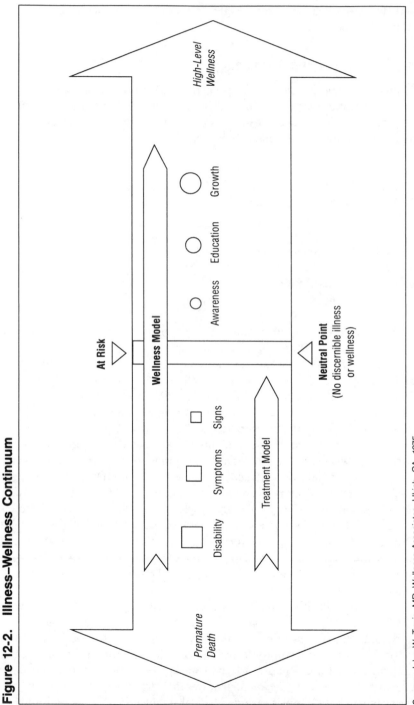

and screening tests. *Tertiary prevention* attempts to forestall the progression of disease once it occurs and to minimize adverse effects, such as pain and disability; examples include disability management, rehabilitation, case management, and work hardening. Most of the current generation of disease management programs focus on tertiary prevention.

Primary prevention is always preferable to secondary or tertiary, if the knowledge and technology exist to put it into place. Primary prevention is sometimes called "working upstream," acknowledging the work of John Snow during a cholera epidemic in London at a time when the disease was thought to be caused by vapors.[7] Noting that individuals who were spared infection lived in certain neighborhoods, Snow painstakingly collected data and tracked the source of infection to the drinking water supply. Those getting water from "downstream" in the Thames became ill; those whose water supply came from "upstream" did not. Snow's profound but simple medical treatment was to remove the handle from the Broad Street pump in order to prevent the water contaminated with sewage from reaching the people.

Disease Trends

Examining causes of death proves insightful in identifying prevention priorities. Much of the public's thinking about medical care emanates from modern medicine's ability to produce dramatic cures of illness, with minimal patient responsibility. Television dramas fuel this perception by portraying heroic measures used to save and extend life. Deaths in the United States during two past years are shown in table 12-1.[8] In 1900, the leading causes of death included not only heart disease but tuberculosis, pneumonia/

Table 12-1. Changes in Cause of Death in the United States

Cause	Rate in 1900 (%)	Rate in 1986 (%)
Heart disease/stroke	17	43.5
Cancer	4	22.3
Accidental injury	4	4.5
Obstructive lung disease	—	3.6
Pneumonia/influenza	12	3.3
Suicide/homicide	—	2.5
Diabetes	—	1.8
Liver disease/cirrhosis	—	1.2
Tuberculosis	11	<1
Intestinal disease	5	<1
Kidney disease	4	<1
AIDS/HIV	—	<1
	57	83.7

influenza, and intestinal diarrhea—all infectious diseases. The successful public health strategy was to provide sanitation, nutrition, and better housing. The best individual strategy was to have access to medical care that could cure acute infectious diseases.

The pattern of death as we approach a new millennium paints a different picture. Seventy percent of people in the United States will suffer a heart attack during their lifetime, and approximately 40 percent will die of cardiovascular disease. One-half of the population will have some form of cancer. By the year 2000, cancer is predicted to overtake cardiovascular disease as the leading cause of death. These chronic diseases require 5 to 30 years to "incubate" through the stages of illness identified earlier.

Chronic diseases are not readily amenable to dramatic cures from medical interventions. In fact, the U.S. Centers for Disease Control and Prevention confirmed findings of the earlier Canadian Lalonde Report, which boldly stated that of all the factors responsible for affecting health status, medical care makes the smallest difference.[9] The 95 percent of our resources spent on medical care yields only about 5 percent of the benefit in terms of improved health outcomes. In fact, 80 percent of medical care dollars are consumed during the last year of life.

Genetic predisposition underpins most illnesses and is a more significant factor than medical care. For example, a far better way to prevent a heart attack is to "pick the right parents." Of even greater importance are environmental factors, which are increasingly being shown to affect the cause and progression of illness. The powerfully significant influences of low-level chemical exposures over decades are only now being understood in occupational medicine and toxicology.

Personal lifestyle is by far the most important factor affecting health status, accounting for more than 50 percent of all attributable deaths. In the United States, more than 70 percent of all the potential years of life lost before age 65 are due to preventable causes. Of these, 75 percent are attributed to tobacco, high blood pressure, and being overweight alone.[10] McGinnis and Foege's 1993 review of actual causes of death in the United States determined the percentage of deaths in 1990 attributable to various lifestyle factors, which are listed in table 12-2.[11]

These studies underscore the paramount importance of personal behavior in determining health status and shaping the patterns of illness in a population. To be effective, population health management efforts must support, and ideally "incentivize," individuals' taking responsibility for their own health largely by adopting and maintaining healthy lifestyles.

Risk as an Integrating Tool for Prevention

Prevention has become a powerful tool—first, because of growing sophistication in understanding precursors (risk factors) for disease, and second,

Table 12-2. **Deaths Attributable to Lifestyle Factors**

Lifestyle Factor	Percentage of Deaths
Tobacco use	19
Diet and inactivity	14
Alcohol	5
Bacteria and other microbes	4
Toxic agents	3
Firearms	2
Sexual behavior	1
Motor vehicles	1

Source: McGinnis, M., and Foege, W. Actual causes of death in the U.S. *JAMA* 270:2207–11, Nov. 10, 1993.

because of growing success of intervention technologies to modify risk. Let us examine each in turn.

Risk factors the general public can now identify and understand were almost always detected first by clinical observation of patients. Clinicians were first to identify most causes of cancer or cardiovascular disease. Once a behavior, exposure, or other risk factor is hypothesized, epidemiologic studies must be performed on populations of people to validate these suspicions. Prospective studies among large populations of healthy people reveal the natural history of disease among those both with and without the risk factors that are being studied.

Once a strong association has been shown and confirmed in other populations, it must then be demonstrated that the risk factor can be modified (for example, reducing cholesterol) and, further, that doing so will reduce the risk of disease. For example, nationwide National Institutes of Health demonstration projects showed that those who reduced mildly elevated blood pressure and serum cholesterol levels over 265 mg/dL significantly reduced their subsequent risk of heart attack. Fortunately, the last few decades have spawned excellent research, validating many risk factors of chronic diseases, as shown in table 12-3.

The concept of *attributable risk* means that a certain proportion of occurrences of a disease can be directly attributed to particular risk factors. Costs can also be attributable to risk factors.[12] For example, 85 percent of lung cancers (and, by inference, the cost of treating these cancers) are directly attributable to tobacco smoking/use.

Well-validated risk factors often increase the risk of an illness by 30 percent to 50 percent. Examples are gross obesity or lack of exercise for cardiovascular disease.[13] Other risk factors, such as smoking, chronic exposure to asbestos, and certain genetic risks for cardiovascular disease, increase the risk of disease 10 or more times. Fortunately, most behavioral risk factors can be modified. Individuals can reduce their blood pressure and cholesterol,

Table 12-3.   Risk Factors for Common Health Threats

Disease	Risk Factor
Stroke	Blood pressure
	Cholesterol (HDL/LDL)
	Stress and personality
Heart attack	Diabetes
	Physical fitness
	Obesity
	Tobacco use
Cancer	Diet
	Rectal bleeding
	Cervical changes
	Breast lumps
Auto injury	Seat belts/air bags
	Driving habits
	Alcohol use
	Stress

increase exercise, quit smoking, reduce alcohol intake and drug use, and make many other changes in lifestyle or use of medical care.

An integrative model, shown in figure 12-3, shows risk identification and risk management to be the cornerstones of the modern era of prevention. Interventions to reduce risk can include health education, disease detection, and primary prevention—all of which are included in health management.

Cost-Effectiveness of Health Promotion and Disease Prevention

A growing literature now documents both the health- and cost-effectiveness of health promotion and disease prevention efforts. The logic of cost avoidance is clear: Health education can increase knowledge, alter health attitudes, and engender more skillful living. Desirable behavior changes usually lead to reduced risk of illness. As a result, the incidence and prevalence of disease drop, as do medical care utilization, hospitalization, medical care costs, and, ultimately, premature disability and death. The dramatic reduction in death from cardiovascular disease over the last two decades is an excellent example of the success of population health management efforts in reducing the prevalence of high blood pressure, elevated cholesterol, physical inactivity, and other risk factors by making these factors known to the public.

The era of managed care is one of cost consciousness and desire for cost-effective health programs. But purchasers and administrators need to recognize that disease management and medical care have not been held to the same high standard as prevention and health education. There is little well-documented scientific evidence that most medical treatments, including many pharmaceutical products, are effective as used today. Furthermore, there is *no* evidence that most medical treatment is cost-effective. Yet when preventive services are discussed, evidence of cost-effectiveness is frequently demanded, whereas it would not even be considered for a new diagnostic tool, laboratory test, or medical treatment.

Despite the dual standard under which prevention must operate, repeated studies during the past decade have shown a 2:1 to 4:1 return on investment. Employers have demonstrated a positive impact on health behavior, absenteeism, hospitalization, or medical care costs among employee populations at Control Data, DuPont, Johnson & Johnson, AT&T, Steelcase, 3M, and dozens of other companies.[14] Not as well quantified is the profound impact that health and illness have on employee productivity, training, and morale. Preliminary studies by the MIT Sloan School of Management and the American College of Occupational and Environmental Medicine suggest that direct medical care costs may be but the tip of a much larger iceberg.[15] Total costs of ill health on employee productivity and the workplace may run 5 to 10 times

Figure 12-3. Integrative Risk Model

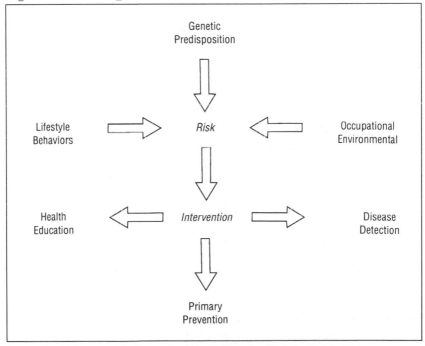

Source: Kent W. Peterson, MD, Occupational Health Strategies, Charlottesville, VA, 1984.

higher than direct measurable expenses. To receive positive returns such as those noted for Control Data and others, a variety of health management tools must be employed in continuing initiatives.

• Health Management: The Tools

Powerful tools can assist population health management efforts. Seven of them are discussed in the following subsections: (1) economic risk analysis, (2) screening and early disease detection, (3) health risk assessment, (4) behavioral approaches to risk reduction and health optimization, (5) economic and other incentives, (6) demand management and self-care, and (7) anti-aging and mind–body–spirit medicine.

Economic Risk Analysis

MCOs are beginning to recognize the value of population health management measures in reducing and preventing costs. Because managed care is measured care, these costs must be measured and well documented. CQI requires ongoing streams of data that can advance evidence-based medicine. Sources of health-related cost data include employers, insurers, third-party administrators, benefit consultants, and a growing number of firms specializing in health data analysis. Domains of cost data include general medical claims, workers' compensation, absenteeism, and short- and long-term disability. Direct health-related costs for most employers range from $3,500 to $5,000 per employee per year.[16] In some industries, such as the railroads, these figures reach $10,000 to $12,000.[17]

Once total costs have been identified, it is useful to ascertain prevalent disease conditions that are both costly and preventable in identified populations. Goals of economic risk analysis include identification of targets for prevention, intervention, and management of illness, productivity, and costs. The end result of economic risk analysis is identification of high-risk intervention areas. These may include particular work sites, jobs, diseases, or behavioral risk factors. Projected cost savings can also be quantified.

In 1990, Occupational Health Strategies in Charlottesville, VA, used a population-attributable risk model to identify the proportion of illness (such as heart attack) attributable to risk factors (such as smoking or hypertension). Attributable cost was calculated in a similar fashion.[18] The results are shown in table 12-4, which reports attributable costs in a large employee population in 1989 dollars. Not surprisingly, smoking accounts for the largest cost impact on the average employee ($176 per year), followed by heavy alcohol use, nonuse of seat belts, lack of exercise, and extreme obesity. Interestingly, because the prevalence in the population is lower, each individual with heavy alcohol intake (six or more drinks per day) added $792. Similarly,

Table 12-4. Cost of Unhealthy Behaviors

Modifiable Risk	Population Prevalence (%)	Cost Average Employee per Year ($)	Cost of High-Risk Employee per Year ($)
High blood pressure	13	95.28	733.32
Smoking	27	176.40	653.16
Moderate alcohol	36	39.24	109.08
Heavy alcohol	14	111.00	792.48
Non-use of seat belts	30	88.56	295.32
Moderate high cholesterol	35	21.12	60.48
Very high cholesterol	15	29.04	193.56
Lack of exercise	50	85.20	170.40
Moderate overweight	23	19.08	84.96
Extreme overweight	13	84.36	69.60
Total		749.28	3,162.36

Source: Unpublished data from Occupational Health Strategies, Inc., Charlottesville, VA, 1989.

each hypertensive whose blood pressure was out of control added $733 to the cost pool.

Similar projected analyses have been reported by Bertera at DuPont and Milliman and Robertson at Control Data Corporation and the Chrysler Corporation.[19,20] These kinds of economic analysis, showing that *personal lifestyle behaviors account for more than $1,000 of medical care expenses per employee per year,* are consistent with the McGinnis/Foege analysis of attributable mortality cited earlier.[21]

The bottom line is that preventable costs are large, and because targets for intervention vary from population to population, there is great value in analyzing morbidity, mortality, and medical cost data.

Screening and Early Disease Detection

Screening is a process in which apparently healthy people in a population are sorted into different categories based on simple screening tools, such as blood pressure, stool for occult blood, urinalysis, or blood tests. Those who screen positive must then undergo diagnostic testing to determine whether they are truly positive or had a false-positive screen. Among those who screen negative, a small percentage really have the disease condition and were screened as false-negative.

In the 1960s, periodic multiphasic screening (people moving sequentially from one station to another to receive a thorough battery of tests) and comprehensive "annual checkup" examinations were considered the cutting edge of prevention. As the understanding of risk factors and risks has become more sophisticated, screening has shifted gradually toward targeted tests tailored by age, gender, and risk. This shift from comprehensive exams to targeted preventive services was heralded by (1) international authorities, such as the Canadian Task Force on the Periodic Health Examination; (2) expert panels at voluntary health agencies, such as the American Cancer Society; (3) specialty societies, such as the American College of Physicians; and (4) governmental bodies, such as the National Cancer Institute, the Centers for Disease Control and Prevention, and most recently the U.S. Preventive Services Task Force.[22] The second edition of the *Guide to Preventive Services* was released in December 1995.[23] Recommendations of the U.S. Preventive Services Task Force are summarized in table 12-5.

Criteria for evaluating screening tests include:

- Preventability of the condition (that is, can intervention truly alter the natural history of disease?)
- High prevalence of the condition in the population to be screened
- An adequate means of detection that is accurate, reliable, sensitive, specific, acceptable, and affordable

Some specialized screening terminology is useful to understand. Let us consider stool occult blood screen done for a population of 100 people, of whom 5 have a hidden colorectal cancer. *Sensitivity* is the rate of detecting true positives, for example, 4 of 5, or 80 percent. *Specificity* is the rate of correctly identifying true negatives, for example, 85 of 95, or 90 percent. *Positive predictive value* is the chance of a positive screen correctly identifying the disease. Positive predictive values for screening tests may range from less than 5 percent to 40 percent but seldom exceed 50 percent. Positive predictive value can be dramatically increased by screening only those at increased risk. Table 12-6 shows that when the prevalence of a condition in the population is 1 per 100, the positive predictive value is 7.5 percent. When the prevalence increases to 25 per 100, the positive predictive value rises to 72.7 percent.

Based on the authorities cited earlier, screening procedures of highest value in the healthy adult population include:

- Medical history
- Blood pressure
- Cholesterol
- Mammogram in women 50 or over
- Pap test for women
- Fecal occult blood testing and/or sigmoidoscopy for those 50 or over
- Oral exam

Table 12-5. U.S. Preventive Services Task Force Recommendations

Intervention	Birth to 10 years	Age 11-24	Age 25-64	Age 65 and older
Screening	Height and weight, blood pressure, vision (3-4 years), hemoglobin-opathy screen (birth) T4 and/or TSH birth	Height and weight, blood pressure, pap test, Chlamydia (females), Rubella serology or vaccination (females > 12 years), problem drinking assessment	Blood pressure; height and weight; total cholesterol (males 35-64, females 45-64); pap test; FOBT and/or sigmoidoscopy (> 50 years); mammogram + clinical breast exam (women 50-69 years); problem drinking assessment; Rubella serology or vaccination (females of childbearing age)	Blood pressure, height and weight, FOBT and/or sigmoidoscopy, mammogram + clinical breast exam (women < 69 years), pap test, vision screening, hearing impairment assessment, problem drinking assessment
Counseling	Injury prevention, diet and exercise, substance use, dental health	Injury prevention, substance use, sexual behavior, diet and exercise, cental health	Substance use, diet and exercise, injury prevention, sexual behavior, dental health	Substance use, diet and exercise, injury prevention, dental health, sexual behavior
Immunizations	DTP, OPV, MMR, Hib, Hep B, Varicella	Td, Hep B, MMR, Varicella, Rubella (females > 12 years)	Td, Rubella (females of childbearing age)	Pneumococcal vaccine, influenza, Td
Chemoprophylaxis	Ocular prophylaxis (birth)	Multivitamin with folic acid (females)	Multivitamin with folic acid (females of childbearing age), discuss hormone prophylaxis (peri- and postmenopausal women)	Discuss hormone prophylaxis (peri- and postmenopausal women)

Source: U.S. Preventive Services Task Force, 1995.

Table 12-6.   Effects on Screening of Population Prevalence

Prevalence in Population	Sensitivity of Screening Test (%)	Specificity of Screening Test (%)	Positive Predictive Value (%)	Negative Predictive Value (%)
25/100	80	90	72.7	93.1
10/100	80	90	47.1	97.6
5/100	80	90	29.6	98.8
1/100	80	90	7.5	99.8

- Well child care
- Immunization
- Lifestyle counseling

In contrast, many excellent diagnostic tests may be of limited value as screening devices in general populations. These include:

- Chest x-ray
- Sputum cytology (for cancer cells)
- Urinalysis
- Spirometry (a lung function test)
- Uric acid (gout)
- Neurimetry (to detect nerve conduction)
- Liver function
- Blood or urine glucose
- Red and white blood counts

Many screening tests have been proven valuable only in targeted, high-risk populations. These include:

- Thyroid-stimulating hormone for postmenopausal women
- Tests for illicit drugs and alcohol in employees working in safety-sensitive positions
- Hepatitis B vaccinations among health care workers
- Occupational medical surveillance among employees exposed to hazards

Finally, there is still controversy among experts about other screening tests. The debate centers on what populations should be screened at what age. Tests in this category include:

- Tonometry (for glaucoma)
- Prostatic specific antigen (PSA)

- Transrectal ultrasound for prostate cancer
- Stress electrocardiogram
- Audiometry for the non–noise exposed
- Hands-on physical examination

David Eddy has analyzed the expected decrease in mortality for selected cancers by using various screening tests in isolation or combination.[24] For example, Pap smears reduce the mortality of cervical cancer by 86 percent if performed every three years, and 87 percent if performed annually. Sigmoidoscopy reduces the mortality from colorectal cancer by 30 percent. Breast self-examination reduces breast cancer mortality by 15 percent, whereas physician breast exam, coupled with mammography, reduces mortality by 39 percent.

Screening services can be delivered by many modalities. These include mass campaigns, such as health fairs, and multiphasic testing, which is often performed in mobile health-testing units. Individual tests can be done as initiatives focusing on blood pressure, cholesterol, oral health, and other areas.

Although authorities usually make blanket recommendations for the general public, technology currently exists to develop personal prevention protocols that would allow an individual to plan individualized preventive care over a period of years. Finally, screening can be integrated into the delivery of other health services, such as vision care, fitness, employee assistance programs, or health promotion efforts. The future holds great promise for home self-test kits and other biotechnology advances, especially as genetic risks become more precisely defined.

Health Risk Assessment

Health risk appraisal (or assessment) (HRA) is a method for estimating an individual's chances of illness or death over a specified period of time. Stated otherwise, an HRA is a way of assessing risk of morbidity or mortality over a 10-, 20-, or 30-year time frame. Its creator, Lewis Robbins, helped initiate the Framingham, MA, prospective study of cardiovascular risk factors. Behind his innovative "health hazard appraisal" was the vision of supplementing the clinician's focus on individual care with population data from prospective epidemiologic studies. Robbins and Hall's 1970 book *How to Practice Prospective Medicine* taught calculation of risk multipliers, which were compared with 10-year cause-of-death tables for men and women at each age range.[25] Subsequent epidemiologic studies and improvements in risk computation methodologies have brought health risk assessment into the mainstream of epidemiology and preventive medicine.[26]

Health risk appraisals are used to help motivate and educate individuals to take personal responsibility for their health, make healthy lifestyle decisions, and appropriately use medical services. Group data provide powerfully accurate estimates of future risk and projected costs, allowing targeting of health education intervention programs, identification of high-risk individuals, and benchmarking baseline data for program evaluation.

Conducting Health Risk Appraisals

There are *five basic steps* to conducting a health risk appraisal program:

1. Enroll participants in the program, using marketing, education, information, and incentives.
2. Collect data. Data are collected by questionnaire or telephone on personal lifestyle behaviors, such as use of tobacco, use of alcohol, exercise, stress, and nutrition, as well as simple physiologic measures, such as height, weight, frame size, blood pressure, and cholesterol. Demographic data are needed, and family and past medical history information are often collected.

    Ryder has described five models of administration of data surveys:[27]
    — The *mandatory group method* encourages employees to attend group orientation sessions (during work hours) at which questionnaires are distributed and returned and clinical data may be collected.
    — The *voluntary group method* invites employees to attend similar sessions either before or after work or during lunch. Depending on promotion, convenience, and social cohesiveness, participation rates may vary widely.
    — The *blanket group method* involves mass mailings of questionnaires to a population, either at home or work, relying on participants to provide clinical data.
    — The *self-administered individual method* can include self-scored questionnaires or interactive computer programs.
    — The *point-of-access individual method* involves people coming to a fitness center, medical clinic, or cafeteria staging area to participate.

    The level of participation and participation rates for these five models of administration are shown in table 12-7.
3. Compute risk. Individuals are assumed to have the average risk of those with the same risk factors, such as smokers of 1 to 10 cigarettes per day. For disease conditions with multiple risk factors, sophisticated logistic, multiple-regression, or log-linear computational algorithms are used. The computational algorithms generate risk multipliers for common conditions, such as having 1.5 times average cardiovascular risk. Risk multipliers are then considered in relation to the average chances of death or disability for people in the same age and sex group. Most health risk appraisals use U.S. population averages.

Table 12-7.   Levels of Participation and Participation Rates for Five Models of Administration

Method	Level of Participation	Participation Rates (%)
Mandatory group	High	75–95
Voluntary group	Moderate	30–70
Blanket group	Low	10–35
Self-administered individual group	Low	2–20
Point-of-access individual group	Low	2–20

Source: Ryder, R. Three common uses and five implementation strategies for health risk appraisals. In: K. W. Peterson and S. B. Hilles, editors. *Handbook of Health Risk Appraisals*. 3rd ed. Omaha: Society of Prospective Medicine, 1996, pp. 47–58.

4. Provide feedback to individuals. Overall risk is often communicated in terms of *health age,* the age at which average total chances of death or disability match the projections from the person's risk profile. *Achievable age* is the age with the same risk that the participant could have if he or she altered modifiable behavior, such as smoking, overeating, and drinking.

   Many individuals find it highly motivational to know their health and achievable ages. Others prefer a health risk appraisal using a health index instead. Top risks are usually presented, both in terms of disease conditions and risk factors.

   Health risk assessments graphically demonstrate the powerful influence individuals can have on their health risks and future health outcomes through lifestyle behavior and preventive care. Risk projections are usually presented for 5 or 10 prevalent diseases, showing current, average, and potential (achievable) risks. Feedback focuses on modifiable risks, suggesting which action steps can be most effective in reducing health risk.

5. Offer assistance with risk reduction and lifestyle change, as described in the next section. Health risk appraisals have been shown to be highly effective in motivating individuals to modify lifestyle behavior, especially when coupled with goal setting, individual counseling, personal empowerment, group support, and periodic reassessment.

Generally it makes sense to provide follow-up health risk assessments that can track progress over time. One schedule is to do these follow-ups every two to three years for everyone, with more frequent reappraisals of high-risk and high-cost individuals. Organizations should not make the mistake of starting HRAs for patients age 40 or over. The time to intervene with chronic disease risk is as early as possible.

Types of Health Risk Appraisals

The 30 HRAs described in the Society of Prospective Medicine's 1996 *Handbook of Health Risk Appraisals* fall into two categories: software and mail-in questionnaires.[28] They range from simple public-domain programs to highly sophisticated commercial products. The best public-domain products are the HealthStyle self-scored questionnaires, developed in the 1970s by the Department of Health and Human Services, and the Healthier People software developed in 1985–86 by the Carter Center of Emory University. The brief Carter Center report is challenging to comprehend, often requiring professional interpretation. Its science base is now somewhat outdated.

Proprietary commercial HRAs vary widely. Most are enhancements to the Carter Center HRA. A few have extended the science of risk assessment, using more up-to-date computational algorithms and better databases created from insured or working populations. They evaluate morbidity as well as mortality and can make 20- and 30-year mortality projections.[29] The most sophisticated HRAs, designed to be highly motivational and educational, include colors, appealing graphics, and positive motivational text written at sixth- to eighth-grade reading levels. One has text that is highly tailored to each individual; in essence, each report is a personal health education booklet.[30] Some comprehensive HRA systems offer comparative risk appraisals that track results year to year, medical record summaries, and a variety of management and aggregate reports.

An HRA is, in itself, only part of a comprehensive health promotion program. The Society of Prospective Medicine guidelines for HRA users are summarized in figure 12-4. The most sophisticated vendors also offer consultation in program planning and evaluation, on-site orientation and group feedback sessions, individual counseling (either face to face or through a toll-free service), and a variety of risk-reduction and lifestyle-enhancement follow-up activities. They can contact high-risk individuals, identify local

Figure 12-4.   Society of Prospective Medicine Guidelines for Health Risk Appraisal Users

- Established instructions for assuring informed consent
- Written statement of program objectives and limitations
- Evidence of science base for risk-appraisal instruments
- Evidence that appropriate risk-reduction resources are available to participants
- Demonstrated staff capability to conduct risk-appraisal/risk-reduction programs
- Evidence that participants receive appraisal results in a form they can comprehend
- Mechanisms to protect confidentiality of individual data
- Evidence of efforts to evaluate program periodically

Source: Guidelines of the Society of Prospective Medicine for health risk appraisal users. In: K. W. Peterson and S. B. Hilles, editors. *Handbook of Health Risk Appraisals*, 3rd ed. Omaha: Society of Prospective Medicine, 1996.

risk resources, and conduct periodic follow-up mailings targeted to each individual.

Health Risk Appraisal Selection

In selecting an appropriate health risk appraisal instrument and designing an HRA program, nine questions should be considered:[31]

1. What services are needed, and what services are offered by the vendor? For example, does the buyer just want mail-in questionnaires, or is extensive assistance needed in designing and marketing the program, conducting orientation sessions, leading risk-reduction programs, and evaluating long-term outcomes?
2. How adequate is the science base of the proposed HRA?
3. How user-friendly are the instruments? How easy is it for users to participate and understand the total process?
4. What is the breadth, quality, appropriateness, and attractiveness of the questionnaires?
5. What is the quality of individual reports, including overall appeal, graphics, individualization, and personalization?
6. How are aggregate and group data treated, including ownership of data and availability of standard and customized group reports and assistance in pooling data for special analysis?
7. How sophisticated are systems, including methods of data entry, central or distributed data processing, and storage and retention of data for future comparison?
8. How good is customer service, including an understanding of the customer's needs, availability and accessibility of vendor staff, turnaround time, confidentiality, and costs?
9. Is the vendor organization stable? What depth and capabilities does it have in scientific underpinnings, measurement, data analysis, information systems, health communications, and client lists and references?

Behavioral Approaches to Risk Reduction and Health Optimization

Many factors influence lifestyle behavior as it pertains to health. Personal behavior is deeply linked to social and cultural norms, personal attitudes, knowledge, and skills. Behavior modification strategies must address each of these aspects. Characterizing behavior change according to stages, as identified by DiClemente and Prochaska, provides a useful framework.[32] An appropriate goal is to move each person from one level of lifestyle behavior to the next, even if it does not lead to immediate changes in health behavior. The different stages are described in the following subsections.

Stage 1. Precontemplation

Although most people do not think about improving their health repeatedly throughout the day, they are influenced subconsciously by the ongoing stream of health information in the environment around them. Health information comes from advertisements and general content in magazines, billboards, radio, television, and other media. It is enlightening to observe how many unhealthy cues are present in, for example, blatant and subconscious messages to smoke, drink, not buckle seat belts, and engage in other risk-taking behavior. Attitudes are often shaped at this precontemplation level.

Because employees spend so many of their waking hours at work, company health programs are strong determinants of health behaviors. Employer policies help to affect people at an unconscious level. Workplace health is influenced by basic company attitudes toward the value of human resources, personnel policies, job design, workers' sense of control over their jobs, and supervisor–employee relations. Interestingly, in studies at Boeing, the latter proved to be the single best predictor of outcomes of acute back injuries, more important than medical risk factors or even medical exam findings.[33,34]

Stage 2. Contemplation

Consideration of changing health and personal lifestyle behavior is brought into consciousness by specific health activities or other trigger events. These events can be carefully planned, such as health risk appraisals, health fairs, education materials, presentations, and discussions. People often start thinking about improving their health because of health concerns among family, friends, and co-workers. The call to action is often triggered by personal illness or threat of disease. What is important is finding or creating "teachable moments" and supporting people when they occur. Health knowledge is often shaped at this level.

Stage 3. Preparation

People in the process of changing lifelong behaviors often need considerable preparation before they act. For example, they may need to master new information (nutrition education); develop new skill sets (how to read food labels, how to measure pulse); structure time (for meditation or aerobic workouts); purchase equipment (vegetable steamers or running shoes); or create a supportive environment around them (meet with friends, coaches, counselors).

Most smokers rate their readiness to quit at about 0 to 3 out of 10. If they had been at 8 to 10, they would have already quit. Smoking cessation programs can support them to (1) identify the positive benefits they derive from smoking, as well as the negatives; (2) understand their many different urges to smoke, reflecting the multiple habits smoking really is; (3) develop nonsmoking skills in stress management; (4) understand the greatest dangers leading them back to smoking—stress, drinking, depression, loneliness; and (5) enroll friends to support their quitting, especially when they fear failure. Smokers compare their relationship with smoking to having a lover who totally controls them.[35]

Stage 4. Action

Actual behavior change is strongly fostered by specific health events. When people are ready to initiate new behaviors, they usually feel a strong sense of confidence and power.

Personal interaction has proven invaluable in supporting decisions to make lifestyle changes. Physicians may be personally frustrated spending time counseling patients about personal lifestyle, but repeated studies have shown physicians to be the *single most influential group* in motivating behavior changes.[36] Nurses, health educators, exercise physiologists, and other trained health professionals can offer valuable assistance in helping an individual to understand his or her own behavior, to explore underlying root causes, to build self-esteem, to provide encouragement, and to schedule follow-up coaching sessions.

Many people are motivated by group activities, such as lectures, classes, self-help groups, and special events. This has been partly responsible for the success of self-help groups or group events such as the Great American Smokeout held each November.[37] Work-site competitions in weight loss, smoking cessation, and fitness have proven popular and successful. Ease and availability are important factors, as evidenced by participation in fitness programs when facilities are available at the job and can be used during working hours.

Health behavior change options need to be available in a variety of forms to appeal to those with different personality styles. Whereas extroverts enjoy social events or group activities, introverts prefer workbooks, journals, self-instructional materials, and electronic communication, such as E-mail or the World Wide Web.

Stage 5. Maintenance

Most behavioral changes are unsuccessful at first, requiring continual persistence from those who are experimenting with new behavior. Maintenance of behavior change requires a focus on relapse prevention, a concept that emerged from the alcohol and substance abuse movement.

It is important to differentiate provision of factual information from education, which emanates from the Latin verb *educare,* meaning "to lead out." It is clear with most smokers that lack of information is not the critical factor in changing their behavior. However, as Farquhar and Wood

demonstrated in the Stanford Three-Community Heart Study, the most effective behavior change among a population of people comes from *combining
multiple media,* each directed simultaneously at bringing attention to desirable health behaviors.[38] Print media, which can create a background for
behavioral change, include posters, envelope stuffers, pamphlets, and newsletters.[39] Excellent health education materials are available in other media as
well, including audiotapes, videos, CD-ROMs, telephone voice-response units,
and 800 telephone lines. In the emerging telecommunication era, people have
access to computer databases, on-line forums, chats, support groups, and other
technologies now emerging through the Internet.[40]

The most fundamental behavioral principle affecting healthy lifestyles
is taking personal responsibility for our own health. Self-responsibility is
particularly important as a patient moves from illness care and rehabilitation into the domains of risk-factor management and high-level wellness.[41]
Wellness is by definition self-initiated; "wellness care" is an oxymoron. Most
important is creating a healthy culture in the home, school, workplace, and
community, with emphasis on the value of healthy lifestyles and the importance of each individual's health, safety, productivity, well-being, creativity,
and self-expression.

Work-site health services programs have been shown to influence health
behavior by (1) making a choice of healthy foods available in vending
machines, during meetings and coffee breaks, and in the cafeterias; (2)
enforcing prohibitive policies for smoking, drugs, and alcohol; (3) providing
posters, newsletters, audiocassettes, videotapes, and other health education
media; (4) sponsoring lunchtime "brown-bag" and other health presentations;
(5) offering or reimbursing for participation in health improvement classes
and courses; (6) sponsoring health fairs and other screening campaigns; (7)
offering health risk appraisals and miniscreenings; and (8) making occupational health nurses or health educators available for counseling.

Employee Assistance Programs

Early in this century, a few pioneering employers created medical programs
to assist employees with alcoholism. After World War II, these employee
assistance programs (EAPs) grew rapidly to help problems among those
returning to the workforce.[42] The programs have subsequently broadened
their initial focus to address a wide range of concerns, including drug abuse,
mental health, family violence, spousal/child abuse, and financial problems.
Employee assistance counselors interview employees and provide definitive
short-term treatment (three to six visits) or make referrals to outpatient or
inpatient therapy. The U.S. Department of Transportation's drug and alcohol testing regulations now require qualified substance abuse professionals
(SAPs) to interview everyone who tests positive for alcohol or drugs, determine their need for treatment, decide when they are ready to return to work,

and determine the frequency of unannounced random follow-up drug or alcohol testing.[43,44]

Many EAPs now also focus on prevention, teaching people how to manage stress, cope with corporate transitions, and enhance mind–body health. Both in-house and contracted models have been shown to be effective and have high participation rates, with each model having strong supporters. Recently, there has been a trend toward contracted programs as vendors have formed regional and national networks of providers. This is providing opportunities for managed care organizations, such as United Healthcare, to include EAP services in integrated health services contracts.

Economic and Other Incentives

Public health efforts have often centered around identifying high-risk populations and targeting services to high-risk individuals. One example is the case method for finding those potentially exposed to tuberculosis or sexually transmitted diseases. Another is identifying subgroups that may be more susceptible to epidemics of infectious disease.

Health promotion efforts also are most effective when concentrating resources on those at highest risk. Yet high-risk individuals tend to have low participation rates in voluntary health screening, health risk assessment, and health education programs. Therefore, the challenge for population based health programs is to motivate voluntary participation. One way to get it is to conduct health events for employees during working hours, inviting everyone to participate. Another is to send follow-up mailings tailored to individuals and based on their personal risk profiles. A third is to urge those at high risk to take advantage of personal health risk counseling or to call a toll-free health information hotline. A fourth is for nurses or health educators to act as case managers for individuals at high risk, scheduling telephone calls or personal appointments every two to six months. Some aggressive programs even call high-risk individuals on the phone. A fifth way is to provide T-shirts, other premiums, and public recognition for those who participate and especially those who make significant strides in reducing health risks. A sixth way is to sponsor competitions or fun runs that reward everyone who participates.

A final way to motivate individuals is to provide economic incentives that reward those at reduced health risk.[45] A growing number of employers are implementing "risk-rated benefits" programs. Their underlying philosophy is to reward individuals who take personal responsibility for their health and medical care costs. Goals include motivating healthy behavior, rewarding those who take steps to be healthy, and requiring that those who do not take care of their health to share a portion of the increased costs they help incur. Incentives vary widely, but include recognition (such as gifts); flexible benefits (such as health days, time off, or purchase of expanded health or life insurance coverage); use of facilities or equipment (such as fitness clubs); cash or drawings (such as lotteries for vacations); and health insurance premiums (such as decreased employee contributions, deductibles, and copayments). Some examples are shown on table 12-8.

Because of potential sensitivity over economic rewards (or perceived punishments), it is important that these programs be based on behaviors or risk factors that are well documented as important contributors to illness and medical costs, and that are well defined, verifiable, modifiable, and practical to measure. Tobacco use, fitness, weight, blood pressure, cholesterol level, alcohol intake, and seat belt use are among the most frequently used risk factors. To ensure conformance with the Americans with Disabilities Act (ADA), individuals with medical conditions who comply with recommended treatment protocols but still have high values are considered as if they are at low risk. Some sponsors accept participants' statements about whether they smoke or exercise; others measure expired carbon monoxide, take blood tests for serum thiocyanate, or do fitness testing to verify the self-reported data.

To simplify measurement and verification issues, some program sponsors base risk-rated benefit programs on participation (for example, completion of a health risk appraisal and enrollment in a risk-reduction program,

Table 12-8. Risk-Rated Lifestyle Incentive Systems

Company	Health Insurance Premiums	Cash	Flexible Benefits	Facility/Equipment
Penrose Health Systems	XX	Vacation		
Baker Hughes	X			
Schneider	X			
Southern California Edison		X		
Quaker Oats		X	X	
Tenneco				X
Mesa Petroleum		X		X
Points Resorts	X			
U-Haul		X		
John Alden Insurance	X			
Coors	X			X
City of Bellvue	XX	X		
Providence Medical Center	XX	X		
Bonne Bell		X		X
Flexcon		X		
Intermatic		X		
Schwartz Meat		X		

XX = Based on health insurance savings

regardless of the result) rather than outcomes. Innovative assessment protocols and educational reports have been designed around the risk-rating concept.[46]

Although some legal controversy has been raised over the degree to which individuals can be penalized based on the results of tests (for example, weight, blood pressure, cholesterol, or fitness), corporate benefits departments are vigorously moving ahead with risk-rated benefit programs.[47]

Demand Management and Self-Care

Disease management efforts focus on providing necessary, appropriate, and carefully monitored care to the 20 percent of individuals who account for 80 percent of medical care costs, as discussed in chapter 2. In essence, disease management is a supply-side approach to managing costs.

Increasing attention is now also being paid to reducing the demand for medical care.[48] Efforts go beyond screening, health risk assessment, health education, and employee assistance. Demand management includes teaching subscribers to become more skilled users of medical care. *Demand management* can be defined as "the use of self-management and decision support systems to enable, educate, and encourage people to improve their health and make appropriate use of medical care."[49] Figure 12-5 shows the remarkable transition we are experiencing from direct reliance on medical authority to widespread access to health information through publications, social support, and the electronic media.

One method of encouraging appropriate utilization of medical care is teaching people to care for their own illnesses through use of self-care manuals for adults and parents.[50] Examples of excess demand are findings that 55 percent of those going to emergency departments in 1992 were not in urgent need of care (National Center for Health Statistics) and that 40 percent of physician office visits could be handled by telephone (Kaiser Permanente). Those trained in using several well-tested self-care guides have been shown to significantly reduce medical care visits and costs, with a positive return on investment.[51] These are good examples of influencing perceived need for medical care.

Another way to encourage appropriate utilization is providing access to nurse telephone health counseling, medical second-opinion services, CD-ROM computer software, and telephone voice-response or PC-based telecommunications information resources.[52] Demand can also be reduced by teaching individuals how to select health professionals and ask questions that help them care for themselves. Self-help groups that share experiences, information, and specialized databases and that may actually invite health professionals to speak with them have also proven effective. Yet another method is to reward employees who review their medical invoices and identify charges for services that were not rendered or other billing errors.

Figure 12-5.   Shifting Health Information Paradigms

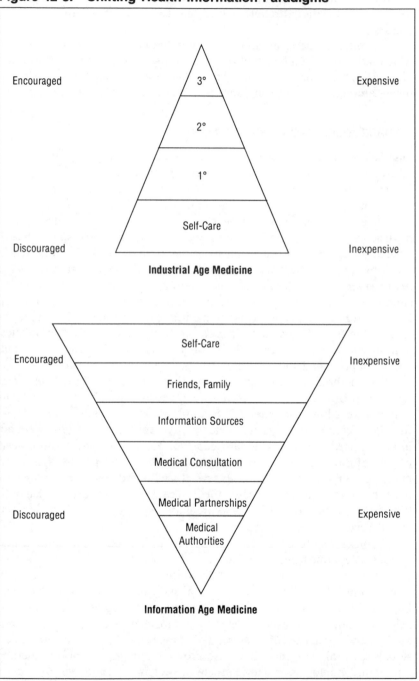

Source: Tom Ferguson, MD, Austin, TX.

An especially helpful approach to reducing medical care use is to help individuals make informed choices about care alternatives. The premise of this shared decision-making model is that medical professionals should assess patient status and outline the benefits and risks of different options. The choice among options is made by the individual and his or her family. One good example is Wennberg's videodisc patient education program about prostate surgery. Another is providing subscribers, patients with chronic illness, those about to have surgery, or those entering hospitals with information about living wills, advanced directives, and durable powers of attorney.[53] Current systems of care too often either fail to educate families about these vital matters or do not provide these documents as part of patient admission procedures. This has been partially remedied by the Patient Self Determination Act of 1991. MCOs can make effective use of ethics committees to address these issues.[54]

Our society, which has idolized youth, demeaned maturity, and denied old age, will soon experience the aging of the post–World War II baby boomers, who will find that many elderly people are astoundingly creative, healthy, and vital. Hopefully, today's wellness movement will help people prepare to age, order their lives, be at peace, and die well. The hospice movement has brought great humanity to the dying process in a remarkably cost-effective manner.

Anti-aging and Mind–Body–Spirit Medicine

Intriguing research has now documented the reversibility of such conditions as coronary artery and peripheral vascular disease.[55] Nutritional support is more than replacing deficiencies, but may be useful in helping the body to deal with stress, detoxify heavy metals and other chemicals, and delay the aging process. The use of antioxidants, such as vitamins C and E and beta-carotene, is being widely recommended.[56] There is a suggestion that "smart drugs," such as priactum, can hold back the common deterioration of mentation in aging. Nutritional supplements, like Coenzyme Q10 and l-carnitine, have also been used to improve energy supply.[57] In addition, previously ignored hormones may play a role in body regulation; dihydroepian-drosterone (DHEA) and melatonin are starting to come into common use, driven by public demand.[58]

Psychoneuroimmunology research is demonstrating the vital linkages between stressor, learned stress responses, mind states, brain wave patterns, neurotransmitters, neuropeptides, and immune system competence.[59] Increasingly, both the healthy and those with chronic disease are turning to body–mind–spirit techniques to improve function and relieve symptoms. Such techniques include meditation, yoga, acupuncture, biofeedback, such martial arts as *akaido*, guided imagery and visualization, art therapy, holotropic breathing, and individual and group prayer. Many of these approaches can teach people to alter their consciousness by regulating brain wave activity, for example, alpha and theta waves. The National Institutes of Health has established an Office of Alternative Medicine to fund academic research in this area.[60]

• Integrating Health Management within Medical Care: The Role of the Employer

Many of the health management tools discussed in this chapter stand alone and can be delivered independent from medical care. In the last two decades the public has made a dramatic shift toward fitness, health promotion, and wellness. This interest in personal health has spawned large publishing, media, clothing, equipment, coaching, and counseling industries.

A growing self-care movement has also emerged throughout the United States among a smaller segment of the population. Although public health and occupational medicine have embraced many population health management tools and programs, most medical care institutions have continued to focus on illness, diagnosis, and treatment of disease, remarkably unaffected by the public's concerns about health. Perhaps this is in part why the marketplace has spawned a host of alternative health and healing approaches.

However, as stated in the introduction to this chapter, the emerging managed care era must incorporate the tools of population-based health management if it is to be fully effective. Managed care organizations must manage health, risk, disease, and costs. Evolving models for delivering integrated, 24-hour health care are the vehicles for doing so.

The final section of this chapter examines the role of employers and the workplace in integrating health and disease management. Employers are particularly important participants in the future of health and medical care because of the following:

- Their responsibility for large, well-defined populations
- Their desire for loyal, healthy, productive employees who are pleased with company benefit programs
- Their extreme concern about the high (and rising costs) of care, especially in light of intense worldwide economic competition
- Their financing of a large portion of employee medical care
- Their concern about escalating workers' compensation costs, which are rising much faster than the medical Consumer Price Index
- Their concern about lost work time, absenteeism, and return-to-work and fitness-for-duty issues
- Their increasingly active roles in setting standards for and restructuring the delivery of health services through group purchasing arrangements

The increasingly proactive role of employers in managing their health care costs has been evident in recent years based on the growth of business health care coalitions. Over 200 active business health care coalitions now manage the health care needs of their employees via direct contracting with health care providers. This trend is expected to continue as employers collectively gain the expertise needed to directly manage their health plans versus offering outside MCOs to their employees. This renewed interest in the hands-on management of health benefit programs by employer coalitions will hopefully lead to increased interest in the promotion of health management to employee populations. As suggested earlier, employers have a number of advantages concerning the "delivery" of health management.

Occupational medicine physicians and occupational health nurses provide employee health, safety, and environmental management services to corporations, as either corporate employees, consultants, or contractors through community-based clinics. Occupational health specialists can be valuable assets to MCOs for many reasons. First, they usually know local employers and their needs. Second, they have established working relationships with employers, as in dealing with workers' compensation cases, and have credibility. Third, as preventive medicine specialists, they understand population-based approaches to health management. Fourth, they are used to working at employer sites. Fifth, they have established referral patterns to other specialists. Occupational medicine physicians understand how the many components of employee health, safety, and environmental management fit together.

Employers are involved in health matters in a variety of ways. Let us examine several models that integrate health management with disease management. These models represent an evolution in the health concerns of employers over the last four decades: from injury care (industrial medicine) to environmental health and safety (occupational medicine) to health promotion and wellness (occupational health) to leadership in organizing integrated health systems (corporate health management).[61,62] These models are summarized in table 12-9.

Industrial Medicine/Disability Management

Disability management is currently a burgeoning sector of the managed care industry, especially that portion directed at work-related injury or illness under workers' compensation, which now costs more than $70 billion annually. Successfully managing disability requires integrating both health and disease management.

Elements of effective disability programs include the following:

- *Primary prevention:* This refers to creating a safe and healthy workplace that is free from safety, chemical, ergonomic, and other hazards, resulting in far fewer work-related injuries and illnesses.

Table 12-9.   Transition from Industrial Medicine to Corporate Health Management

Industrial Medicine	Occupational Medicine	Occupational Health	Corporate Health
Urgent care focus	Examinations (preplacement, medical surveillance)	Wellness/health promotion	Integrated management of overall health risks and health services (personal and organizational)
Injured worker		Clinical disease prevention	
Efficient follow-up exams	Hazard communications	Ergonomics	
Specialty referrals			Continuous quality improvement
Testing/screening	Toxic exposures	Case management	
	Hearing conversation	Organizational health assessment	Outcomes management
	Industrial hygiene		
	Regulatory compliance (OSHA/EPA/EEOC/ NIOSH)		

Source: Kent W. Peterson, MD, and Ronald R. Loeppke, MD, 1990.

- *Promoting personal health:* Employees who are fit, flexible, at their ideal body weight, not using illicit drugs, and able to manage stress have fewer accidental injuries. Ensuring that employees are properly qualified for their jobs is also important.
- *Testing for illicit drug and alcohol use:* A majority of employers with more than 250 employees now require drug testing as part of the employment process. Many employers conduct periodic or random drug testing among workers in safety-sensitive positions, including more than 7 million workers covered under Department of Transportation mandatory drug and alcohol testing regulations.[63]
- *Acute injury management:* This involves early identification, triage, and referral of illness and injury. Many employers teach employees CPR and first aid, and ensure that qualified "first aiders" are available at all building sites on all work shifts. Industrial sites often employ occupational health nurses or physicians to ensure rapid initial evaluation, treatment, and appropriate medical referral as necessary. It is helpful to communicate with the treating physician early in the care process, for example, to convey the availability of modified work duty.
- *Acute illness management:* This can often be built around self-care protocols, use of information resources, and other employee assistance programs.

- *Appropriate acute care:* Managed care workers' compensation programs often designate primary care "gatekeeper physicians" who provide acute diagnosis and treatment using treatment guidelines or protocols.
- *Rapid and effective communication:* Supervisors need to know quickly the severity of an employee's condition and an estimated date of return to work. This allows filling in or securing temporary replacements. Communication should require no longer than 24 hours. Given the many psychosocial, legal, union, and political issues involved in workplace illness and injury, effective communication with the employer, supervisor, insurer, or third-party administrator can be invaluable.
- *Case management:* Many industries now employ in-house rehabilitation specialists or contract for case management. Case managers — usually occupational health nurses or rehabilitation specialists — will contact an injured employee and offer assistance in obtaining access to prompt, high-quality medical care. They will monitor treatment, verify that the treatment plan is reasonable, and facilitate early return to work. Acute case management is usually more helpful than that begun only after an employee has been out of work one to four weeks or a cash reserve has been assigned above a cutoff, such as $25,000. Coordination of care for complex cases can include visits with the patient, family, physician, rehabilitation facility, and others.
- *Appropriate specialist referrals:* Gaining rapid access to specialists can often be a challenge, especially in HMOs and other managed care organizations where patients must often wait until appointments are available. A skilled case manager can often expedite a specialty referral.
- *Use of diagnostic, treatment, or case management guidelines.* Protocols are now being used not only for disease management, but also to help manage the flow of cases from primary care physicians to specialists. Disability duration guidelines can be helpful in creating realistic expectations of when an individual should be able to return to work.[64]
- *Rehabilitation:* Acute rehabilitation involves early evaluation to identify and minimize all abnormalities that could lead to chronic problems. Work conditioning involves symptom management directed at functional activities and individualized tests or procedures to quantify work-related musculoskeletal and neurologic restoration. Independent community rehabilitation and work-hardening centers have sprung up, offering both prevention and rehabilitation. Many facilities are associated with hospitals. Finally, given the litigious nature of work-related injury, disability assessment examinations are frequently performed.
- *Work hardening/return to work:* Work hardening is the last step in the rehabilitative process. It is oriented to functional activity centered around job tasks. The individual is put through work simulation and conditioning, with gradual increases in time and intensity of effort. Work-hardening techniques are also used to help condition noninjured employees to perform their jobs more efficiently and to reduce risk of accidental injury.

- *Modified duty/reasonable accommodation:* Employers that encourage early return to work by offering modified duty positions, have far better outcomes in terms of reduced costs and disability. Many companies require a return-to-work medical evaluation for employees absent five or more days. These evaluations ensure that the individual is able to return to his or her essential duties, identify temporary work restrictions, and ensure appropriateness of private medical care.
- *Use of independent medical evaluations (IMEs):* These are comprehensive medical assessments of complex cases undertaken by a physician not previously involved in the diagnosis, treatment, or management of the case. They include thorough review of previous medical records and test results, as well as complete medical history, physical examination, and additional tests and procedures as necessary. IMEs are usually requested where there is dispute over the actual diagnosis, the extent to which the findings are work related, the extent of impairment and disability, ability to return to work, and long-term prognosis. An IME follows an objective standard such as the AMA's *Guides to the Evaluation of Permanent Impairment.*[65]

Occupational Medicine

The transition from an industrial medical to an occupational medical perspective incorporates awareness of the profound impact of work environments on human health. A host of environmental health issues require going beyond management of illness (disease management). Several components illustrate the scope of health management in this area:

- *Preplacement and medical surveillance examinations:* Preplacement exams ensure that an individual can adequately perform job tasks, document preexisting conditions, and confirm that preexisting illness will not be aggravated by workplace exposures. Medical surveillance exams are designed to ensure that employees are not adversely affected by workplace exposures. In addition to performing the right tests of the right people at the right periodicity, population data must be analyzed. For example, the finding that 10 percent of workers in a particular job have elevated liver function tests cannot be interpreted without knowing the expected rates in unexposed populations.
- *Toxicologic risk managment:* Study of the long-term effects of low-level exposure to potentially toxic chemicals has revealed a growing list of hazardous substances that are regulated by the Occupational Health and Safety Administration, Environmental Protection Agency, and other agencies. Hazardous chemicals, dusts, noise, heat, and vibration must be identified, labeled, monitored, and employees must be trained, given protective equipment, and otherwise protected. Industrial hygienists play an active

role in monitoring exposure levels, complying with regulations, and assuring a safe workplace. Hazard communication regulations (so-called "employee right to know") require that every employee have access to material safety data sheets that identify known hazards of all chemicals with which they work.

- *Ergonomics:* In recent years, understanding has grown of the adverse health effects of repetitive motion, such as bending and lifting (back pain), or grasping and manipulating (carpal tunnel syndrome). Although there is still controversy about whether these conditions constitute medical pathology or symptom complexes, there has been an epidemic rise of workers' compensation claims in these areas. Among health care workers, back strain is one of the most common causes of illness or injury. As a result, the health management process must include assessment of the relationship between people, job tasks, and the work environments.

Occupational Health

A further step toward integrated health management occurs by acknowledging the powerful influences of personal fitness, wellness, and lifestyle behavior, as described earlier. Interestingly, visionary businesspeople led the way to creating integrated population health management programs in the 1970s, long before research documented the cost-effectiveness of health promotion.

Several models have emerged for providing wellness in industry. Many employers discovered that on-site fitness programs will gain participation from employees who would not do so if it were less convenient. Fitness is also a good way to mobilize cardiovascular risk reduction because it tends to trigger weight loss, cholesterol and blood pressure reduction, and stress management.

A different model is used by health promotion programs operated by health education or fitness staff separate from a medical department. Here, limited risk factor detection is done (for example, blood pressure and cholesterol checks), followed by health risk assessment. Results can be communicated in group feedback sessions, personal sessions, or by mail, with remote telephone follow-up. Individuals are encouraged to participate in health education and risk-reduction programs, often with an incentive.

A third model is an integrated employee medical program where health risks are identified at the time of employment and managed on an ongoing basis. Periodic health evaluations often combine focused screening, health risk appraisal, and medical surveillance procedures as appropriate. Employees are referred to their personal physicians for treatment of non-work-related illness. Risks are managed by continuing health education; personal counseling with a physician, nurse, or health educator; and reassessment.[66] As discussed earlier, companies that have evaluated health promotion programs

have found a consistent positive return on investment of 2:1 to 4:1 in terms
of reduced absenteeism, medical care utilization, and medical costs.

Corporate Health

Corporate health includes all of industrial medicine and disability management, environmental health and safety, and health promotion and wellness.
But it combines them in an organized system of care that also integrates
concerns for high-quality employee medical care and cost management. The
principles that underlie corporate health management include CQI and outcomes management.

In a corporate health management framework, lifestyle and occupational health risks are addressed as well as medical costs. This is important
because workers do not leave their personal health risk on their doorsteps
when they go to work in the morning. And they do not leave their occupational health risks at their place of business when they go home. From
this vantage point, both individual health and organizational health are
addressed. A continuum of care needs to be built into an organized delivery system for providing truly integrated health services. It was from this
framework that business leaders helped to form the National Commission
on Quality Assurance (NCQA), which has spawned a set of data bench-
marks by which the integrated delivery of clinical and preventive services
can be measured.[67]

A visual portrayal of the integrated components of an employee health,
safety, and environmental management program are presented in figure 12-6.
The occupational health hierarchy typifies the challenge of integrating health,
disease, and cost management. At the base of the pyramid is acute treatment and management of ill or injured workers. Once these concerns have
been addressed, medical care cost issues become the pressing issue. After
this, a company moves to create a safe and healthy work environment that
goes beyond minimal regulatory requirements. Only on top of this foundation will employees be willing to support health promotion and lifestyle
health issues. As the productivity benefits of healthy workers become apparent, a corporation can then address the final aspects of organizational
health — creating a healthy culture that supports individual creativity, adaptability, and change. Just recently, several management texts have begun to
address these issues.[68,69]

• Conclusion

Although the workplace is only one setting in which population health issues
can be addressed, it provides an excellent model for integrated health risk
management, demand management, disease management, and outcomes

management. Employers have the opportunity to make a very important statement concerning the value of health management. Other areas of integration include public health and community health systems and the growing managed care market. There is some evidence that community health models are rapidly gaining recognition as a viable means to influence the health of society. For example, the Greater Detroit Area Health Coalition is but one example of a major community/business effort to proactively address the health needs/problems of the community. Concurrently, the development of community health information networks (CHINs) also raises the hope that health management initiatives will be supported by an appropriate health information system. Hopefully, the health services delivery organizations of the future will continue to combine the best features of occupational health, public health, and managed care.

The success of today's disease management initiatives is important in this evolution toward population-based health management in that it will hopefully foster the beginning of a new viewpoint/attitude on how health care is addressed in this country. The mere phrase "health care delivery system" has negative connotations in that it reflects our entrenched entitlement

Figure 12-6. Occupational Health Hierarchy

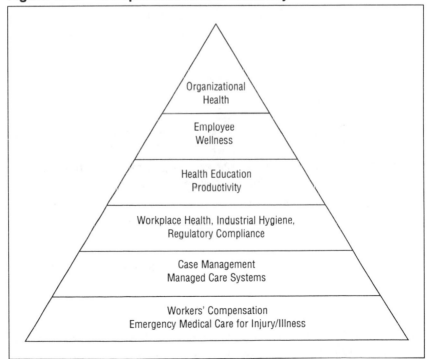

Source: Ronald R. Loeppke, MD, PhyCor, Nashville, TN.

attitude that "someone is supposed to deliver health care to us." The ultimate success of both disease management and health management will rest
on the value that society places on health care and whether each member
of society is held responsible for his or her own lifestyle. Despite the variety
of positive factors that support the potential expansion of both disease
management and health management, both concepts will succeed only if
we as a society change.

References and Notes

1. Travis, J. W., and Callander, M. G. *Wellness for Helping Professionals: Creating Compassionate Cultures.* Mill Valley, CA: Wellness Associates, 1990, pp. C-1,
   C-6.

2. Dubos, R. *Man Adapting.* New Haven, CT: Yale University Press, 1965, pp.
   321–22.

3. Travis, J. W., and Ryan, R. S. *Wellness Workbook.* Berkeley, CA: Ten Speed
   Press, 1988, p. xvi.

4. J. W. Travis, personal communication with author, 1979. Travis first found the
   term *high-level wellness* in a pamphlet by that name written by Halbert Dunn,
   MD (Arlington, VA: Beatty, 1961).

5. Constitution of the World Health Organization. *WHO Chronicle.* 1:29, 1947.

6. Last, J. M. Scope and methods of prevention. In: J. M. Last, editor. *Maxey-
   Rosenau Public Health and Preventive Medicine.* 12th ed. Norwalk, CT:
   Appleton-Century-Crofts, 1986, p. 3.

7. Snow, J. *On the Mode of Transmission of Cholera.* 2nd ed. 1855. Reprint, New
   York City: Commonwealth Fund, 1936.

8. Office of Disease Prevention and Health Promotion, U.S. Department of Health
   and Human Services. *Prevention '93–'94. Federal Programs and Progress.*
   Washington, DC: U.S. Government Printing Office, 1994, pp. 11–37.

9. Report to the Honourable Marc Lalonde, Minister of National Health and Welfare, Canada. Ottawa: Health and Welfare Canada, 1976.

10. Amler, R. W., and Eddins, D. L. Cross-sectional analysis: precursors of pre-
    mature death in the United States. In: R. W. Amler and H. B. Dull, editors.
    Closing the Gap: The Burden of Unnecessary Illness. New York City: Oxford
    University Press, 1987, pp. 181–87.

11. McGinnis, M., and Foege, W. Actual causes of death in the U.S. *JAMA*
    270:2207–11, Nov. 10, 1993.

12. Thar, W. E. *A Model for Calculating Population Attributable Risk and Costs.*
    Atlanta: Centers for Disease Control and Prevention, 1983.

13. NIH Consensus Development Panel on Physical Activity and Cardiovascular
    Health. Physical activity and cardiovascular health. *JAMA* 276(3):241–46, July
    17, 1996. See also Blair, S. N., Kampert, J. B., and others. Influences of cardio-

respiratory fitness and other precursors on cardiovascular disease and all-cause mortality in men and women. *JAMA* 276(3):205–10, July 17, 1996.

14. Leavenworth, G. Preventive medicine: strategies for quality care and lower costs. *Business & Health* 13(3):Supplement A, 1995. See also Chapman, L. *Proof Positive: An Analysis of the Cost-Effectiveness of Wellness.* Seattle: Corporate Health Designs, 1995. K. Pelletier has provided some valuable material on this subject. See the following: Pelletier, K. A review and analysis of the health and cost-effective outcome studies of comprehensive health promotion and disease prevention programs at the worksite: 1993–1995 update. *American Journal of Health Promotion* 10(5):380–88, May–June 1996. His 1991–1993 update appeared in *American Journal of Health Promotion* 8(1):50–62, Sept.-Oct. 1993. His original article by the same title appeared in *American Journal of Health Promotion* 5(4)311–15, Mar.-Apr. 1991. See also Wilson, M. G., Holman, P. B., and Hammock, A. A comprehensive review of the effects of worksite health promotion on health-related outcomes. *American Journal of Health Promotion* 10(6):429–35, July-Aug. 1996.

15. Greenberg, P. E., Finkelstein, S. N., and Berndt, E. R. Economic consequences of illness in the workplace. *Sloan Management Review,* Summer 1995.

16. Rice, D. P., Hodgson, T. A., and Kopstein, A. N. The economic costs of illness: a replication and update. *Health Care Financing Review* 7:61–80, Fall 1985.

17. K. W. Peterson, unpublished studies by Occupational Health Strategies, Charlottesville, VA. Peterson analyzed health-related costs among five Class I railroads during 1991–1995.

18. Peterson, K. W., Thar, W. E., and Brosius, D. *Preventable Costs and Lifestyle Behavior: An Analysis Using Population Attributable Risk and Cost.* Charlottesville, VA: Occupational Health Strategies, 1990.

19. Bertera, R. The effects of workplace health promotion on absenteeism and employee costs in a large industrial population. *American Journal of Public Health* 80(9):1101–5, Sept. 1990.

20. *Health Risks & Behavior: The Impact on Medical Costs.* Preliminary study by Milliman and Robertson, Inc., and Control Data Corporation, 1987. See also *Health Risks: Their Impact on Medical Costs.* Study by Milliman and Robertson in conjunction with the Chrysler Corporation and the International Union, UAW, 1995.

21. McGinnis and Foege.

22. Canadian Task Force on the Periodic Health Examination. The periodic health examination. *Canadian Medical Association Journal* 121:1194–1254, 1979.

23. U.S. Preventive Services Task Force Report. *Guide to Clinical Preventive Services: An Assessment of the Effectiveness of 169 Interventions.* Baltimore: Williams & Wilkins, 1995.

24. Eddy, D. M., editor. *Common Screening Tests.* Philadelphia: American College of Physicians, 1991.

25. Robbins, L. C., and Hall, J. H. *How to Practice Prospective Medicine.* Indianapolis: Methodist Hospital of Indiana, 1970.

26. Breslow, L., and others. *Risk Factor Update Project: Final Report.* Atlanta: U.S. Department of Health and Human Services, Centers for Disease Control, Center for Health Promotion and Education, 1985.

27. Ryder, R. Three common uses and five implementation strategies for health risk appraisals. In: K. W. Peterson and S. B. Hilles, editors. *Handbook of Health Risk Appraisals.* 3rd ed. Omaha: Society of Prospective Medicine, 1996, pp. 47–58.

28. Guidelines and ethical considerations for HRA users. In: K. W. Peterson and S. B. Hilles, editors. *Handbook of Health Risk Appraisals.* 3rd ed. Omaha: Society of Prospective Medicine, 1996, pp. 15–21.

29. One example of such an assessment is the Personal Health Evaluation Health Risk Assessment, created by Occupational Health Strategies, Inc., Suite 400, 901 Preston Avenue, Charlottesville, VA 22903-4491.

30. How to select an HRA: guidelines from the Society of Prospective Medicine. In: K. W. Peterson and S. B. Hilles, editors. *Handbook of Health Risk Appraisals.* 3rd ed. Omaha: Society of Prospective Medicine, 1996, pp. 23–29.

31. How to select an HRA.

32. DiClemente, C. C., Prochaska, J. O., and others. The processes of smoking cessation: an analysis of precontemplation, contemplation, and preparation stages of change. *Journal of Consulting and Clinical Psychology* 59:295–304, 1991.

33. Bigos, S. J., and others. Methodology for evaluating predictive factors for the report of back injury. *Spine* 16(6):669–70, June 1991. See also Bigos, S. J., Battie, M. C., and others. A prospective study of work perceptions and psychosocial factors affecting the report of back injury. *Spine* 16:1–6, 1991.

34. Bigos, S. J., and others. Back injuries in industry: a retrospective study. III. Employee related factors. *Spine* 11:252, 1986.

35. Ferguson, T. *The No-Nag, No-Guilt, Do-It-Your-Own-Way Guide to Quitting Smoking.* New York City: Ballantine Books, 1987.

36. *A Report on Lifestyles/Personal Health Care in Different Occupations.* Kansas City: American Academy of Family Physicians, 1979.

37. The Great American Smokeout occurs the third Thursday of November and is sponsored by the American Cancer Society.

38. Farquhar, J. W. Heart disease: the message gets across. *Medical World News,* Feb. 10, 1975, p. 8.

39. The consumer health education literature is vast. Pamphlets are available from hundreds of sources including government agencies (for example, the National Heart, Lung, Blood Institute; U.S. Dept. of Health and Human Services), voluntary health associations (for example, the American Cancer Society; American Lung Association), and commercial publishers (for example, Krames Communications, San Bruno, CA; Hope Publications, Kalamazoo, MI; Channing L. Bete Co., South Deerfield, MA; Journeyworks, Santa Cruz, CA; Health Promotion Publications, Park Nicollet Medical Foundation, Minneapolis).

Newsletters include: *Berkeley Wellness Letter,* University of California at Berkeley; *Employee Health & Fitness,* American Health Consultants, Atlanta; *Harvard Health Letter, Harvard Heart Letter,* and *Women's Health Watch,* Harvard Medical School, Boston; *Hope Health Letter,* International Health Awareness Center, Kalamazoo, MI; *Nutrition Action Health Letter,* Center for Science in the Public Interest, Washington, DC; *Tufts University Diet and Nutrition Letter,* Boston; *Vitality,* Vitality, Dallas.

40. Ferguson, T. *Health Online.* New York City: Addison-Wesley, 1996.

41. Travis and Ryan.

42. Stockman, L. V. Employee assistance programs. In: R. B. Swotinsky, editor. *The Medical Review Officer's Guide to Drug Testing.* New York City: Van Nostrand Reinhold, 1992, pp. 141–42.

43. U.S. Department of Transportation. Limitations on alcohol use by transportation workers (part II: final rules, common preamble). *Federal Register* 59(31):7302–38, Feb. 15, 1994.

44. Substance abuse professional procedures guidelines for transportation workplace drug and alcohol testing programs. Washington, DC: U.S. Department of Transportation, Office of the Secretary, Drug Enforcement and Program Compliance, June 1995

45. Peterson, K. W. Practical issues in establishing risk rated health incentive programs. In: S. Muchnik-Baku, editor. *The Challenge of Financial Incentives and Risk Rating: A Collection of Essays and Case Studies.* Washington, DC: Washington Business Group on Health, May 1992, pp. 38–40.

46. One example is the HealthMax Risk Rated Benefits Program, created by Health Examinetics, Inc., San Diego.

47. Mercer survey of benefits departments about risk rated benefits.

48. Fries, J. F., Koop, C. E., and others. Reducing health care costs by reducing the need and demand for medical services. *The New England Journal of Medicine* 329(5):321–25, July 29, 1993.

49. Vickery, D., and Lynch, W. Demand management: enabling patients to use medical care appropriately. *Journal of Occupational and Environmental Medicine* 37(5):1–7, May 1995.

50. Self-care manuals include Kemper, D. *HealthWise Handbook.* Boise, ID: HealthWise, 1991; Vickery, D., and Fries, J. *Take Care of Yourself.* New York City: Addison-Wesley, 1993; *Healthy Life.* Farmington Hills, MI: American Institute for Preventive Medicine, 1995; Eisenberg, A., Merkoff, H. E., and Hathaway, S. E., *What to Expect When You're Expecting.* New York City: Workman, 1991. Pantell, R., Fries, J., and Vickery, D., *Taking Care of Your Child.* New York City: Addison-Wesley, 1994.

51. Employees who self-care when sick cut health care costs by nearly 25%; one program's return investment is 19 to 1. *Employee Health and Fitness* 17(12):133–34, Dec. 1995.

52. Examples of on-line telephone health information services include Access Health, Rancho Cordova, CA; Employee Managed Care Corporation (EMC2), Bellevue, WA; Health Decisions International, Golden, CO; HealthWise, Boise, ID; Informed Access Systems, Boulder, CO; Informed Health, Aetna, Hartford, CT; National Health Enhancement Systems, Phoenix; Optum Nurseline and Informed Care, Center for Corporate Health, Oakton, VA.

53. Hibbard, D., and Hibbard, C. *The Patient–Family–Physician Guide.* Louisville, CO: Family Medical Center, 1996.

54. Excellent materials on the formation and operation of ethics committees in health care institutions are published by the Hastings Center for Bio-Ethics, Briarcliff Manor, NY.

55. Ornish, D. *Dean Ornish's Program from Reversing Heart Disease.* New York City: Random House, 1990.

56. Cooper, K. H. *Antioxidant Revolution.* Nashville: Thomas Nelson, 1994.

57. Clatz, R., editor. *Advances in Anti-Aging Medicine.* Larchmont, NY: Mary Ann Liebert, 1996.

58. Books for the public include: Sinatra, S. *Optimum Health.* Gatlinburg, TN: Lincoln-Bradley, 1996; Carper, J. *Stop Aging Now.* New York City: Harper Collins, 1995; Kugler, H. *Tripping the Clock: A Practical Guide to Anti-Aging.* Reno, NV: Health Quest, 1993; Griscom, C. *The Ageless Body.* Galisteo, NM: Light Institute Press, 1992; Weiner, M. *Maximum Immunity.* Boston: Houghton Mifflin, 1986; Schachter-Shalomi, Z. *From Age-ing to Sage-ing.* New York City: Warner Books, 1995.

59. Dacher, E. S. *Intentional Healing.* New York City: Marlowe, 1996.

60. *Alternative Medicine: Expanding Medical Horizons.* NIH Publication 94-066. Washington, DC: U.S. Government Printing Office, Dec. 1994.

61. Peterson, K. W. Corporate health programs: what they are, where they've been, where they're going. *Benefits Law Journal* 9(1):117–44, Spring 1996.

62. Loeppke, R. R. Prevention and managed care: the next generation. *Journal of Occupational and Environmental Medicine* 37(5):558–62, May 1995.

63. U.S. Department of Transportation.

64. Reed, P. *The Medical Disability Advisor: Workplace Guidelines for Disability Duration.* 2nd ed. Horsham, PA: LRP Publications, 1994.

65. *Guides to the Evaluation of Permanent Impairment.* 4th ed. Chicago: American Medical Association, 1993.

66. Woolf, S. H., Jonas, S., and Lawrence, R. S., editors. *Health Promotion and Disease Prevention in Clinical Practice.* Baltimore: Williams & Wilkins, 1996.

67. Sennett, C. An introduction to HEDIS—The Health Plan Employer Data and Information Set. *Journal of Clinical Outcomes Management* 3(2):59–61, 1996.

68. Richards, D. *Artful Work: Awakening Joy, Meaning, and Commitment in the Workplace.* San Francisco: Berrett-Koehler, 1995.

69. Costs, J. D. *Working Wisdom.* Toronto: Stoddart, 1995.

Index